Trust and Incidents

Katja Beitat

Trust and Incidents

The Dynamic of Interpersonal Trust between Patients and Practitioners

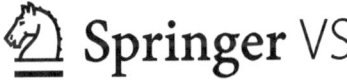

Katja Beitat
Leipzig, Germany

This book is an updated version of a PhD thesis submitted at the University of Leipzig (2014)

ISBN 978-3-658-09669-4   ISBN 978-3-658-09670-0 (eBook)
DOI 10.1007/978-3-658-09670-0

Library of Congress Control Number: 2015937268

Springer VS

Printed on acid-free paper

Springer VS is a brand of Springer Fachmedien Wiesbaden
Springer Fachmedien Wiesbaden is part of Springer Science+Business Media
(www.springer.com)

Acknowledgement

This book is adapted from a dissertation, which would not have been possible without the generous support from many people and organisations. The book includes some minor updates and amendments in response to the examiners' reports.

Firstly, I'd like to thank Professor Dr Günter Bentele for his guidance throughout the process despite being located on the other side of the world for most of the time. I also thank Professor Roderick Iedema for the invaluable discussions we had, his support and guidance.

I'd like to thank Kieran Pehm, the Commissioner of the NSW Health Care Complaint Commission, who not only offered practical support that allowed me to write this book, but also his insight that had an influence on the way I approached the topic. Ideas from discussions with other colleagues at the Commission over the years have also influenced this book and particularly the conclusions I offer.

I extend my greatest gratitude to the participants of the empirical studies – those patients and practitioners who were willing to share their experiences, despite in many cases being linked with emotions and unpleasant memories. Without them, this work would never been possible and I hope that their voices can be heard through this book.

I'd also like to thank Dr Gunnar Dittrich and the Kassenärztliche Vereinigung Sachsen for their assistance in distributing the survey to medical practitioners in Saxony/Germany, as well as the Royal Australian College of General Practitioners and the Royal Australasian College of Surgeon for their support in promoting the survey to practitioners in NSW/Australia. I would like to thank the University of Technology, Sydney for giving me access to excellent research facilities.

In addition, there were many wonderful and collaborative people who directly and indirectly supported this journey, including Dr Lakshman de Silva and Dr Günter Plum who proofread the original dissertation.

To my family – I thank you for raising me with the belief that effort and hard work will bring good ideas to fruition. Finally, and most importantly, I thank my beloved husband, Suresh de Silva, and my beautiful daughter, Isabella, for their patience, love and support. This book is dedicated to you – the two most important people in my life.

Foreword

Health care delivery in Australia and Germany, the two systems that are the focus of this book, is characterised by a high level of complexity. Patient trust is required on several levels of the health care system in order for it to work efficiently and effectively and provide safe health care of a high quality.

The book takes an interdisciplinary approach to conceptualising interpersonal trust between patients and medical practitioners, considering it the elemental level of other trust relationships, and offers a unique model to describe the dynamics of trust building and deterioration.

The empirical work, consisting of two separate studies, is guided by the model and looks specifically at situations where something has gone wrong in the patient's care or treatment to inquire about the impact of the incident on the relationship and trust levels and the practitioner's willingness to disclose medical errors to patients. The trust model is placed into the context of patient-practitioner communication and specifically the open disclosure of health care incidents.

The first study, consisting of explorative interviews with patients and practitioners who had been involved in a formal complaint that resulted from an incident, gives an insight in what both sides consider relevant for the building of trust and the deterioration of trust in the patient-practitioner relationship. Comparing the accounts reveals a disconnection between the perceptions and expectations of patients and practitioners, which is associated with the deterioration of trust after incidents.

The second study, an anonymous survey about the attitudes and experiences of medical practitioners regarding medical errors, shows a gap between practitioners' general willingness to be transparent about errors, and the actual actions they take after having been involved in an error. The survey outlines common barriers that exist in practice that prevent practitioners from openly communicating with patients about errors, but at the same time provides some insight as to possible strategies how these barriers could be overcome.

The discussion of the results from both studies in the context of the overall research question – What is the relationship between interpersonal trust in the doctor-patient relationship and communication in the context of health care incidents? – concludes that trust facilitates open communication after incidents, but in return is restored as a result of successful open disclosure.

The empirical findings broadly support and expand the proposed dynamic model of trust, consisting of a cycle of information, expectation and evaluation of outcomes which is influenced by communication, competence and care related aspects. A key finding that emerged was that open, timely and responsive communication about incidents poses a unique opportunity to restore the patient's trust and thus is an additional reason why practitioners should be open about incidents, beyond considering it an ethical obligation; an extension of obtaining informed consent from the patient; a response to patient wishes; or a strategy to prevent costly and lengthy complaints and legal proceedings. In return, trust appears to be a facilitating force in open disclosure, as it ensures goodwill on both sides striving to be aware of and align the differences in their perceptions, which need to be addressed in order to find a common understanding of what happened and how to move forward.

Given that the findings suggest that the trust relationship is formed at the first encounter and builds or deteriorates with every interaction, the prevailing view on incident management requires extension to consider the overall quality of the relationship between patients and practitioners and the overall quality of their communication, with a view that incidents are part of the patient's journey rather than something separate from it.

The book concludes with reflecting on the findings of the empirical studies and offering some recommendations to practitioners, patients, researchers and policy makers.

Table of Contents

List of Figures

List of Tables

List of Charts

Glossary of Key Terms

Expectation   An anticipation of an event, behaviour or action that is re-
garded as likely to happen or occur in future.

General practitioner (GP)
A medical practitioner who provides basic general medical
services, mainly in community-based primary health care settings. In Australia, general practitioners have undergone specialist training and are fellows of the Royal Australian College
of General Practitioners. In Germany, general practitioners are
specialist practitioners (Facharzt für Allgemeinmedizin) or
practitioners of a different speciality, for example paediatrics,
who provide general medical services in a community-based
setting (hausärztlich tätige Ärzte).

Health care   Medical and other services provided for the maintenance of
health, or prevention of disease.

Incident   An unexpected occurrence or event, related to the health care
provided to a patient that harms or has the potential to harm
the patient physically or psychologically, or both.

Interpersonal trust
A dynamic and voluntary process, involving both cognitive and
affective elements that shape a positive expectation about a
future outcome and thus enables cooperation by accepting
vulnerability posed by associated risks.

Medical error   The failure of a planned action to be completed as intended or
the use of a wrong plan to achieve an aim. A medical error includes serious errors, minor errors and near misses.

Medical practitioner

A person providing medical care and treatment who is registered as a medical practitioner with the relevant registration authority and thus authorised to provide medical services, including prescribing medication and referring patients for specialist medical services.

Minor error   An error that causes harm which is neither permanent nor life-threatening.

Near miss   An error that could have caused harm but did not, either by chance or timely intervention.

NSW   New South Wales, state of the Commonwealth of Australia.

Patient   A person who receives medical or surgical care or treatment. With reference to the empirical studies in this book, all patients were adults with full capacity to provide consent.

Open disclosure

Is the open and timely communication with patients about incidents in their health care that includes an explanation of what had happened, an apology, and measures taken to prevent future occurrence of similar incidents. Given the broad definition of incident used in this book, open disclosure would relate to communication about any perceived deviation from expected health care and treatment.

Patient-practitioner relationship

The connection between a patient and their treating medical practitioner in medical professional encounters.

Perception   The result or product of a subjective process of gathering information about something or someone through senses. People's perceptions of the same object, situation or person may differ. For the purpose of this book, perception is the individual view of a situation or information.

Serious error   An error that causes permanent injury or transient but potentially life-threatening harm.

Surgeon   A medical practitioner who underwent specialist training in
surgery, enabling them to undertake invasive operational procedures on patients. In Australia, surgeons are fellows of the
Royal Australasian College of Surgeons.

Trust dynamic The process of interpersonal trust development or deterioration over time.

Chapter 1   Introduction

Trust takes years to build, seconds to break, forever to repair.
(Unknown)

This book is an adapted version of my dissertation that explores interpersonal trust in the context of incidents in health care. The topic is set in a highly complex environment of diverse theoretical conceptualisations of interpersonal trust and a variety of different factors in practice that relate to health care incidents. Ultimately, I[1] aim to bring these concepts together in order to gain an understanding of the relationship between interpersonal trust in the doctor-patient relationship and communication in the context of health care incidents.

When I started this journey, it became quickly clear that trust appears to be a complex phenomenon involving cognitive and affective, conscious and subconscious processes and elements. Nevertheless, it seemed crucial for the effective delivery of health care in general, by bridging uncertainties, risks or incomplete information (Luhmann, 1979), so common in modern health care processes, to allow cooperation (Gambetta, 1988). My approach to understanding trust was rooted in communications – my primary background – but dipped into many other areas, including psychology, social science, governance, law and medicine.

In this book, I argue that while trust may not be essential for health care delivery in short term, one-off encounters, it nevertheless fosters their effectiveness and efficiency. When dealing with health care incidents, however, I view trust

---

1   This book is written in a personal style, using the pronoun 'I' to reflect my approach, understanding and interpretation of relevant information. This style of writing might be perceived by the German academic reader as an unusual choice, but it is a style more commonly used in contemporary academic publications in social science in the Anglo-Saxon countries. I personally believe that the style enhances the attribution of ownership of ideas and conclusions, as well as is more readable, in general, due to the active voice used. In choosing to write in this personal style, I have been influenced by the work of my fellow PhD students at the Centre of Health Communication at the University of Technology in Sydney, where I was located as a visiting scholar during most of the time I worked on this book.

to be essential to prevent or resolve conflicts and continue the patient-practitioner relationship. Fostering and restoring trust after health care incidents is important for both patients and practitioners. Without some level of residual interpersonal trust, it appears impossible to find closure after an incident and to develop renewed confidence in one's own judgement as well as health care delivery in the future.

Trust and its influence on open communication is also relevant to the broader improvement of health care delivery, in that incidents that are disclosed and resolved can lead to measures designed and implemented to prevent them from recurring in the future. Considering trust as one of the building blocks of a responsive and learning health care system, I link the interpersonal level to an organisational and systemic approach to patient safety and quality of health care. Highlighting the link between trust and open communication and illustrating the wider implications for improvements in the quality and safety of the health care system, I endeavour to support the call for increased transparency in health care overall (Leape, Berwick, Clancy, Conway, Gluck, & et al., 2009), and particularly after incidents (Hobgood, Tamayo-Sarver, Elms, & Weiner, 2005; Truong, Browning, Johnson, & Gallagher, 2011).

I approach the topic by establishing my understanding of interpersonal trust in health care encounters derived from a review of relevant literature and develop a dynamic model that summarises the process of how trust is built or deteriorates in the patient-practitioner relationship. I then specifically explore the interdependence of communication and interpersonal trust in such relationships before turning my attention specifically to incidents and their aftermath. I inquire about the impact of open communication about incidents – known as open disclosure – on interpersonal trust between patients and providers and the willingness of practitioners to be open about incidents.

I choose to explore the dynamic of interpersonal trust in the aftermath of health care incidents in this book (a) because I identified a gap in existing research on interpersonal trust, and (b) because incidents challenge existing trust in patient-practitioner relationships and thus appear to offer a unique opportunity to gain insight into the dynamics of interpersonal trust and factors associated with its increase or deterioration. Trust, as presented in this book, is closely related to communication – they are interdependent, impacting on each other. Successful and appropriate communication can be viewed as both the source and the result of trust and vice versa. When attempting to understand both interpersonal trust and communication, conscious and subconscious elements and different levels of influencing factors will be considered.

Ultimately, the aim of this book is a) to gain an understanding of the role, functions and dynamics of interpersonal trust after medical incidents, b) to understand its interaction and interdependence with communication and particularly open disclosure of incidents, and c) to offer support for increased transparency in dealing with incidents to enable the restoration of trust which has a wide ranging impact on the ethics, effectiveness and efficiency of health care delivery in general.

1.1 Why this topic?

There are several factors that played a role in my decision to write this book and I believe it might be useful to introduce these to the reader. I migrated to Australia from Germany and in early 2007 started to work for the NSW Health Care Complaints Commission. At that time, health care, and the Australian system in particular, were foreign to me and I often compared structures and processes to the German system. Having had a background in communications and a professional ethic that strove for transparency and simplicity to the greatest extent possible, I was initially surprised by the opaqueness and complexity of health care delivery in this country. After a few years with the Commission, I wondered how practitioners were expected to know and follow a myriad of rules and regulations, continuously develop their clinical skills and monitor those of peers, and, in addition, be good communicators and have a sense of caring for people from the most diverse backgrounds with their diverse expectations and needs. All of these expectations were reflected in the policies, codes of conduct and legislation that applied to the work of medical practitioners. While I acknowledged that holding this complex balance might have been achievable in routine daily work, I saw this fragile balance under pressure in situations when something went wrong.

Although patients desire open communication about incidents (Gallagher, Waterman, Ebers, Fraser, & Levinson, 2003; Hobgood et al., 2005) and most practitioners support it in principle (Gallagher, Waterman, Garbutt, Kapp, Chan, & et al., 2006), my experience with the Commission suggested that in practice, often disclosure did either not happen or was inadequate in the patient's perception (Hobgood et al., 2005). Patients made complaints with the intention of getting the information and explanation they needed to understand what had happened, and in some cases, to reprimand the practitioner for their handling of the incident. Working for the Commission, which deals with complaints in an independent and impartial manner, placed me in a unique position where I understood the difficulty in establishing a mutual understanding of what happened, amid a multitude of emotions, fears, anxieties and misunderstandings. I came to this topic from a practical perspective and with respect for both the patients' and the practitioners' side in their mutual quest to understand and find closure when something had gone wrong, while navigating a complex environment with the inherent risks of serious consequences and dealing with their own and others' emotions.

In Australia, and the state of New South Wales (NSW) specifically, a legislative and policy framework has been established since 2002 that supports the open disclosure of incidents to patients that, in principle, enables practitioners to safely disclose incidents and errors to patients. In Germany, open communication about incidents was only officially recognised in 2013, with the introduction of the Patientenschutzrecht (patient protection legislation) (Bundesministerium für Gesundheit, 2013). While in Australia the focus of incident communication has shifted from whether to do it to how to do it properly, in Germany more action is required to implement the new patient rights of openness about medical errors in practice. In both countries, a balance between the regulatory framework and the existing medical culture that commonly links incidents to a perception of failure or incompetence appears to not have been fully achieved.

Despite this overarching framework of influencing factors, I personally saw the relationship between a patient and a practitioner as the place where health care – in the sense of caring for the patient's health – eventuated. Understanding this unique relationship and its dynamics I hoped would give me some insight into how it could survive being challenged and often shattered through an incident. Given that health care as such, but particularly immediately after incidents, harbours a multitude of uncertainties and risks, trust appeared to be particularly relevant when understood as a mechanism to reduce complexity and accept risk (Luhmann, 1979).

With my background and understanding of health care delivery in both countries, I intend to offer a unique perspective on the topic, and aim to assist in achieving a better understanding of the links between interpersonal patient trust in medical encounters, open communication and incident management. A better understanding of how those factors are intertwined I hope could assist in changing practice and facilitating greater transparency after incidents.

Given the lack of existing research in this particular area, my approach to fieldwork was explorative and I conducted semi-structured interviews with patients and practitioners who had been involved in a complaint to the NSW Health Care Complaints Commission. The fact that there had been a complaint meant that the incident was known to both sides. This is important considering that many incidents in health care may not be recognised by patients and, if not voluntarily disclosed by the practitioner, will never be known to the patient.

From the narratives provided through my fieldwork, it emerged that where incidents lead to complaints, trust had deteriorated to a point where the continuation of the relationship seemed untenable. Interestingly, for practitioners, it was the fact that the patient made a complaint that often triggered their goodwill towards the patient to subside. What also emerged were the differences in perceptions of certain aspects in the patient-practitioner interaction and the different priorities assigned to those that contributed to the deterioration of trust. I considered that to restore trust in a situation where perceptions differ considerably required the willingness to attempt to find a mutual understanding which in return necessitated open communication not only about facts, but also about assumptions, perceptions and emotions. Such open communication, however, appeared to require a level of trust that at least at the time of the complaint no longer existed.

When exactly did it deteriorate and how? The narratives suggested it was the direct aftermath of the incident that was a critical point in the relationship and both sides agreed that at that point in time there may have been the opportunity to salvage the relationship. What patients wanted was foremost openness (Hobgood et al., 2005), but practitioners were often guarded in their communication after incidents (Gallagher, Garbutt, Waterman, Flum, Larson, & et al., 2006).

I decided to complement my explorative fieldwork and look specifically at this aspect, the willingness of practitioners in practice to disclose an incident. I hoped that understanding their attitudes and experiences would assist me in examining how any remaining barriers that existed in practice could be overcome.

Ultimately, this book was born in practice and aims to apply its insight in the practice of daily medical encounters between patients and practitioners. I also attempt to discuss the reality of the Australian experience, which is closely related to developments in the Anglo-Saxon systems, in order to assist the emerging discussion about open communication about incidents in Germany and what that may mean for patient-practitioner relationships.

1.2   Structure of this book

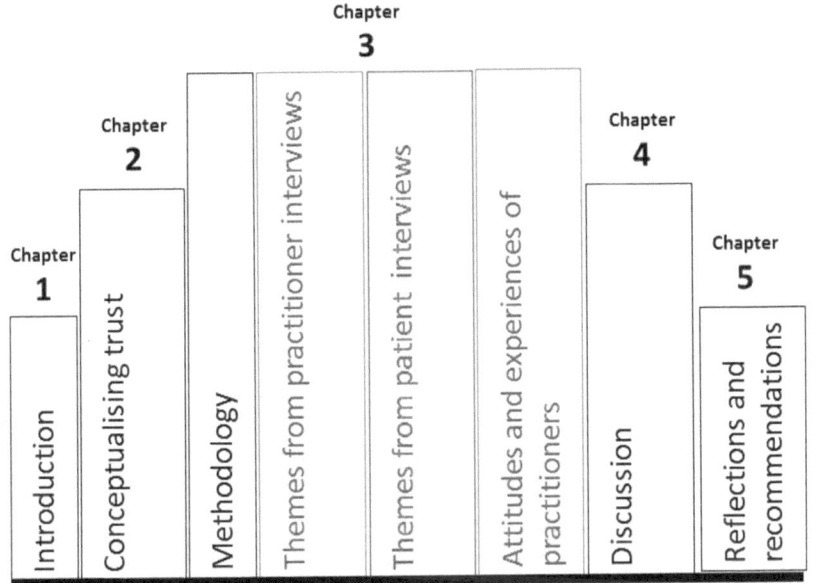

Figure 1.1   Structure of the book

In Chapter 1, I introduce the topic of my book and my personal background as far as it is related to this book. I emphasize my close relationship to the practice of dealing with health care incidents and my explorative and practical approach to the topic. In the second part of the chapter, I outline the structure of the book which follows a classical scientific approach of introduction, review of relevant literature to identify research gaps, methodology and presentation of findings, followed by discussion and concluding remarks including recommendations for future research, policy, the medical profession and patients.

In Chapter 2, I set out different conceptualisations of trust (Gambetta, 1988; Luhmann, 1979) and in particular interpersonal trust (Coleman, 1990; Jones, 1996) to derive my own understanding of the term for the purpose of this book. I then discuss related concepts, including trustworthiness, credibility,

risk and mistrust and present my understanding of how they relate to interpersonal trust between patient and practitioner, specifically after incidents. I will
introduce a dynamic model of trust that will assist in explaining my understanding of how trust is established or deteriorates in a relationship.

I will then describe the relationship between communication and trust in
the patient-practitioner relationship and the relevance of trust for the implementation of open disclosure, incident management and complaint management. Open disclosure, the open and transparent communication about incidents in the treatment or care of a patient, is a concept that has been widely
adopted internationally and in Australia in the past few years. The focus in the
relevant literature and research appears to have shifted from initially concentrating on why open disclosure should happen (Berlinger, 2005; Hobgood et al.,
2005; Woods, 2007) and what barriers prevent it from happening (Levinson,
2009) to looking at the quality of its implementation in practice and the practitioners' willingness to engage in the process (Truong et al., 2011). The chapter
closes by summarising my understanding of the relation between incidents,
open disclosure and complaints and their relevance to interpersonal trust between patients and practitioners after something went wrong in the care or
treatment of a patient, which sets the groundwork for my empirical studies.

Chapter 3 is the core of my book summarising my methodological approach and the key results of two empirical studies exploring the relationship
between trust and incidents in the treatment and care of patients. The topic
and my access to it are not limited to one specific discipline, and hence my
approach is interdisciplinary drawing on communication studies, psychology
and sociology, law and governance studies.

In the first part of the chapter, I summarise my research design and approach to data collection, analysis and interpretation. My explorative approach
to the fieldwork shapes both the way I conduct the interviews, trying to limit
imposing my pre-conceptions on the participants, as well as the way I analyse
the participants' narratives. My approach is founded in a constructivist view of

what empirical fieldwork can or cannot achieve. I am interested in the perceptions, which I acknowledge are subjective and may differ in the way they are presented to me. Ultimately, I assume that perceptions shape expectations and behaviour and thus are relevant in trying to understand trust dynamics.

In the second part of the chapter, I present themes emerging from explorative interviews with practitioners, while the third part contrasts these with the themes that emerged in interviews with patients. I present the emerging narratives in three broad categories, namely communication, competence and care-related, to compare practitioner and patient experiences of a health care incident. I use a number of direct excerpts from the interviews to give the reader the opportunity to form their own impression and to enable the transparent discussion of my findings, which I will offer in Chapter 4.

Lastly, I present the results of an anonymous survey of medical practitioners about their attitude and experiences with medical errors (adapted from Gallagher, Waterman et al., 2006). The survey focussed on issues from a practitioner's point of view that either prevented them from disclosing a medical error or impacted on their attitude to disclosing and dealing with medical errors, in general.

In Chapter 4, I relate the findings of the interview and survey study to my research questions and relevant literature. The aim of the discussion is to elicit what is the relationship between the interpersonal trust in the doctor-patient relationship and communication in the context of health care incidents. The discussion recalls relevant findings from the literature that informed the development of the dynamic model of trust which functioned as a framework for the empirical work before moving to compare themes that emerged in the interviews with patients and practitioners that are associated with the building and maintaining of interpersonal trust, as well as those associated with the deterioration of trust. I will look more specifically at the role of apologies after incidents and emotions associated with incidents and their aftermath.

I will show that the empirical findings broadly support and expand the dynamic model of trust consisting of an ongoing cycle of information, expectation and evaluation of outcomes that is influenced by communication, competence and care related aspects.

In response to my research question – What is the relationship between interpersonal trust in the doctor-patient relationship and communication in the context of health care incidents? – I conclude that trust facilitates open communication after incidents, but is also restored as a result of successful open disclosure.

The results strengthen the importance of a local, open and timely response to incidents. Any delay in open communication increases the risk of the patient's trust in the practitioner deteriorating, which in turn will influence negatively the way the patient perceives information or explanations provided at a later stage. Similarly, where the open disclosure is inadequate in responding to associated emotions and acknowledging the broader impact the incident had on the patient's life, the same dynamic will apply, decreasing the opportunity to prevent and resolve conflicts.

With this in mind, the results from the anonymous survey of medical practitioners are particularly relevant to understand the key areas that influence the willingness of practitioners to engage in open disclosure processes. Practitioners' remaining fears of negative consequences of disclosure for their professional life and the perceived lack of support after incidents stood out.

In Chapter 5, I conclude the book by describing the implications of my findings for further research, as well as any relevance it may have for medical practitioners, patients, policy makers, educators and regulators of the medical profession. Linking back to my original motivation to start this research, I will concentrate on making suggestions for practical measures that can be taken to improve open communication after incidents, which correlates with re-building and strengthening the interpersonal trust between patients and practitioners in such situations.

Chapter 2   Conceptualising Trust

2.1   Introduction

The aim of this chapter is to discuss the different ways trust, specifically in interpersonal relationships, has been conceptualised in the literature to derive
my own understanding for the purpose of this book. I will critically discuss general approaches to interpersonal trust as well as those specifically relating to
health care, adopting some elements and rejecting others while developing my
own, integrated approach to interpersonal trust.

Existing literature on interpersonal trust has mainly concentrated on routine health care situations; trust after health care incidents has played no, or
only a marginal, role in existing studies. It is unclear whether trust dynamics in
those circumstances differ from routine encounters. Based on the review of the
literature, I will develop a dynamic process model of trust that could be applicable to both routine situations as well as after incidents. The model will guide
my empirical work that inquires into factors related to the maintenance or deterioration of trust after health care incidents. As will become clear from the
model, communication is particularly relevant to the trust dynamic and, vice
versa, trust is relevant for the quality of communication between practitioners
and patients.

In the second part of the chapter I discuss related terms and their relevance to interpersonal trust. I will firstly discuss the open disclosure concept
that has been widely adopted internationally and in Australia in the past few
years and its relation to interpersonal trust dynamics after incidents. Following
on, I look closely at the practical implementation of open disclosure and identify
key incentives and barriers that can influence the willingness of practitioners to
engage in open disclosure. Lastly, I will briefly outline how incidents in health

care are currently being dealt with in Germany and Australia, including the complaint avenues available to patients.

The chapter will close with a summary of my understanding of the relation between incidents, communication, open disclosure and complaints and their relevance to interpersonal trust between patients and practitioners after something went wrong in the care or treatment of a patient.

2.2   Definitions of trust

Conceptualisations of trust can be found in the contemporary literature across a broad range of disciplines, including psychology (Earle & Siegrist, 2006; Rotter, 1967, 1971, 1980), sociology (Coleman, 1990; Giddens, 1990, 1991; Luhmann, 1973, 1979, 2000; Misztal, 1996), organisational studies (Dirks, 2006; Gambetta, 1988), economics (McKnight & Chervany, 2006), media studies (Bentele, 1998, 2008; Bentele & Seidenglanz, 2005) and health care (Benedetti, 2011; Entwistle & Quick, 2006; Hall, Dugan, Zheng, & Mishra, 2001; Thom, Hall, & Pawlson, 2004; Trachtenberg, Dugan, & Hall, 2005).

Trust in today's sense became established in the mid-seventeenth century. At around the same time, trust entered the lexicon of political philosophy with a meaning closely related to promise keeping (Seligman, 1997, p. 169). As such, trust was understood as a two-sided process: where one person trusts the other, they will base their behaviour on the assumption that the other person will act as promised. The other person has an implied obligation to keep the promise to honour the trust that was placed in them. This understanding of trust implies a conscientious and rational decision to trust; an understanding that has been adopted by Coleman (1990), whose conceptualisation I will discuss in more detail later in the chapter.

The layperson's intuitive understanding of trust appears to be commonly linked to both confidence in the competence (technical skills and abilities) of a person and trust in the goodwill of a person, often because of their character. The German term 'Vertrauen' appears to combine these two perspectives, illustrated by its translations into English as either trust or confidence. Trust is commonly used to describe the belief that a person or organisation will act with goodwill based on their nature or character, while confidence is foremost used to describe the belief in a person's skills and abilities. I will argue that both aspects are closely related to interpersonal trust, and depending on the circumstances, their importance will vary.

'Trust' is a term with overall positive connotations. Synonyms suggested by the Duden (2014), the most widely used German dictionary, include: belief, optimism, confidence, reliance and assuredness. A Google search[2] offers similar synonyms of trust: confidence, belief, faith, freedom from suspicion/doubt, sureness, certainty, certitude, assurance, conviction, credence and reliance. An overall positive connotation of trust can also be found widely in the literature (Gambetta, 1988; Lewis & Weigert, 1985). Some authors, however, have suggested that very high levels of trust could turn into 'blind faith' and could lead to the person who trusts being taken advantage of (Deutsch, 1958; Kramer, 1996, 2006; Langfred, 2004). Niklas Luhmann (1979) accordingly argues that both trust and distrust to some extent are functional in social interactions. While blind trust can be dysfunctional, informed or (at least partially) rationalised trust appears to have a positive function in social interactions.

The increase in literature relating to trust since the late 1950s, and particularly since the 1990s, can be attributed to changes in society during those periods. The increasing specialisation and fragmentation across a wide range of professions together with the onset of the information and technology age have brought with them a shift in social interaction and communication from primarily face-to-face and personal to more impersonal and technology-based forms. Indirect communication increases the risks of misunderstanding and with it the risk of non-cooperation. Trust has been viewed as an increasingly important

---

[2] www.google.com

factor to enable relationships and cooperation amid higher risks brought about by the increasing use of and reliance on technology and a decline in face-to-face interactions. Christopher Candlin and Jonathan Crichton, both linguists, introduce their book on discourses of trust (2013) outlining the importance and scope of trusts in modern societies:

> *Issues surrounding trust are foundational to people's lives in contemporary societies, a fact not merely and sharply highlighted by the recent history of interrelational practices associated with the financial markets, international security, marketing and public relations, but even more persuasively and ever-presently in the formation and maintenance of relations among partners in the delivery, for example, of health and welfare services and in the public and private arenas of political and religious institutions. (Candlin & Crichton, 2013, p. 1)*

With the growth in the importance of trust in modern society overall, specifically in the past two decades, research on trust has increased (Bachmann & Zaheer, 2006; Lewicki, Tomlinson, & Gillespie, 2006; McKnight & Chervany, 2006).

2.2.1   Levels of analysis

Before outlining relevant approaches to trust in more detail, I will distinguish different levels of analysis, as the understanding of trust varies depending on the chosen level of analysis.

While Candlin and Crichton (2013) distinguish two levels at which trust can be directed, firstly towards social/institutional orders and secondly towards individuals relating to each other, I will differentiate between a) interpersonal trust, b) trust in organisations or processes, and c) trust in systems. Opinions vary whether to consider trust in technology a distinct fourth type of trust (McKnight & Chervany, 2006), or subsuming it under trust in organisations and processes, with technology merely a facilitator. I adopt the latter view and hence will not refer to trust in technology as a distinct form.

On a systemic level, one of the most influential approaches to trust has been Luhmann's (1973, 1979) sociological definition of trust as a 'social mechanism' which reduces complexity. Essentially, in his view, trust is a tool to reduce the complexities of reality and as a result enables actors within the system to act. Similar to the role Luhmann assigns to communication, which is considered essential for both the coordination within one system as well as between different systems, trust enables development within a particular system, as well as cooperation between different systems. He argues that 'trust, in the broadest sense of confidence in one's expectation, is a basic fact of social life' (Luhmann, 1979, p. 4).

Although Luhmann did not explicitly define health care as a unique system, adapting his definition that a system needs to be functionally unique, health care could be considered a distinct system in modern society with its foremost and specific function being to ensure the health of the public and its members, by providing care and treatment to sick people, but also by preventing illness. Applying Luhmann's views on trust to his understanding of system theory (Luhmann, 1984), trust plays a significant role in the modern health care system, in that it is a mechanism that reduces complexity and fosters cooperation in the highly specialised, complex and fragmented delivery of health care, as well as in the interaction with other systems, including the legal and political systems.

Luhmann's conceptualisation of trust has followed a 'top-down' approach to explain social interaction and behaviour. Other sociologists, including Diego Gambetta (1988, 2000), have chosen a 'bottom-up' approach concentrating on interpersonal trust and its implications for cooperative behaviour. Similarly, James Coleman (1990) considers interpersonal trusting relationships the building blocks for other forms of trust, including trust in organisations, processes and systems. In his view, the relationship a person has with other persons shape their trust in an organisation or system to which the known person is related.

To visualise the different analytic levels of trust and the relations between those, I adapted a layer model that Günter Bentele (2008) developed to illustrate his understanding of credibility.

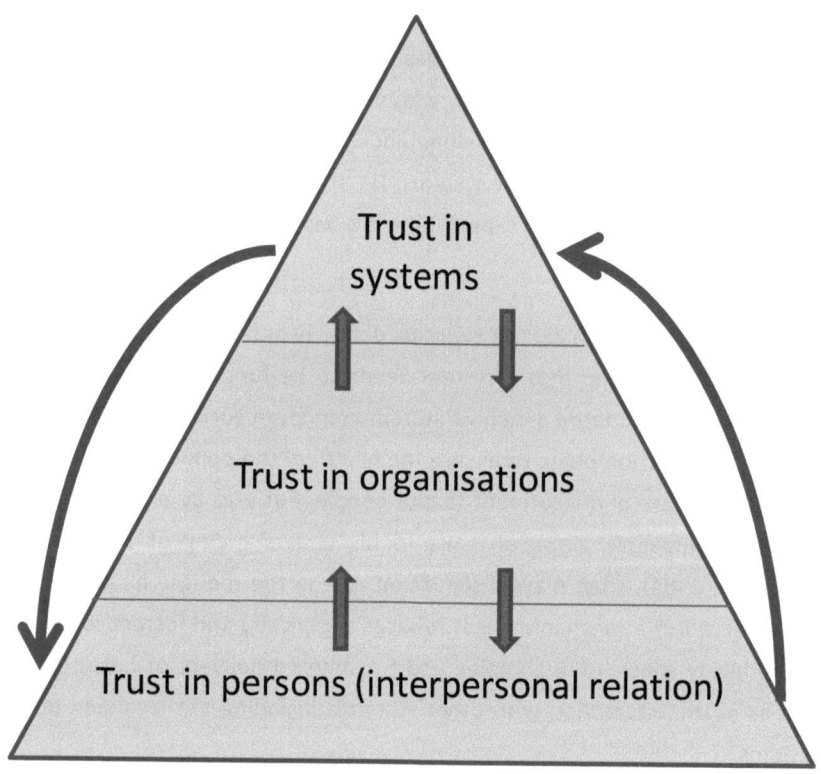

Figure 2.1   Layer model of trust (adapted from Bentele, 2008)

Bentele developed his layer model of credibility to explain public trust in persons, as well as organisations and systems (Bentele, 1998). Replacing credibility with trust, in the above adapted model, the base level is interpersonal trust. The next layer is trust in processes or organisations (Grey & Garsten, 2001), and on the third level, there is trust in systems. The arrows represent that, in my conceptualisation of trust, every layer includes elements of the layers underneath, meaning that trust in systems is related to some extent to interpersonal and/or organisational trust. In the opposite direction, the higher levels can also influence the ones below in that a person's perception and experience of a system and/or organisation can influence their expectation of a person representing the system and thus their interpersonal trust levels. In more practical terms, if I have a positive experience and rapport with my bank manager, it is very likely that I consider the bank as a whole as a trustworthy institution. Similarly, I would argue that if a patient has a good relationship with their general practitioner, they are likely to view positively the practice or hospital that doctor works for. In return, where a patient has only had limited personal interactions with the health system, but reads a lot about failures in the health system, poor patient outcomes and unprofessional conduct of practitioners in the media this may shape a negative perception, particularly in the absence of personal interaction with it. However, I will argue that the influence of organisational and systemic trust on the relationship between patient and practitioner will decrease with an increase in their interactions on a personal level.

In summary, I argue that trust is a phenomenon that can be understood by looking at different layers of analysis, but which ultimately cannot be understood without considering its most basic level – trust in interpersonal relationships. Karen Jones (1996) states that '[o]ne can only trust things that have wills, since only things with wills can have goodwill' (p. 14). According to her, only persons or agents acting on behalf of an organisation can act in good faith, and as such be trusted. On the surface, Jones's approach may sound limited, as in the modern world we often do not have a direct experience or interaction with a person who is related to an organisation. So how could we ever trust a process, system or organisation?

To answer this question, it might be helpful to refer to Coleman (1990) who introduces the concept of interpersonal 'mediated' trust. He distinguishes three types of intermediaries: advisers, guarantors and entrepreneurs (Coleman 1990, p. 180). In essence, the trustor trusts the intermediary's judgement about another person, assuming that the intermediary has more information about the third party than the trustor themselves. If the trust placed in the third party based on the intermediary's advice is not honoured, the trustor does not only lose trust in the third party, but more importantly in the intermediary's judgement as well. For example, a patient asks their general practitioner for a suitable specialist for their heart check. The patient trusts in the judgement of their general practitioner who will recommend the most suitable cardiologist. The risk for the general practitioner is that he loses the patient's trust in his judgement if the cardiologist turns out to be less competent in treating the patient's condition. The patient might still see the general practitioner, but may consult other sources when looking for a specialist in future, or the patient may decide to cease their relationship with the general practitioner.

While Coleman uses trust in intermediaries to explain how trust in organisations and systems occurs, Anthony Giddens (1990) distinguishes two types of trust in organisations and systems. He argues that where there have been no previous encounters with an organisation or system, trust relies on the interaction with a representative of the system at the 'access point'. Such encounter could be between a patient and nurses in the emergency department. According to Giddens (1990), continuing trustworthiness of an organisation or system requires face-to-face interaction with representatives of the system, which remind people that systems are operated by people.

Having distinguished the different levels at which trust can be analysed, from here onwards, I will concentrate on interpersonal trust.

2.2.2   Conceptualising interpersonal trust

There have been a number of different approaches to conceptualising interpersonal trust. Kurt Dirks (2006) distinguishes between a relationship-based and a
character-based perspective. While in a relationship-based perspective trust is
built by the behaviour and interaction between the person who trusts and the
person trusted, the character-based view suggests that trust depends on the
evaluation of the trustworthiness of a person based on their perceived characteristics. In a relationship-based view, trust is based on goodwill and mutual
consideration and obligation, while in a character-based view trust is based on
characteristics of the trusted person, such as competence, integrity and reliability.

Another way to categorise different types of interpersonal trust is introduced by Candlin and Crichton (2013) who refer to Maguire, Phillips and Hardy
(2001) when they distinguish between 'calculus-based trust', 'knowledge-based
trust' and 'relationally based trust' (pp. 7-8). While this categorisation refers to
the primary source of trust, it implies some level of cognitive choice people
make when deciding whether or not to trust, be it because they calculate risks;
have prior knowledge that allows predicting future behaviour, or by endorsing
or sharing values and needs when interacting with each other. This implied
choice to trust is an approach closely linked to rational choice theory and has
been adopted by Morton Deutsch (1958), Dale Zand (1972), James Coleman
(1990) and Russell Hardin (1992, 2001). The underlying assumption of such an
approach is that a person is self-interested and acts purposefully and rationally
when trusting another person, selecting the option with the greatest utility to
them.

Coleman (1990) expands Deutsch's and Zand's conceptualisations beyond
a single transaction and takes into account the gain or loss related to future
transactions when making the decision to place and honour trust. Trust levels
grow with every successful transaction, meaning trust was placed by one person and honoured by the other person by behaving in the way it was expected

(Coleman, 1990). In contrast to Deutsch (1958) and Zand (1972), Coleman (1990) also includes situations where someone potentially acts irrationally by not placing trust in a trustworthy person. Coleman argues that material resources are always limited, and actors or persons have an interest in or want control over these limited resources. As no person has complete control over all desirable resources, actors attempt to access their desired resources by giving other actors access to other resources (Coleman, 1990). This exchange of access to resources reflects a market based understanding of trust, where trust results from the successful completion of transactions.

This conceptualisation does not account for affective elements in the decision-making process. Coleman pre-empts such criticism by introducing elements of threat and power to explain more complex exchanges. He also qualifies his understanding of rational behaviour as being subjectively, as opposed to objectively, rational, meaning a choice is rational to a particular person. He argues that when something appears to be irrational, it is only a lack of information and knowledge about the facts being taken into consideration by the person who makes the choice that make that choice appear irrational from the outside. He argues that rational behaviour is individual, but through communication one may better understand the choices made by another actor. Implicitly, communication becomes essential to understanding the other person's rationale and is thus fundamental to establishing and maintaining interpersonal trust.

Although the conception of trust as a rational choice may appeal, particularly in the fields of business and economics, it is limited in that it does not explain why people often recognise whether or not they trust another person only when the trust is being challenged. In other words, in routine situations, trust is often not the result of a consciously made decision, but unconsciously formed. According to Joseph LeDoux (1996):

[w]hile conscious control over emotions is weak, emotions can flood consciousness. This is so because the wiring of the brain at this point of our evolutionary history is such that connections from the emotional systems to the cognitive systems are stronger than connections from the cognitive systems to the emotional system. (p. 19)

This view is contrary to the rational choice approach, which assumes that people can rationally evaluate factors that are relevant to their decision (Bhattacharya, Devinney, & Pillutla, 1998). Coleman (1990) himself concedes that people are selective in their awareness of facts and information, hence, even if they had access to all relevant information, they would not base their decision on all facts, but only on the ones that they have selected. Another aspect is that some people may have cognitive impairments that make it impossible to make rational choices or to communicate adequately the factors they base their choices upon. But do these people not trust others?

Explaining why people trust by referring to their rational decision-making appears limited, as it does not take into consideration that, often subconsciously, emotions can play a role in the formation of interpersonal trust (Becker, 1996; Damasio, 2005; LeDoux, 1996). Demonstrating the complexity of factors to be considered when capturing the development of trust, McKnight, Cummings and Chervany (1998) introduced a model of initial trust that separates a range of factors and processes that may influence the initial establishment of trust. According to their model, relevant to the formation of trust are the following:

- the person's overall disposition to trust (Rotter, 1980)
- cognitive processes, such as in-grouping or stereotyping
- institution-based trust
- belief in existing structures such as legislation that guide or frame what is considered 'normal' in the given situation

- the person's trusting beliefs regarding benevolence, competence, honesty predictability

These then form their intention to trust. Although the model is limited to initial trust, which according to McKnight and Chervany (2006) relates to the situation where the persons or parties involved did not have the opportunity to know each other through prior interactions or transactions, it shows both rational and affective processes play a role in establishing trust. While the dynamics of initially forming trust may differ from those in maintaining trust, I will adopt the view that a multitude of factors, both rational and affective, play a part in explaining how interpersonal trust is formed, maintained and destroyed. Figure 2.2 illustrates that trust appears to be psychologically generated from an individual person's point on a spectrum ranging from pure emotion, or blind faith, to pure rationality. Following this view means that each person differs in the way they trust, and the same person may differ in the way they trust depending on the particular person they are forming a relationship with and the particular situation.

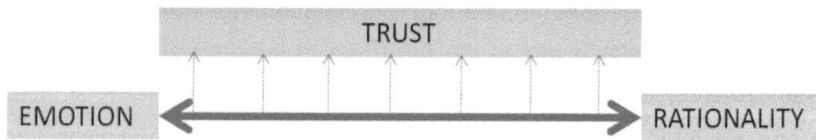

Figure 2.2   Psychological basis of trust

Jeffrey Braithwaite, Rick Iedema and Christine Jorm (2007) explain why people trust from an evolutionary psychology view, suggesting that behaviour and thinking is shaped by millions of years of natural selection. In their view, people trust members of their 'tribe', people who are in some way familiar to them. In other words, patients primarily trust their families, and clinicians trust their peers. Such conceptualisation may not be suitable to explain how people can trust others outside their 'tribe' in situations of uncertainty.

Karen Jones (1996) defines interpersonal trust as being:

composed of two elements, one cognitive and one affective or emotional ... to trust someone is to have an attitude of optimism about her goodwill and to have the confident expectation that, when the need arises, the one trusted will be directly and favourably moved by the thought that you are counting on her. (p. 11)

She clarifies that optimism does not mean a general positive outlook, rather a situation specific and directed attitude; it is being optimistic – meaning to interpret available facts by excluding negative options – about the goodwill and competence of another person in a particular situation (Jones, 1996). Contrary to Jones, I argue that negative influences can be present in a trust relationship, but may influence the extent to which people trust.

Referring to the above approaches, each appears to conceptualise interpersonal trust from a unique point of view. Each of the approaches discussed so far has some limitation in explaining why, when and how people trust. At this stage, I adopt a broad working definition of interpersonal trust and will look more closely at specific elements and associated concepts to form a suitable definition for the purpose of this book.

A broad definition is suggested by Denise Rousseau, Sim Sitkin, Ronald Burt and Colin Camerer (1998) in their multidisciplinary review that states that 'trust is a psychological state comprising the intention to accept vulnerability based upon positive expectations of the intentions or behaviour of another' (p. 395). By referring to 'a psychological state', the definition acknowledges that there may be a multitude of factors leading to the positive expectations about another person's future behaviour or action. As any future action inherently has the risk of not eventuating, the person who trusts accepts their vulnerability that this could happen.

In the next section I will more closely look at some of the associated concepts that this definition implicitly relies upon, including risk, trustworthiness and credibility. In addition, I will briefly discuss the concepts of mistrust and interpersonal communication and their relation to trust. The section will culminate in a definition of trust that I adopt for this book.

2.2.2.1 Elements and dynamics of trust

Risk

Looking at the origins of the German term 'Vertrauen', part of the word is 'trauen' which can mean to overcome an obstacle or accept a risk in order to do something. Conceptually, trust is commonly linked to the risk that a promised or expected action or behaviour may not eventuate. Trust is a mechanism to mitigate this risk (Luhmann, 1973, 1979, 2000) and to enable social transactions (Coleman, 1990) and cooperation (Gambetta, 1988) in situations that involve risks or uncertainty (Becker, 1996). According to Coleman (1990), many social transactions are not immediate and the asymmetry in time introduces a risk. Contracts and legally enforceable sanctions can mitigate some, but not all risks. For example, transactions relating to non-material or hard to value goods often involve risks that require trust to succeed (Coleman, 1990). Ragnar Löfstedt (2005) points out that trust should not be overly relied upon to manage risk in a 'post-trust' society, but should be integrated with other risk reducing mechanisms, depending on the specific situation.

Trust on an interpersonal level is the result of confidence[3] placed in another person to act or behave in a certain way towards them in the future. A person who trusts assumes that any risk that an undesirable action or outcome will eventuate is minimal to non-existent (Beitat, Bentele, & Iedema, 2013).

---

[3] Different to the approach I take, Timothy Earle and Michael Siegrist specifically distinguish confidence from trust, defining trust as the 'willingness to make oneself vulnerable to another based on a judgement of similarity of values. Confidence is defined as the belief, based on experience or evidence that certain future events will occur as expected' (Earle & Siegrist, 2006, p. 386). In my view, their distinction is an attempt to separate the affective and rational elements of trust.

The link between risk and trust has been well-established (Coleman, 1990; Luhmann, 1973; Seligman, 1997). Some have argued that a higher risk or higher level of uncertainty is associated with higher levels of trust and that in situations where there is no risk a person will behave other than intended, for example through coercion, trust is not required (Gambetta, 2000).

Trustworthiness and credibility

Another concept that is closely linked to trust is trustworthiness – the perceived quality of a person to be honest (Bentele & Seidenglanz, 2005). Interpersonal trust requires a person to trust another person and that in return, the person trusted honours the trust placed in them by behaving the way they were expected to (Kramer, 2006). But what is the motivation or incentive for a person to honour the trust placed in them?

According to the rational choice theory (Coleman, 1990), a person behaves trustworthily when they expect a future return from the transaction. Where it is unlikely that there will be another interaction in future, it appears there is limited motivation for a person to be trustworthy. Coleman (1990) suggests that the motivation in such situation would be that if a person breaches the trust of another, their reputation will be damaged and other members of the social environment may no longer perceive the person as trustworthy, impacting on their ability to have transactions with a wider group of people. Implicitly, this explanation of a motivation to trust refers to social identity theory that suggests that people derive their social identities from identifying with a specific group (Tajfel, 1978; Tajfel & Turner, 1986). Coleman (1990) gives the example of a close, small group of diamond traders, where transactions are mainly agreed to verbally. Members share the understanding that if someone should breach the trust placed in them, the other members would know about it and would exclude this person from any future transaction. The potential loss for the trustee to breach the trust far outweighs the potential momentary gain.

The dynamic he describes may be suited to small, homogenous groups that have direct communication to build and share a common understanding about a person's reputation and trustworthiness. However, people re-construct reality differently: similar facts may be evaluated and perceived differently by different persons based on their selection processes, influenced by their awareness, prior experience, preferences and situational circumstances (Hardin, 1992). Even in a small group, the same fact can be perceived differently by different people, or the same facts can be perceived differently by the same person in different situations.

Closely related to trustworthiness is the concept of credibility. Credibility is the perceived expertise of a source of information and the trustworthiness of the message (Hargie, Saunders, & Dickson, 1994). When evaluating the trustworthiness of a person, people may consider external information from different sources, including from other people or the media. The credibility, or believability, of that source will impact on how the person will interpret the information. When there are discrepancies between information from different sources, people tend to select the information from a trustworthy source that is perceived to be more credible than others. Even if a person has never met the other person before, the available information and how much credibility is assigned to it will influence whether the person will trust the other person and to what extent. Relying on information from a range of sources also explains why someone can trust a person without any prior interaction.

Credibility is based on perceptions. According to Bentele (2008), perceived discrepancies in the credibility of a communicator can result in a deterioration of trust. Such discrepancies can relate to contradictions between the following:

- information and experience
- verbal statements and action
- different information or action by similar persons or institutions
- different statements by the same person or organisation at different times

- norms/law and actual behaviour

Although Bentele's discrepancy hypothesis primarily relates to the c124onstruction of reality through media, it is also relevant to interpersonal relationships, where perceived discrepancies can have a negative impact on trust.

Credibility and trustworthiness are qualities that people attribute to a person or source of information (Deppermann, 1997). People's perceptions may be influenced, but they cannot be controlled. Similarly, trust is voluntary in a sense that, whether a person trusts another person and whether a person accepts to be trusted, are both voluntary. The latter is described by Karen Jones (1996, p. 9) who defines 'unwelcome trust' as a situation where the trustee feels uncomfortable with the 'obligation' to honour the trust that was placed in them, as they might feel unable to perform to the expectations placed in them, or may feel that it is a burden to them.

According to Leon Festinger's (1962) cognitive dissonance theory, people act to achieve a balance between their perception of others and behaviour towards them. Applying this theory, it could be argued that people trust where they perceive the person as being trustworthy to achieve a balance between their perception and the behaviour of the trustee. In addition, people will act as is expected of them where they perceive that the trust placed in them is warranted. Extrapolating this dynamic, trust becomes self-affirming, a view shared by other authors (Dirks & Ferrin, 2001; Murray & Holmes, 1999). Where a person trusts another person, they have a certain positive expectation. If that expectation is fulfilled, they continue trusting – there is no dissonance between their perception and the actual behaviour or outcome. However, if their expectations are not met, there is a dissonance between the expectation and the actual behaviour or action of the other person. As a result, the person who trusted will try to limit or decrease this dissonance, which they can achieve by either (a) re-interpreting the unexpected behaviour so that it becomes consistent with the existing picture or perception they have of the other person, or

(b) by removing their trust. By evaluating actual outcomes against earlier expectations, trust becomes the result of a retrospective 'check' of the trustworthiness and credibility of a person.

To summarise, trust involves elements of the past (experiences), the present (available information) and the future (predictions). Expectations are shaped by one's own or others' past experiences, available information (Earle & Siegrist, 2006) and a calculation of risk. In the absence of absolute certainty about future action, behaviour or outcome, the perceived trustworthiness of a person or source of information and the credibility assigned to information provided by them are fundamental in the formation of trust.

The opposite of trust

While interpersonal trust is based upon positive expectations, negative expectations can explain mistrust. I use 'mistrust' and 'distrust' interchangeably, acknowledging that the German opposite of 'Vertrauen (Trust) is the term 'Misstrauen', which can be translated into English using both 'mistrust' and 'distrust'.

When people say, 'I do not trust this person', there usually is a negative connotation that implies that they distrust the person. In this sense, it is not a neutral expression. Jones (1996) describes distrust as trust's contrary. In her view, distrust is the 'pessimism about the goodwill and competence of another' (Jones, 1996, p. 7). In that understanding, distrust is conceptualised as an expectation of negative action or behaviour. Luhmann (1979) on the other hand describes distrust as functional in that it allows a person to identify the potential for undesirable behaviour and offers the opportunity to manage it.

Accepting the idea that trust is self-affirming, the same could be said about distrust. Where a person has the expectation that another person will act or behave in a negative manner, they will distrust the other person. Referring back to Festinger (1962), distrust could be overcome where there is a dissonance between the negative expectation and the actual behaviour or outcome. In such situations, people will attempt to address the dissonance by either re-interpreting the action of the other so it fits into their negative perception, or by changing their negative expectations into a neutral or positive one.

Different to both views on distrust is the absence of trust, which includes situations where trust is simply not required for interacting with each other, either because there are no risks that are perceived as substantial by the trustee, or where any associated risks have been mitigated by other means, for example through a legal contract. These situations can be described as trust neutral.

2.2.2.2 Proposing an integrating definition of interpersonal trust

The discussion of relevant approaches in the literature up to this point has revealed some key elements of interpersonal trust, which I consider relevant for defining interpersonal trust in this book. Specifically, I assume that interpersonal trust:

- is foremost an interpersonal phenomenon. Trust in organisations or systems is usually mediated through interpersonal trust (Coleman, 1990; Jones 1996);
- has both rational and affective elements (Damasio, 2005; Jones, 1996; LeDoux, 1996; Rousseau et al., 1998);
- is closely related to risk, trustworthiness and credibility, all of which rely upon an individual's perception of a unique situation (Deppermann, 1997; Lewicki et al., 2006)
- is voluntary, i.e. it cannot be forced or controlled (Calnan & Rowe, 2006; Gambetta, 1988, 2000; Jones, 1996);
- enables or fosters cooperation (Calnan & Rowe, 2006; Gambetta, 1988); and
- is a dynamic process that is influenced by a person's perception of their own or other's past experiences (Hardin, 1992), present information

and future predictions, all of which impact upon a person's expectations, which ultimately will be evaluated, retrospectively.

Based on the above points, I propose the following definition:

Interpersonal trust is a dynamic and voluntary process, involving
both cognitive and affective elements that shape a positive expec-
tation about a future outcome and thus enables cooperation by
accepting vulnerability posed by associated risks.

Clarifying this definition, I conceptualise trust as neither cause nor effect,
but a process that influences people's behaviour. Where there is interpersonal
trust between people their behaviour and actions are likely to be cooperative
and mutually confirming. Trust is strengthened or diminished depending on the
consistency between prior expectations and the evaluation of actual outcomes
or behaviour of a person in a relationship. As I will outline in more detail later in
this chapter, a core part of any such interaction is communication. This view is
shared by Gambetta (2000) who comments that '[t]he problem, therefore, is
essentially one of communication: even if people have perfectly adequate motives for cooperation, they still need to know about each other's motives to
trust each other' (p. 216).

2.2.3   Interpersonal trust in health care settings

After having looked at different conceptualisations of trust in the literature and
having developed a working definition, I now focus on interpersonal trust between patients and medical practitioners and will discuss the dynamics of trust
in routine situations, before moving to situations when something has gone
wrong.

Health care delivery in Germany and Australia, as in most developed countries, is highly complex and trust on various levels is essential (Calnan & Rowe,
2004, 2006; Entwistle & Quick, 2006; Mechanic, 1998). Conceptualisation and

research of trust in health care settings overall has concentrated on the interpersonal level between clinicians and patients (Benedetti, 2011; Calnan &
Rowe, 2004, 2006). Patient trust in their medical practitioner has been linked to
patients being more willing to seek care, higher patient satisfaction, greater
levels of compliance and return visits (Krupat, Bell, Krawitz, Thom, & Azari,
2001; Lee & Lin, 2009; Trachtenberg et al., 2005) and overall better health care
outcomes for the patient. It is widely recognised that patient trust is fundamental to an effective patient-provider relationship (Benedetti, 2011) in that it enables open communication between patients and practitioners (Macintosh,
2007), and cooperation (Gambetta, 1988).

The organisational and systemic level can influence the interpersonal relationship between patients and practitioners by providing a framework for reasonable and safe health care through relevant legislation, directives, policies,
guidelines and checklists. In an ideal health care system, these levels complement each other. However, as Trachtenberg et al. (2005) conclude, 'patients'
views about particular physicians are substantially (but not entirely) independent from their views about the medical system in general' (p. 351).

Applying the layer model I introduced above for health care, I suggest that
trust in the interpersonal relationship between patients and practitioners is
fundamental for other forms of trust in health care organisations and the health
care system overall. In return, trust at higher levels of the model can influence
trust at the interpersonal level, as trust in health care processes and systems
appears crucial for patients to seek treatment in the first place (Trachtenberg et
al., 2005). Systems and frameworks can support the work of individual health
care providers, but do not replace professional judgement and behaviour.
Where there are inconsistencies between trust on different levels, the model
suggests that interpersonal trust is the most relevant to the patient's decision-
making, whether or not to continue care after the initial stage, whether to increasingly rely on the practitioner's judgement and what level of involvement
the patient prefers to have in their care (Trachtenberg et al., 2005).

2.2.3.1 Patient-practitioner relationship

Up to this point, I have referred to the 'patient', the 'practitioner' and their relationship in a general sense. In reality, every patient and every practitioner are unique, bringing with them their own unique combination of past experiences, current information and strategies to predict future action and behaviour – they are individuals interacting in unique situations. For example, patients' experiences in primary health care settings when consulting their long-term general practitioner in a non-emergency situation are distinctly different from their experiences of emergency departments with their often foreign and complex environment. In the former situation, the patient is able to maintain a level of independence and control in relation to dealing with their health issues, while in the latter, the patient's independence and sense of control is limited. However, where a patient suffers from a chronic disease that requires regular hospitalisation, they may be more familiar and confident in hospital settings. How do the characteristics of the patient, the practitioner and the health care environment influence interpersonal trust?

In attempting to answer this question, I will distinguish three types of patient-provider relationships and their relevance to interpersonal trust. The three types of relationship[4] can be described broadly as:

- Expert relationship
- Equal partnership
- Patient-led relationship

Patients differ in their level of involvement in their treatment (Arora, Ayanian, & Guadagnoli, 2005; Ende, Kazis, Ash, & Moskowitz, 1989; Lee & Lin, 2009). Each of these relationships is characterised by typical role expectations

---

[4] Allen & Brock (2000) distinguish 16 personality types using the Myer-Briggs type indicator and discuss the relevance of adjusting communication to suit the patient's personality to be effective. I will more broadly summarise three typical relationship types.

and preferences that determine specific communication and trust dynamics in interpersonal relationships.

Expert relationship

An 'expert relationship' is characterised by a power and knowledge asymmetry between the patient and practitioner, with the practitioner taking on a paternalistic role. Typically, the patient trusts and relies on the professional judgement and expertise of the practitioner. The underlying belief is that the practitioner will act in a patient's best interest taking into consideration their unique circumstances and preferences, which is not an unreasonable expectation given the well-known Hippocratic Oath requires practitioners to 'use treatments for the benefit of the ill in accordance with [their] ability and [their] judgment, but from what is to their harm and injustice [to] keep them' (Sokol, 2008). This expectation of a practitioner is also reflected in modern professional ethics and guidelines, such as the European and Australian codes of professional conduct (Australian Medical Board, 2010; Bundesärztekammer, 2006).

Patients in an expert relationship expect the practitioner to fix their problem, without being necessarily interested in fully knowing and understanding the details of different treatment options and associated risks. The patient trusts the practitioner's expert judgement and advice. While intuitively it may appear trust becomes more prevalent In such relationships to address the gaps in information and the less active role of the patient in the decision-making process, Das and Teng (1998) suggest that control and trust in a relationship are parallel concepts, meaning that more control in a relationship does not correlate with less trust and vice versa. Macintosh (2007) goes further when he suggests that patients 'who trust too easily, or refuse to take any responsibility for their own actions, diminish the relationship' (p. 164) with their practitioner. He argues that with such patients, the practitioner would lose their sense of obligation and this would potentially lead to carelessness and indifference. This argument is in line with Luhmann's view on distrust being functional to identify potentially undesirable behaviour and the ability to manage it (Luhmann, 1979).

However, as Macintosh (2007) clarifies, a high level of distrust, particularly over a period of time, can destroy the patient-practitioner relationship. He argues that '[if] we feel we are not trusted, we often respond with anger, at least partly due to a sense of loss and the feeling we are not appreciated, but eventually this anger cools and is replaced with indifference' (p. 165).

A challenge for the practitioner in expert relationships is to ensure that they obtain valid informed consent from the patient, which requires the patient to fully understand the proposed treatment and relevant associated risks. Referring to a decision of the High Court of Australia (Rogers v Whitaker, 1992), the majority of judges found that:

> [a] doctor has a duty to warn a patient of a material risk inherent
> in the proposed treatment; a risk is material if, in the circum-
> stances of the particular case, a reasonable person in the patient's
> position, if warned of the risk, would be likely to attach signifi-
> cance to it or if the medical practitioner is or should reasonably
> be aware that the particular patient, if warned of the risk, would
> be likely to attach significance to it. (paragraph 16)

In particular, the second interpretation of 'material risk' offered in the judgement as one that would be significant to this particular patient poses a challenge for practitioners in expert relationships, where the communication with the patient can be one-sided and less commonly a dialogue. The judgement commented that the patient does not have to express that a certain risk is significant, as long as it can be inferred from other statements or preferences the practitioner is aware of, a requirement many practitioners may not be fully aware of (Skene & Smallwood, 2002). In a relationship where the patient is rather passive, the practitioner may (subconsciously) revert to their preferred style of transmitting information, which often focusses on communicating accurate medical facts rather than placing them into the individual context of the patient's life (McWhinney, 1989). Effective communication in an expert relationship appears to rely upon an aware and reflective practitioner (Longhurst, 1989).

Equal partnership

The second type of typical patient-practitioner relationship is characterised by a more equal role of both sides. In these relationships – also referred to as patient-centred care (ACSQH, 2011; Say, Murtagh, & Thomson, 2005) – the patient expects to be involved in any decision-making about their care and treatment. The practitioner's role is to provide relevant information so that the patient is able to weigh up their options, taking into account their own preferences, needs and values.

Patient-centred care has been associated with better patient compliance (Schneider, Kaplan, Greenfield, Li, & Wilson, 2004; Stewart, Brown, Donner, McWhinney, Oates, & et al., 2000), higher levels of patient involvement in their care and treatment and greater satisfaction (Beach, Sugarman, Johnson, Arbelaez, Duggan, & Cooper, 2005) and an awareness of risks and ultimately greater acceptance of complications and side effects (Arora et al., 2005).

In equal relationships, trust is relevant in that the patient trusts the practitioner will select information that is relevant for the patient's decision-making and present it in a way that the patient can understand. To do so, a practitioner is not only required to ascertain medical information from the patient, but also to some extent has to understand the patient as a person with their unique capacities, life experiences and preferences. It is equally important to understand and acknowledge how the patient perceives their own illness. Weston and Belle Brown (1989) comment that the 'physician need not believe that the problem is the way the patient sees it, but the doctor's explanation and recommended treatment must at least be consistent with the patient's point of view and make sense from the patient's world' (p. 83).

The implementation of a shared decision-making relationship requires skilled communication that is commensurate with the health literacy and possible level of impairment of the patient (Levinson, Lesser, & Epstein, 2010; Son-nenmoser, 2004). Studies have shown that the information needs of patients are rarely met (Coulter, Entwistle, & Gilbert, 1999; Healthcare Commission, 2005; Tang, Newcomb, Gorden, & Kreider, 1997). The same information may have to be delivered in different formats to different patients, taking into account their literacy levels and cognitive abilities.

In addition to providing relevant information to patients in a way that they understand, the patient also needs to be actively involved in the decision-making process (Loh, Simon, Kriston, & Härter, 2007; Richards, 1998). Practitioners also have to take into account issues related to gender, cultural or social backgrounds that can impact on the patient's preferences and their trust (Boulware, Cooper, Lloyd, LaVeist, & Powe, 2003). To give some examples, female patients with a traditional or religious background may not be comfortable to consult on their own with a male practitioner. People from some foreign language and cultural backgrounds may not feel comfortable sharing their personal health information with an interpreter they do not know personally, while in other cases the use of a family member as an interpreter may impact on the quality of information given to the patient, when the family member not only translates, but also interprets the information based on their own understanding and preferences. In addition, patients from different cultural backgrounds may perceive differences in the delivery of health care differently. Boll-Palievskaya (2005) refers to Russian patients in Germany who culturally prefer a practitioner to be an authoritative figure and perceive the reliance on tests and instruments to reach a diagnosis as a sign of the practitioner's lack of competence.

An equal relationship is the result of an ongoing dialogue between the patient and the practitioner that requires openness and responsiveness on both sides. Trust is both an enabling factor and can also be a result of such a relationship. Patients who trust their practitioner will feel more comfortable in speaking up on their own behalf (Sun, Zhang, & Dong, 2011), which in turn makes it easier for the clinician to ascertain the patient's preferences and expectations (Hall et al., 2001; Thom et al., 2004).

Patient-led partnership

The third type of patient-practitioner relationship is broadly characterised by an active patient and a reactive practitioner. Examples may include where patients themselves have medical knowledge, either because they are practitioners themselves or because they have had extensive interaction with the health care system, such as patients suffering from chronic conditions that require regular treatment. In patient-led relationships, it is the patient who primarily steers the relationship and confidently expresses their treatment preferences with the expectation that the practitioner will be responsive to these.

The literature on such relationships has focused on patients demanding prescriptions (Britten, 1995; Ganther, Wiederholt, & Kreling, 2001). The lack of wider studies about this type of relationship and its effects on interpersonal trust may be an indication that it applies to only a small proportion of patient-practitioner interactions, or that interpersonal trust in such relationships may not be as prevalent. It could be argued that in those relationships it is less the patient's trust in the practitioner that is of relevance, but also the practitioner's trust in the patient's health literacy and being able to make decisions that are in their own best interest. Given that, for example, the understanding of risks of medication and procedures vary among trained medical practitioners depending on the way the information is presented (Gigerenzer & Edwards, 2003), it may be detrimental to assume a patient has a sufficient level of health literacy to make their own decisions without thorough consultation.

The above categorisation of typical patient-practitioner relationships is intentionally broad. The aim is to illustrate that different types of relationships are characterised by different roles, different expectations and communication styles, which in turn are all directly or indirectly related to interpersonal trust.

Any relationship is dynamic and a specific patient-practitioner relationship can evolve from one type to another. An expert relationship at the initial stage can evolve towards a more equal relationship with repeated interaction or encouragement (Arora et al., 2005). In turn, a patient may be active in treatment relationships regarding a condition they are familiar with, but revert to a more passive role concerning the treatment of new or unfamiliar conditions.

In essence, when researching interpersonal trust in the patient-practitioner relationship it is important to acknowledge that any understanding is necessarily limited to a unique relationship at a singular point in time. Although certain general patterns may be identified, any generalising must be done with caution. I will discuss this point further in relation to my empirical data in the methodology section of Chapter 3. As indicated in the discussion above, communication preferences and patterns may differ depending on the type of patient-practitioner relationship and appear to be relevant in understanding trust dynamics. I will now turn my attention to the relationship between communication and trust in the patient-practitioner interaction.

2.2.3.2 Interpersonal trust and communication

As discussed above, different types of relationships between patients and practitioners require different styles of communication to be effective. Communication is not only necessary to exchange information about the medical facts, but it is equally important to establish what both sides' preferences are regarding their roles in the relationship and to ascertain contextual information that may be relevant to the patient's decision-making in medical encounters.

> Many health professionals think that effective communication means giving patients clear, unambiguous information in a timely manner. This is true, but it is only part of the story. Communication involves listening as well as talking. (Levett-Jones, Macdonald-Wicks, & Oates, 2014, p. 4)

Effective communication begins with listening (Lange, 2007) and is tailored to the other person's needs (Leavitt & Leavitt, 2011) and thus underpins the development or maintenance of trust in such encounters. In return, trust in practitioners allows the patient to make decisions amid more or less incomplete information and considering that information already provided to the patient is often recalled incompletely (Leavitt & Leavitt, 2011).

To guide the following discussion on what is required to effectively communicate, I introduce a dynamic process model of trust that applies to personal interactions between patients and practitioners and visualises the factors that influence the process of building and destroying trust.

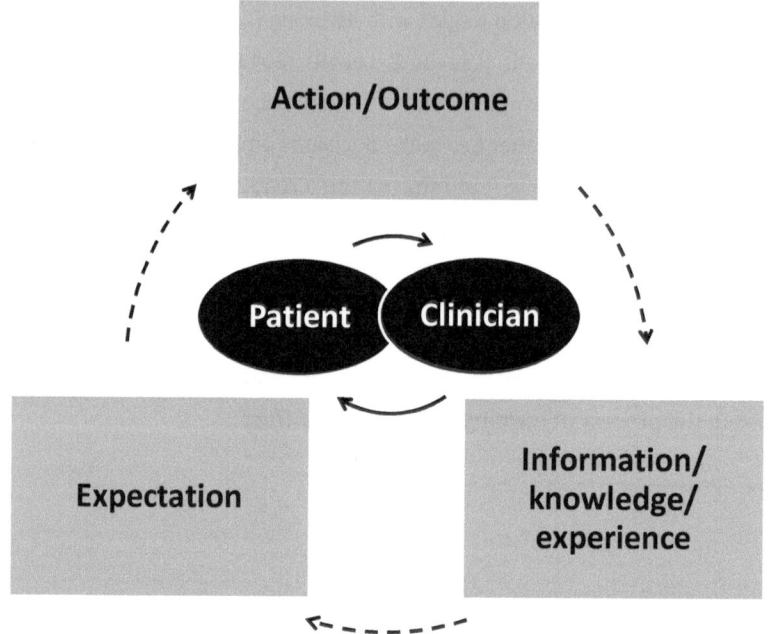

Figure 2.3   Dynamic process model of trust
(adapted from Beitat et al., 2013, p. 81; reprinted with permission)

At the core of interpersonal trust between clinicians and patients is their relationship and ongoing interaction, which is indicated by the inner circle in Figure 2.3. These interactions are facilitated through verbal and non-verbal communication (Friedman, 1979). Where communication is effective and successful, it influences the elements in the outer circle that represent the trust dynamic.

Communication influences the information and knowledge levels of both patient and practitioners, in that where the communication takes the form of an open and responsive dialogue, both sides can attempt to understand each other and build a shared knowledge that is relevant for the medical decision-making. The source of information can be the other partner in the relationship;

it can be prior knowledge; it can also be external sources. For example, the rise in patients using the internet to gain information and a preliminary understanding of their conditions is widely recognised (Kirschning, Michel, & von Kardoff, 2004; Prokosh, 2008). Other external sources may include friends and family, or other health practitioners. Open communication offers the opportunity to identify and address possible inconsistencies between information from different sources, and develop a shared understanding of its relevance in a particular situation.

In the trust process, illustrated as the outer circle, expectations are formed referencing the information and knowledge a person has that is influenced by prior experience. Where patients do not have prior information about a practitioner's abilities, skills, competence or character, their communication with the practitioner becomes fundamental for the trust relationship (Thom et al., 2004). Communication also enables the opposite partner in the relationship to be aware of one's own expectations and where there is a mismatch between the expectations held by the patient and those held by the practitioner, successful communication can identify and address these. In cases of incomplete or unsuccessful communication, a mismatch of expectation may lead to conflict in the next stage, the outcome or action stage of the trust process. In this stage, the actual outcome or action is evaluated against the previously held expectations. Where expectations and outcomes broadly match, trust is re-enforced. Where there is a mismatch, it may impact on the trust relationship between the patient and the practitioner.

Continuing the outer circle of the model, perception of the outcome and the associated evaluation of the relationship based on the outcome itself becomes new information that shapes future expectations. The process is continuous.

In my understanding, where the inner and outer circles – both facilitated through communication – are unbroken, trust develops and strengthens over time. In cases where the outer circle is interrupted, either through issues in the relationship or issues in the communication between patient and practitioner, trust deteriorates. Repeated interruptions will eventually lead to a complete breakdown of trust and usually end the relationship.

Particularly relevant to the initial stages of trust formation in the patient-practitioner relationship is that, compared to other professions, doctors are generally considered to be trustworthy (GfK Verein, 2014; Readers' Digest, 2013). This may be due to people ascribing overall positive attributes to members of the medical profession (Beitat et al., 2013), including that practitioners:

- are qualified experts who have experience helping patients relieve the health problem they present with;
- understand patients' suffering;
- do not (intentionally) harm;
- act in the patient's interest; and
- are ethical and act morally.

Generally, high levels of initial trust foster open communication in medical encounters. During the further development of the relationship, which happens even within a single encounter, patients then, partly consciously, partly subconsciously, evaluate the communication with the practitioner and adjust their expectations accordingly.

The influence communication has on interpersonal trust levels cannot be underestimated and both appear to impact on each other. Indeed, effective interpersonal communication and interpersonal trust in health care encounters have been associated with similar effects on patient outcomes including higher compliance rates (Harms, 2007), patient empowerment in self-managing their health care (Goleman, 2006), as well as enhanced patient satisfaction (Leavitt & Leavitt, 2011; Stewart, 1995) and better care coordination (Mickan & Rodger, 2005).

To illustrate the relationship between patient-practitioner communication and interpersonal trust, I introduce the following model in Figure 2.4.

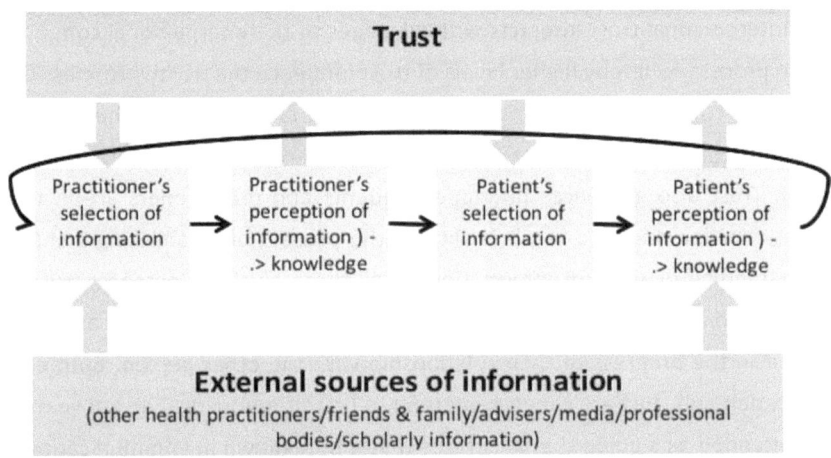

*Figure 2.4   Model of communication and interpersonal trust between pa-
tients and health practitioners*

The oval shaped arrow illustrates the continuous interpersonal communication between practitioner and patient. Both sides select relevant information
from all the information that is available to them in a particular situation and,
depending on their perception, will form certain expectations. In the (often
subconscious) selection process, patient and practitioner may consider information that is already known to them, information from external sources, and
information from the other partner in the conversation. The communication
can be considered effective where both sides achieve a shared understanding of
information that is relevant to both. In most cases, this not only means sharing
the relevant information, but sharing an understanding of how it is perceived by
both sides and what relevance each person attaches to it. In other words, effective communication builds a shared understanding of (a) the facts, (b) each
side's emotions associated with the event and (c) the perception of the rela-

tionship, and in some instances may require communicating on a meta-level about the latter two levels.[5]

Interpersonal trust interacts with all stages of the interpersonal communication process, whereby higher levels of trust influence the trustworthiness that is ascribed to information from a particular source and impacts on the selection (Erdem & Harrison-Walker, 2006; Hesse, Nelson, Kreps, Croyle, Arora, & et al., 2005). Trust also influences how open patients and practitioners are in their communication and as a result facilitates the process of establishing a shared understanding of relevant information on all three levels. In essence, trust influences what people hear, how they hear (perceive) it and how they are acting upon it in the progress of their relationship with the other person. Both communication and trust are circular and tend to be self-enforcing. The above model is intended as a guide that illustrates that a breakdown in communication or a misunderstanding may negatively impact on interpersonal trust and vice versa.

While up to this point I have described interpersonal trust in health care encounters in routine situations, I now turn to situations where something has gone wrong in the patient's treatment or care. It is important to note that, in some instances, it is not a treatment issue, but an issue relating to the communication between patient and doctor that forms an incident and may be grounds for a patient complaint (Kable, Farmer, & Beitat, 2014).

---

[5] I distinguish three levels of interpersonal communication. There are other approaches to interpersonal communication, including the 'problematic integration' theory by Austin Babrow (2001). Babrow argues that people deal with uncertainties when selecting information using their individual probabilistic orientation based in cognition and their evaluative orientations based in emotions. Another model is the Friedemann Schulz von Thun's communication quadrant model that distinguishes four levels of communication: the factual level, the relationship level, the self-disclosure level and the appeal or plea level. He argues that interpersonal communication conveys information on all four levels. The recipient needs to decipher all four levels for the communication to be successful, which may require some level of meta-communication (communication about communication) to avoid errors in the interpretation (Schulz von Thun, 2014).

In the next section, I focus on communication after incidents and the concept of 'open disclosure' that, among other intentions, aims to restore the patient's trust in the provider after something has gone wrong through open and transparent communication.

2.3 Communicating about health care incidents

> A trusting relationship between provider and patient is the bedrock of medical care. Following an adverse medical event, patient and provider relationships face their greatest test. The key to success is open patient-provider communication and a true sense of caring. (Duclos, Eichler, Taylor, Quintela, Main, & et al., 2005, p. 485)

The above quote illustrates that an incident interrupts and tests the 'normal' patient-practitioner relationship. Incidents, broadly understood as something unexpected that happened in the care or treatment, pose a physical and emotional challenge for the patient's and often their families' expectations (Leape, 2011). Incidents can be a physical challenge, because of the related prolonged or additional suffering the patient has to endure; they can also emotionally challenge people coming to terms with the fact that something unexpected has happened, which creates a sense of uncertainty about what will happen in future. The understanding of incidents that I adopt for this book is very broad by defining an incident as *anything that is unexpected in the care and treatment of a patient and could have or did harm a patient*, including communication incidents that did not harm the patient physically, but psychologically. This goes beyond the definition proposed by the World Health Organisation (2005) that in its definition of an incident includes errors, preventable adverse events and hazards.

An incident is a deviation from what is expected and can cause an emotional reaction on both the patient's and the practitioner's side. Despite statistics suggesting that a significant number of patients will experience an incident in their health care, neither the patient nor the practitioner appear to start their relationship with such an expectation (Blendon, DesRoches, Brodie, Benson, Rosen, & et al., 2002). Incidents challenge the positive notion associated with trusting the practitioner to act in the patient's best interest. Incidents create uncertainty and therefore challenge existing trust, but at the same time require trust to overcome such situations of uncertainty in order to continue the relationship and to cooperate. Incidents are powerful determining factors in a relationship, and in general have a more powerful effect than events that were perceived as positive (Earle & Siegrist, 2006).

Estimates about the number of incidents vary significantly, which may partially be due to the difference in definitions used to describe incidents. Since the publication of the US landmark study 'To err is human' by the Institute of Medicine (2000), the prevalence of incidents in health care has entered public discussion and has coincided with a focus on health policy to improve patient health and safety. Studies of the prevalence of adverse incidents have focused on hospital admissions (Baker, Norton, Flintoft, Blais, Brown, & et al., 2004; Barach & Cantor, 2007; Schiøler, Lipczak, Pedersen, Mogensen, Bech, http://europepmc.org/search;jsessionid=NeY0meKdapEH5kO6Kopd.2?page=1&query=AUTH:%22Stockmarr+A%22& et al., 2001). Estimates vary, but roughly one in ten patients who are admitted to hospital will be involved in an incident with adverse outcomes (World Health Organisation, 2014). Many incidents are considered preventable (Cave & Dacre, 2008) and often incidents are associated with longer hospital stays and increased health care costs (Encinosa & Hellinger, 2008).

There is a well-established link between incident disclosure and improving the safety and quality of the health care system (NSW Health, 2007a; World Alliance for Patient Safety, 2004). However, any clinical governance response to incidents relies on the clinician's willingness and ability to disclose the incident. Health care systems have established reporting systems that allow clinicians or staff to report incidents anonymously without the fear of being penalised, so that the data can be used for quality and safety improvement measures (World Alliance for Patient Safety, 2004). While such reporting systems can support safety improvements, they do not address the need of patients who would like to know when something went wrong (Gallagher et al., 2003; Mazor, Simon, Yood, Martinson, Gunter, Reed, & Gurwitz, 2004).

When incidents are disclosed to patients and their families, this is referred to as open disclosure. With the recent shift in focus from *safe* health care to a more holistic understanding of *better* health care that is patient-centred (ACSQH, 2011) and respects a patient's rights (ACSQH, 2008), both patient-directed open disclosure and clinical governance directed incident management are considered important in the improvement of health care delivery. This integrated view is reflected in the Australian safety and quality framework for health care (ACSQH, 2012).

While it is important to set the framework and acknowledge the interdependence between internal and external disclosure processes, from here onwards, I will concentrate on the patient-directed open disclosure of incidents.

2.3.1   Open disclosure

When something goes wrong, patients want their clinician to tell them immediately what happened and how (Gallagher et al., 2003; Hobgood et al., 2005). Respecting and responding to the patients' preference for open communication about the incident – known as open disclosure – is essential to maintain trust. According to the Australian Open Disclosure Framework (ACSQH, 2013a), open disclosure is:

> [an] open discussion with a patient about an incident(s) that resulted in harm to that patient while they were receiving health

care. The elements of open disclosure are an apology or expression of regret (including the word 'sorry'), a factual explanation of what happened, an opportunity for the patient to relate their experience, and an explanation of the steps being taken to manage the event and prevent recurrence. (p. 4)

One of the earliest known adopters of open disclosure was the Veteran Affairs Medical Centre in Lexington in the United States, which changed its procedures in relation to medical incidents in 1987 and adopted a proactive approach to openly disclose errors, to offer an apology and financial compensation when the error resulted in physical harm or loss of earning capacity. The changes were prompted by comparatively high claim pay-outs, and have since resulted in a significant decrease in pay-outs (Clinton & Obama, 2006; Kraman, 2010).

Other successful examples in the United States include the University of Michigan Health System (Clinton & Obama, 2006), the Dana Farber Cancer Institute in Boston, the Johns Hopkins University in Baltimore, and the Children's Hospital in Minneapolis. Even some professional indemnity insurance companies, such as the Denver based COPIC, have adopted a proactive approach to disclosing and settling medical errors and have since substantially decreased their pay-outs (Berlin, 2006; Gallagher, Studdert, & Levinson, 2007; Iedema, 2014; Truong et al., 2011; Woods, 2007). However, what appears from the literature is that open communication about errors does not result in a drop in the number of liability claims per se (Studdert, Mello, Gawande, Brennan, & Wang, 2007), rather it is associated with on average lower compensation payments being sought by patients and their families (Mazor et al., 2004). An explanation might be that patients and families, especially in the US, may face substantial costs associated with additional care and treatment required after an incident and hence seek to recover these costs through liability claims. Open communication after serious incidents may facilitate patients not seeking further damages beyond reimbursement of additional medical costs (Guijarro, Andrés, Mira, Perdiguero, & Aibar, 2010).

While open disclosure of medical errors appears to make sense from an economic point of view, the discussion has evolved to support open disclosure as an 'ethical practice seeking to re-establish trust by meeting patients' needs and expectations following an incident and to improve the quality of care' (McLennan, Beitat, Lauterberg, & Vollmann, 2012, p. 23). Nancy Berlinger's book *After harm* (Berlinger, 2005) became an influential narrative in the ethical debate about why open disclosure of medical errors is necessary not only for the patient's benefit, but also the benefit of involved clinicians. Berlinger argues that being open and truthful about medical errors is the right thing to do moral-ly. Coupled with a genuine apology and care it can also be a way to achieve forgiveness and ultimately closure for both sides.

Others have argued that disclosing errors is a professional obligation, in the sense that it can be considered an extension of obtaining informed consent from the patient (Bismark & Micalizzi, 2011). Valid consent requires the patient to fully understand their treatment and care and hence would require the dis-closure of errors and the impact on the patient's condition and care.

In Australia, open disclosure formally became part of health care delivery through the publication of the Australian Open Disclosure Standard in 2003. At that stage, it was the only nationwide standard for open disclosure in the world (ACSQH, 2014). The original national standard was not mandatory, and was adopted by the different states and territories in different ways. In NSW, the Department of Health issued an open disclosure policy in 2007 that required staff in the public health system to openly communicate with patients about errors (NSW Health, 2007b). The policy was underpinned by the *NSW Civil Lia-bility Act 2002* (s. 69) that provides that apologies are not considered an admis-sion of liability in civil litigations. While in NSW apologies are afforded full legal protection, the degree of protection in other Australian jurisdictions varies (Madden & McIlwraith, 2008), a fact that continues to contribute to a degree of uncertainty and confusion among clinicians. A simple 'I am sorry' appears to be protected in all Australian jurisdictions. The full statutory protection for apologies in NSW means that an apology, whether it includes or implies an admission of fault or not, will not be relevant for the determination of liability or fault during civil legal proceedings (*NSW Civil Liability Act* 2002).

Although clinicians support disclosure of incidents in principle, a twofold gap exists between what patients want, what clinicians are willing to disclose and actual disclosure rates (Gallagher, Garbutt et al., 2006; Gallagher, Waterman et al., 2006; Levinson, 2009). A range of potential barriers to disclosure are discussed in detail below.

2.3.1.1 Barriers to open disclosure

Firstly, I will describe commonly cited barriers for practitioners to actually disclose an error; and secondly, I will describe barriers to a successful open disclosure by identifying issues with the way it is being implemented. In other words, firstly, I look at why open disclosure may not happen, and secondly, what can go wrong when it happens. Barriers include legal, organisational, cultural and personal barriers.

One of the most commonly cited barriers for practitioners that prevents them from disclosing errors or incidents to patients is their fear of being sued or held liable for the incident (Gallagher, Waterman et al., 2006; Studdert & Brennan, 2001). Notably, a study of Australian doctors that was undertaken in 2007 (Nash, Walton, Daly, Kelly, Walter, et al., 2010) found that practitioners who actually had experienced a medico-legal claim or complaint against them in the past were more likely to agree that patients were more likely to sue a doctor who had told them about an error. In contrast, another study suggests that full disclosure was associated with no increased likelihood of patients seeking legal advice (Mazor, Reed, Yood, Fischer, Baril, & Gurwitz, 2006). The difference may be explained by a discrepancy between what practitioners think will happen after disclosure and what patients actually do, or by a mismatch between the extent of the disclosure that is desired by patients versus the disclosure that is provided by practitioners. While some clinicians believe that only adverse events that cause significant harm need to be disclosed (Barach & Cantor, 2007), patients want to know about errors regardless of their severity and impact (Hobgood et al., 2005).

Studies have shown that where patients perceive a lack of communication about errors they often want the practitioner punished (Hickson, Clayton, Githens & Sloan, 1992; Hobgood et al., 2005; Mazor et al., 2004). In contrast, an honest and accountable approach to disclosing incidents that is respectful of the patient's feelings and needs has been linked to the patient being less likely to seek punishment of the practitioner (Kraman & Hamm, 1999; Schwappach & Koeck, 2004) or intending to sue the practitioner (Hickson et al., 1992).

A second barrier to practitioner's willingness to disclose relates to professional pride and cultural factors. Practitioners are trained and expected to help, not harm. This expectation is mutually shared among practitioners and patients (Guijarro et al., 2010). When there is an error, it challenges the self-perception of the practitioner's competence, as well as the way they think they will be perceived by patients and peers. Attributing errors to a lack of competence of a practitioner is still common (Reason, 2000; Tasker, 2000).

Lastly, for any person, including practitioners, it is difficult to admit an error and take responsibility. Most practitioners never have had any training in how to disclose an error to a patient (Gallagher, Waterman et al., 2006; Stroud, McIlroy, & Levinson, 2009) or how to deal with their own and the patient's emotions that will most likely be associated with the disclosure.

While the above reasons may prevent a practitioner from disclosing an error to the patient, I will now turn my attention to barriers to the successful implementation of open disclosure. Although in principle disclosing incidents can be a way to maintain or re-establish trust, where it is not responsive to the individual patient's needs, it may in fact result in a further deterioration of interpersonal trust.

In Australia, the national Open Disclosure Framework was updated in 2013 (ACSQH, 2013a) and has been incorporated in the mandatory national standards for the accreditation of public health services (ACSQH, 2012). Mandating open disclosure is intended to ensure that open disclosure happens rather than relying on the practitioner's willingness. In practice, the implementation rate and success vary (Iedema, Mallock, Sorensen, Manias, Tuckett, & et al., 2008b). From my experience working with the NSW Health Care Complaints Commission, complaints can eventuate when patients are dissatisfied with the way they were treated by the practitioner after an incident and in some cases the main issue for the patient is no longer the incident, but the way it was handled. This experience concurs with findings by Duclos et al. (2005), Guijarro et al. (2010) and Lamb (2004).

I will highlight some of the key reasons that can hinder the successful implementation of open disclosure in the Australian, and specifically NSW, context, drawing partially on discussions I had as a member of the panel responsible for the review of the open disclosure policy and guide that applies to all public health staff and facilities in NSW. The following discussion highlights the complexities in implementing open disclosure despite a broad consensus to openly manage incidents.

While, in the context of civil proceedings, practitioners are protected from liability when they say sorry for errors that occurred in the patient's care (*NSW Civil Liability Act 2002*, s. 69), the law does not protect them from being sued or from having to respond to a patient's complaint. The practitioner's fear of being sued referred to above does not only relate to the possible outcome of the proceedings, but also to having to enter a prolonged and often adversarial process.

Practitioners may disclose an incident and apologise, but they cannot admit liability without the prior agreement of their medical indemnity insurer (Doms, 2010). Where a practitioner admits liability to the patient, they may risk losing their indemnity cover due to a common non-cooperation clause in indemnity contracts (AVANT, 2013). In addition, there are competing legislative provisions that may require practitioners to withhold certain information from the patient. In NSW, when there has been a serious incident, a root cause analysis must be undertaken by an appointed team. All information prepared during the course of this analysis attracts an absolute privilege according to the *NSW Health Administration Act 1982* (s. 20P, 20Q) and therefore cannot be disclosed to the patient, or be accessed by subpoena. The patient can only have access to the final report of the root cause analysis, which in practice can take some time to be completed and does not address specific questions the patient might have in the timeframe they expect. In practice, legal and insurance considerations contribute to practitioners remaining cautious in their disclosure to patients.

Another aspect of successful open disclosure that can preserve or reinstate trust is compensation where warranted. In the US, so called 'disclosure-and-resolution' programs have been adopted by several health services (Mello, Senecal, Kuznetsov, & Cohn, 2014), which, where appropriate, offer compensation after an error has been disclosed. Although it appears that this approach has reduced liability costs overall, a recent study by Murtagh, Gallagher, Andrew and Mello (2012) examines offers of compensation in more detail. In one scenario the offer of compensation was made together with the apology and disclosure, and in another scenario the compensation discussion was held separately. Their findings suggest that the offer of full compensation can be perceived as an attempt to avoid litigation, and it may be beneficial to separate open disclosure from discussions of compensation. Nevertheless, it was important for the majority of patients that an offer of compensation was made. It appears that in both scenarios discussed in the study, patients would not relinquish their right to take legal action by accepting compensation. Such compensation agreements may have a different impact on patients' perceptions.

Disclosing an error is a difficult psychological challenge for any person, but specifically for practitioners (Wears & Wu, 2002) who have been trained in a culture that commonly associates errors with the perception of incompetence or can threaten someone's professional reputation (Engel, Rosenthal, & Sutcliffe, 2006). Where a practitioner discloses an error, a lack of experience or training in how to do it appropriately can result in the relationship to the patient or their family deteriorating after the disclosure. Specifically, the emotional impact of and reaction to the incident that is experienced by both the practitioner and the patient can be underestimated. As mentioned above, few practitioners have been trained specifically in open disclosure (Gallagher, Waterman et al., 2006; Stroud et al., 2009), and if they were trained, they may not have access to support at the time of subsequent, actual disclosure. To ensure relevant training, support and resources are available to practitioners involved in open disclosure, it needs to be given priority by senior management of the health service (Levinson & Gallagher, 2007). The review of the Open Disclosure Policy in NSW will introduce dedicated open disclosure coordinators and advisors to support practitioners during the actual open disclosure process (NSW Health, 2014b).

Practitioners have sometimes been described as 'second victims' (Wu, 2000) of the incident and lack of support, in some cases, had a significant impact on practitioners' personal and professional lives, with some practitioners stopping practising after incidents (Gallagher, Waterman et al., 2006). Lack of support and a negative impact on personal and professional lives can act as a deterrent to be frank, open and honest to patients, colleagues and peers, and may mean a retreat to defensive practising of medicine or non-disclosure of future incidents.

In summary, although open disclosure of incidents is what patients want, there are a number of personal, cultural, organisational and legal barriers that can prevent practitioners from engaging in open disclosure. Where practitioners do disclose, the disclosure can go wrong if communication is partial or defensive, or does not address the patient's expectations and needs. I argue that only where (a) open disclosure takes place and (b) is fully transparent and responsive to the patient's expectations and needs can it be a mechanism to regain or maintain trust (Woods, 2007; Wojcieszak, Saxton, & Finkelstein, 2007). Both the practitioner's willingness to speak about the incident and the quality of communication between the practitioner and patient are critical factors that influence whether their trust continues or breaks down after incidents (Beitat et al., 2013).

Before I summarise the findings from the literature review and their applicability to my own research, I would like to turn my attention specifically to the German and Australian health care environments to highlight some relevant differences in the way health care incidents are being dealt with.

2.3.2 Broader context – dealing with health care incidents in Australia and Germany

Germany is the biggest European economy and has the highest health care spending in the European Union. In 2012, about 80.5 million people lived in Germany (Statistisches Bundesamt, 2014a), compared to just over 23 million people in Australia (Australian Bureau of Statistics, 2014). Germany is a federal system with 16 states (Bundesländer) and medical practice is regulated at federal and state levels (Bundesministerium für Gesundheit, 2014a, b). Similarly, Australia is a Commonwealth union of two territories and six states, and medical practice is regulated both at federal (Australian Department of Health, 2014) and state levels (NSW Health, 2014a).

The health sector in both countries is structured into different levels. For the purpose of comparison, I focus on medical services provided by medical practitioners. General services are mainly provided by general practitioners in the community, while specialist services can be provided by both community and hospital based practitioners (Hurley, Baum, Johns, & Labonte, 2010; King & Green, 2012; Powell-Davies, McDonald, Jeon, Krastev, Christl, & Faruqi, 2009). Unlike in Australia, in Germany there is a legislated freedom of choice for patients (Bundesministerium für Gesundheit, 2014c), which means that patients can directly access specialist care. In Australia, every patient is required to be referred to a specialist by a medical practitioner who considers that specialist treatment is required (Health Insurance Act 1973, s. 132A; Health Insurance Regulation 1975 (Commonwealth), s. 29). Often the general practitioner acts as the patient's gatekeeper to the specialised health care system.

In general, the complexity of health care delivery increases once a patient accesses specialist care. With increasing complexity, the risk of something un-expected happening also increases. At the same time, the relevance of trust in the interpersonal relationship between a single patient and their practitioner decreases, and interpersonal trust is dispersed onto multiple interpersonal interactions.

In relation to health care incidents, Australia and NSW in particular, has relevant legislation and policy directives that require serious incidents that happen in the public health system be investigated to determine their root cause (*NSW Health Administration Act 1982*, division 6C; NSW Health Admin-istration Regulation 2010, part 3); that incidents be reported for quality and safety improvement (NSW Health, 2007a); and that incidents be disclosed to the patient and/or their family (NSW Health, 2007b).

In contrast, in Germany, until 2013 when the Patientenschutzrecht (patient protection law) was passed (Bundesministerium für Gesundheit, 2013), there was no legislation that directly required the investigation, reporting and disclo-sure to patients of serious incidents. Although it had been argued that German practitioners already had a duty to disclose serious incidents as an extension of the contractual agreement they have with their patients to treat them (Thomeczek, Hart, Hochreutener, Neu, Petry, & et al., 2009), in practice, exist-ing measures to deal with incidents were mainly local and voluntary. Although there is some willingness to anonymously report incidents for quality and safety improvement (Tuffs, 2005), the disclosure to patients is less well supported. According to a survey undertaken by the University of Bonn, 57% of the hospital respondents currently have no standard and have no plans to develop a standard about informing patients or their relatives about serious medical errors (Immel-Sehr, 2011).

With the introduction of the Patientenschutzrecht in March 2013 (Bundesministerium für Gesundheit, 2013), practitioners are required to inform patients about medical errors under certain circumstances; patients have the legal right to access their medical records; health insurance organisations are obliged to support patients in making complaints or claims regarding medical errors; and the burden of proof for claims has mainly shifted to the practitioner.

As outlined above, one potential barrier to openly disclose incidents and errors can be the practitioner's fear of losing their medical indemnity insurance cover. In Germany in 2008, a specific provision was added to the relevant legislation (*Versicherungsvertragsgesetz*, section 105, see Deutscher Bundestag, 2007) that declares 'non-cooperation' clauses in insurance agreements invalid. Non-cooperation clauses can be commonly found in all types of insurance contracts (Banja, 2005), also in Australia (AVANT, 2013, p. 37), and operate to release the insurance company from its obligation to pay costs if the insured person admits liability without the prior consent from the insurer. While the German legal amendment appears to provide security to practitioners to freely speak to their patients about medical errors and even admit liability, they still risk losing their insurance cover (Ärzte Zeitung, 2008). If the practitioner accepts liability, they may have to prove this claim to their liability insurer to remain covered. Effectively, although practitioners are free to talk to patients about errors without admitting liability, given the current insurance provisions, most will first check with their indemnity insurers, which in some cases will lead to delays in talking to the patient about an error or incident.

On a professional level, the code of conduct for medical practitioners in Australia includes a section that states:

> [w]hen adverse events occur, you have a responsibility to be open
> and honest in your communication with your patient, to review

what has occurred and to report appropriately. (Australian Medical Board, 2010, p. 7)

By contrast, the relevant federal (Bundesärztekammer, 2011) and state level codes of conduct (Sächsische Landesärztekammer, 2011) that apply to practitioners in Germany do not include comparable provisions. With the introduction of the Patientenschutzrecht in 2013, it is anticipated that a specific provision around the disclosure of medical errors would be reflected in these professional codes in the future.

In summary, in Australia a legislative and policy framework has been established since 2002 that supports the open disclosure of incidents to patients. Although there are some remaining issues with competing interests in the legislation and insurance provisions, in general, it can be said that the regulators have created a supportive basis on which Australian practitioners can safely disclose incidents and errors to patients. In contrast, in Germany open disclosure has only been recognised in the Patientenschutzrecht in 2013, and more steps are required to include new patient rights regarding open disclosure of medical errors in relevant professional standards and organisational policies. In both countries, changes in the medical culture are required to challenge the common perception that incidents are a sign of a practitioner's failure or incompetence, and to provide practical help and support to both patients and practitioners to engage in open disclosure after incidents.

Following on from the above discussion, although open communication about incidents is desired by patients and supported in principle by practitioners (Gallagher et al., 2003; Gallagher, Waterman et al., 2006), in practice disclosure may not happen or be inadequate in the patient's perception. These situations can trigger a patient complaint about the health care provider to get the information and explanation they seek, and in some cases, to reprimand the practitioner for their handling of the incident, which in the patient's eyes was deficient. Patients also complain because they do not want what happened to them to happen to anyone else (Hobgood et al., 2005), indicating that open disclosure, if it took place, did not address adequately how to prevent similar incidents from occurring in future.

I will briefly outline existing avenues available to patients in Germany and Australia to make a claim or complaint about an incident. Understanding patients' options and the transparency afforded by the regulatory system is important in understanding the discrepancy between patients' wishes for open and honest information after incidents in general, and possible measures in practice. I argue that the greater the discrepancy between what patients want and what they can actually achieve within the given systems, the more likely there will be a negative impact on the patient's trust in the practitioner after incidents.

2.3.2.1 Patient avenues for complaints and claims

In Germany, patients who are concerned about their health care can complain directly to the provider who can inform their indemnity insurer. Patients can also complain to the relevant state's medical board; they can initiate civil proceedings against the provider or, in serious cases of alleged physical assault, the police can investigate and, if evidence is found, initiate criminal proceedings.

Where patients complain to the medical board alleging a medical error, the board will usually refer this complaint to one of the twelve Gutachterkommissionen (expert assessor commissions and mediation bodies)[6]. These expert assessor commissions are estimated to deal with approximately one quarter of all claims of medical error or negligence, or over 12,000 claims in 2012 (Bundesärztekammer, 2013b, p. 2). The expert commissions found no evidence of error or negligence in over two thirds of claims it assessed in 2012 (Bundesärztekammer, 2013b, p. 5). In cases where the commission finds evidence of an error or negligence, the patient can take this result to the indemnity insurer of

---

[6] Twelve expert assessor commissions and mediation bodies exist in Germany (Bundesärztekammer, 2013a).

the practitioner and in many, but not all cases, the insurer will reach an agreement with the patient. Expert commission reports are not binding and there are no formal appeal options against determinations made by the assessment commission. Where patients disagree with the commission's finding, they are free to initiate civil proceedings against the practitioner (Bundesärztekammer, 2013a). The advantage for patients is that the expert commission proceedings come at no costs to them and if the commission finds some evidence, it enhances the patient's claim to the indemnity insurer and possibly in civil litigation against the practitioner (Bundesärztekammer, 2013a).

At its core, the German system of expert assessor commissions is a system of self-regulation of the medical profession, with proceedings relying on voluntary engagement of the practitioner and outcomes lacking legal authority. In 2009, the chair of the permanent association of the expert assessor commissions, Dr. Andreas Crusius, said at a press conference that the German system of dealing with claims is unique and no comparable institutions exist in the world:

> Die Gutachterkommissionen und Schlichtungsstellen sind in gewisser Weise einzigartig. Es gibt nirgendwo auf der Welt vergleichbare Einrichtungen, die den Patienten ein derartiges Angebot der Begutachtung und Schlichtung unterbreiten.[7] (Crusius, 2009, pp. 1-2)

Australia, and specifically NSW, went further than the German model and established by legislation independent health complaints commissions in the early 1990s, including in NSW in 1993 (*NSW Health Care Complaints Act 1993*). Similar to Germany, patients in Australia have multiple avenues to complain about the treatment and care they have received. Patients can complain directly to the practitioner seeking direct resolution; or to the management of the

---

[7] Translation: 'The expert assessor commissions and medication bodies are in a certain way unique. There are nowhere in the world comparable bodies that make patients such an offer of assessing and mediating a claim.'

health facility where the practitioner works. They can make a complaint to the independent Health Care Complaints Commission or the medical board, or they can initiate civil proceedings. In cases of criminal conduct, patients can report to police who may investigate and bring criminal charges against a practitioner. The main difference between the German and Australian systems, and the NSW system in particular (HCCC, 2014a), is the role and functions of the independent Health Care Complaints Commission, which acts as a co-regulator in conjunction with the registration authorities. Where either body receives a patient complaint, they must notify the other body and consult with each other to determine how to most appropriately deal with the complaint. There is a balance of power between the self-regulatory registration system and the independent commission, and patients have the legislated right to request a review of decisions. A second difference is that the Health Care Complaints Commission has as its core function the protection of the health and safety of the public; its jurisdiction is protective, not punitive. In some cases that can mean that the perspective the Commission takes when assessing complaints and the conduct of a practitioner can be different to the patient's view and what they want to achieve. The Commission takes into account complaint histories of practitioners when assessing complaints, while the German assessor commissions look at each case individually. While some patients primarily seek compensation or punitive actions against a practitioner, the NSW Commission's aim is to protect the public from unsafe practitioners. In the most serious case, investigations by the Health Care Complaints Commission can lead to prosecutions before a disciplinary body, a Tribunal or Professional Standards Committee, which can result in the Tribunal cancelling a practitioner's registration or suspending the practitioner for a specified period, as it considers the practitioner practising a risk to the health or safety of the public. In Germany, the state based medical boards can initiate disciplinary action to seek de-registration of a practitioner.

Overall, the multitude of complaint avenues in both countries can be confusing for patients to navigate. Patients who have experienced an incident or who are dissatisfied with the care and treatment they received may not raise their concerns because they fear retribution by the practitioner or they find the complaint system too confusing to navigate on their own. Especially where patients primarily seek information to understand what had happened or where they wish to receive an apology, they may be disheartened to enter into a formal complaint process, particularly given that the outcome they seek may not be achievable.

Despite the differences in systems, patient expectations after incidents are unlikely to be met by complaint bodies in the majority of cases. Patients expect to be informed of incidents as soon as possible, offered support, receive an apology and be assured that the provider will take action to prevent a future occurrence (O'Connor, Coates, Yardley, & Wu, 2010). Formal complaint processes can only ever achieve the requested outcomes after a lengthy process, which can have a negative impact on acceptance by the patient. However, formal complaint processes can complement open disclosure in cases where error or misconduct did occur to ensure that appropriate action is being taken against the practitioner or provider to ensure the health and safety of patients in general.

In summary, complaint processes cannot replace open disclosure of incidents, which I have discussed above as a measure to maintain or restore the patient's trust in the practitioner. Complaint processes may be a mechanism to restore trust in the regulatory and medical system, and as such may have some influence on the interpersonal trust relationship between patient and practitioner according to the layer model, I outlined at the beginning of this chapter.

2.4 Summary

In this chapter, I discussed different approaches to trust by firstly distinguishing three levels of analysis, before focussing on the interpersonal level and describing elements and related concepts, including risk and trustworthiness, in more detail. I then derived my understanding of interpersonal trust for the purpose of this book as:

Interpersonal trust is a dynamic and voluntary process, involving both cognitive and affective elements that shape a positive expectation about a future outcome and enables cooperation by accepting vulnerability posed by associated risks.

I then looked specifically at the relationship between patients and practitioners and developed a model to illustrate the dynamics of interpersonal trust being a continuous circle consisting of information and knowledge, expectations and outcomes, all of which constantly influence and are influenced by the relationship between the patient and practitioner and their communication. I then applied my understanding of the interpersonal trust dynamics to situations where something has gone wrong, where an incident in the care or treatment of the patients occurred.

Incidents constitute something unexpected and undesirable and thus test patients' trust in practitioners. Having established the importance of patient expectations being met to sustain trust, open disclosure appears to be a mechanism to be responsive to patient expectations and thus restore trust. However, in practice, barriers exist that may prevent practitioners from disclosing incidents, or where they do disclose, the communication and action may not meet the patient's expectation. Where open disclosure is successful in restoring the patient's trust, patients may abstain from taking further action against the practitioner. In contrast, where there is a lack of or inadequate disclosure, this may become the trigger for the relationship between patient and practitioner to deteriorate with significant impact on trust levels. Where patients decide to take further action, for example by making a formal complaint against the practitioner, these processes may bring closure to the patients, but rarely can restore trust. I argue that restoring trust is essential for the continuation of the relationship and for effective care and treatment of the patients, due to its close association with openness of communication, patient compliance and satisfaction.

The dynamics of trust between patients and practitioners appear to be the same in routine situations and after incidents. What appears to differ are the patients' and their families' expectations and the actions required to meet them.

In the next chapter, which is the core of this book, I will attempt to find empirical evidence that would support this statement.

Chapter 3   Experiences of Patients and Medical Practitioners

3.1   Introduction

This chapter is the core of my book, summarising my methodological approach and the key results of two empirical studies exploring the interaction between trust and incidents in the treatment and care of patients. I present this information in one chapter to facilitate the reader's understanding by cross-referencing the key results and explaining how they relate to the overall research aim. A separate discussion chapter will include my interpretation of the results and place them in the broader context of relevant literature.

The chapter consist of four parts. The first part – the methodology section – summarises my research design and approach to data, collection, analysis and interpretation.

In the second part, I present themes emerging from explorative interviews with practitioners, while the third part contrasts these with the themes that emerged in interviews with patients. I present the emerging narratives in three broad categories, namely communication, competence and care related, to compare practitioner and patient experiences of a health care incident.

In the fourth section of this chapter, I will summarise the results of an anonymous survey of medical practitioners regarding their attitude and experiences with medical errors. The survey focussed on issues from a practitioner's point of view that either would have prevented them from disclosing a medical error or have impacted on their attitude to disclosing and dealing with medical errors in general.

3.2   Measuring interpersonal trust

The review of the relevant literature in Chapter 2 showed that there is a broad understanding that interpersonal trust in the relationship between patients and their medical practitioner is positively associated with open communication, higher levels of patient compliance and satisfaction and overall better health care outcomes.

What remained unanswered was what exactly happens to interpersonal trust between patients and practitioners after an incident in the care or treatment of a patient? Do higher trust levels influence the practitioner's willingness to disclose the incident to the patient? What is the impact of the incident on the trust levels in the relationship?

Before I describe my approach to fieldwork and my methodology in more detail, I will briefly summarise the empirical research on interpersonal trust in patient-practitioner settings to date and identify a gap that I aim to at least partially address with my own fieldwork.

Although there are numerous theoretical conceptualisations of interpersonal trust in the patient-practitioner relationship, there are fewer empirical studies, most of which have concentrated on interpersonal trust in routine health care settings (Anderson & Dedrick, 1990; Kao, Green, Davis, Koplan, & Cleary, 1998; Kao, Green, Zaslavsky, Koplan, & Cleary, 1998; Thom, 2001; Thom et al., 2004; Thom, Kravitz, Bell, Krupat & Azari, 2002; Thom, Ribisl, Stewart, & Luke, 1999).

One early, influential study was Anderson and Dedrick (1990) in which they developed a 'trust in physician' scale. Initially, they developed a survey with 25 items derived from theoretical considerations that were later reduced to 11 items that fell into five categories: fidelity, competence, honesty, confidentiality and global trust, the latter functioning as a connector between the other four categories. The survey used a 5-point Likert-scale ranging from *strongly agree* to *strongly disagree*. All participants of the study were male, suffered from diabetes and were treated as primary health care or outpatients. Anderson and Dedrick made some assumptions, including that trust and patient satisfaction would be correlated. They also assumed that higher levels of interpersonal trust would be associated with a lesser degree of the patient's wish to have control in their relationship with the practitioner. In relation to the latter assumption, I outlined above when distinguishing different types of patient-doctor relationships that active or passive patient roles may be the result of patient personality types and preferences, and therefore unsuitable to indicate lower or higher levels of interpersonal trust.

Anderson and Dedrick's trust-in-physician-scale was further validated in a study by Thom, Bloch, et al. (1999) that included primary health care patients who were followed up after six months. Participants were surveyed using the trust-in-physician-scale, as well as about their demographic data, their preferences for and satisfaction with care. Results further validated the scale and indicated that interpersonal trust increased with the length of the relationship patients had with the practitioner. Results also indicated that trust levels were higher among patients who had actively chosen their practitioner, preferred their practitioner to be more involved in the decision-making and other aspects of their health care. Patients who reported trusting their practitioner also more commonly reported continuing to consult with that practitioner, adhering to medication schemes and generally were more satisfied with their practitioner. Based on data from the same study, Thom (2001) related certain practitioner behaviour to higher levels of self-reported patient trust. According to Thom, patients' trust in their practitioner was most strongly associated with perceiving the practitioner as caring, technically competent and being a good communicator.

Building on the findings from the earlier study, Thom, Bloch, et al. (1999) attempted to change practitioners' behaviour to see whether it would influence the trust levels reported by patients. Practitioners underwent a one day training workshop. However, reported trust and satisfactions levels of patients of practitioners who had undergone the intervention were not significantly different from those for patients of a control group. Thom (2001) concluded that the intervention was not strong enough to achieve the anticipated result.

A British study among primary health care patients that was undertaken by Tarrant, Stokes and Baker (2003) reached similar findings to Thom (2001), namely, that the quality of the patient-practitioner relationship, specifically where the patient perceived the practitioner's communication, care and knowledge to be of a high level, was strongly associated with the patient's reported trust in the practitioner.

There have been a number of other survey studies using different types of scales to assess the interpersonal trust a patient reported to have in their practitioner (Hall et al., 2001; Kao, Green, Davis, et al., 1998; Kao, Green, Zaslavsky, et al., 1998; Mechanic & Schlesinger, 1996; Safran, Kosinski, Tarlov, Rogers, Taira, & et al., 1998; see also Pearson & Raeke, 2000; Turjalei, 2008). These studies researched interpersonal trust in various types of health care routine situations using quantitative surveys based on different pre-defined scales to obtain the self-reported levels of interpersonal trust of patients. I did not find any studies that specifically referred to incidents and the impact of an incident on the patient's reported trust levels.

Looking at relevant research about incidents in health care and open disclosure, I found a great number of studies that looked at patient experiences of and expectations after incidents (Gallagher et al., 2003; Iedema, Sorensen, Manias, Tuckett, Piper, & et al., 2008; Schwappach & Koeck, 2004; Wu, Huang, Stokes, & Provonost, 2009) and studies that researched practitioners' experiences with incidents and open disclosure and attitudes towards those (Chan, Gallagher, Reznick, & Levinson, 2005; Gallagher, Studdert, et al., 2006; Gallagher, Waterman, et al., 2006).

The study of Gallagher, Waterman, et al. (2006) mentions interpersonal trust as a side issue, asking participating practitioners whether they believe that disclosing an error would damage the patient's trust in their competence. Wu et al. (2009) looked at patients' reaction to disclosure and as part of that study found a high association between practitioners offering a full apology and patients' trust in their practitioner. Duclos et al. (2005) explored patient perspectives of the interpersonal communication after adverse events and found that the patient's perceived trust in the practitioner was associated with the practitioner communicating well after an incident.

In summary, research of medical incidents did either not include trust at all or referred to it as a side issue, assuming a common and shared understanding of what is patient trust in physicians. I could not locate studies that specifically looked at the impact of incidents on interpersonal trust.

Given the lack of studies about trust development after incidents and my understanding of trust as a holistic phenomenon, including partly subconscious, psychological processes, my approach to the fieldwork was exploratory. I did not assume that the factors associated with higher patient trust that emerged from the studies in routine situations above would be the same after incidents. Rather than using a set of pre-defined categories of factors I believed from theoretical considerations to influence or be influenced by interpersonal trust levels after incidents, I used an explorative approach that attempted to minimise preconceptions and used the data gathered from my fieldwork to identify factors that were relevant to practitioners and patients after incidents and their relationship to interpersonal trust development after incidents. I will outline my approach and methodology in more detail below.

3.2.1   Approach to fieldwork

I conceptualised that patient trust in their medical practitioner, in most cases, subconsciously exists without people rationalising or thinking about it. Existing studies on interpersonal trust related to routine situations. The common use of pre-defined scales to measure trust made them unsuitable to explore the dynamic of trust after incidents, because of the risk of missing new or unexpected aspects. To reflect the explorative nature of my approach, the following broad question guided my fieldwork: What is the relationship between interpersonal trust in the doctor-patient relationship and communication in the context of health care incidents?

I considered that an incident constitutes a period in the patient-practitioner relationship that is non-routine and unexpected and may therefore cause the patient to reconsider or reflect on their trust in a practitioner. This may affect the dynamic of the interpersonal trust in the relationship, which may differ from routine situations.

Having rejected the idea of positivism and the associated notion that as a researcher I could have direct access to an 'objective' reality, my approach to researching trust can be broadly described as a constructivist, following Crotty's (1998) understanding of constructivism:

> There is no objective truth waiting for us to discover it. … There is no meaning without the mind. Meaning is not discovered, but constructed. In this understanding of knowledge, it is clear that different people may construct meaning in different ways, even in relation to the same phenomenon. (pp. 8-9)

My access to understanding what trust means to patients and practitioners was indirect through the way people describe how they perceived and experienced a particular event or incident. Any knowledge about trust would be the result of multiple construction processes. Participants in my research would have re-constructed an event or incident by categorising the information they saw, heard, smelled or otherwise experienced in a way that made sense to them (Dervin, 1998). Participants would then communicate their perception to me (or another person), aiming to achieve a mutual understanding, and I would assign meaning to the information I receive with reference to my own prior knowledge. Participants and researcher would attempt to mutually construct a shared understanding of the incident and related action by constantly (and often subconsciously) categorising the information using their own existing knowledge in addition to checking back whether the information provided was understood as intended. In the progress of this multi-layer construction process, the person may adjust their initial perception of the incident.

Ultimately, I could only research a person's perception of an event at a particular point in time. Perceptions of the same event may change over time. Similarly, my interpretation and sense making of the narratives provided would depend on my own knowledge and preconceptions at a particular point in time when analysing and interpreting the data.

Although I could not have direct access to the 'objective' world, understanding a person's perception of a situation was most relevant in order to understand what trust means to them. Referring to Leon Festinger's (1962) theory of cognitive dissonance, I considered that the way someone perceives something would ultimately influence their behaviour. The access to the 'objective truth' of what trust is became irrelevant, as I was interested in how people perceive others or certain events and how that related to interpersonal trust. The constructive approach to fieldwork also had implications for the way I analysed and interpreted the collected data.

Derived from the review of literature, I theorised that both the quality of the patient-practitioner communication as well as the practtioner's willingness to disclose and discuss an incident with the patient would influence whether interpersonal trust between both sides would be able to be maintained or rebuilt after an incident.

Designing my research study, I wanted to combine an explorative, flexible approach to what trust after incidents means for patients and practitioners with inquiring about the willingness and experiences of practitioners in disclosure of incidents to patients. In my understanding, such willingness was fundamental to maintaining or rebuilding trust after incidents. I chose a mixed method approach consisting of a qualitative, explorative interview study (see also Silverman, 2005) that aimed to identify themes and dynamics of trust and communication after incidents, followed by a descriptive, quantitative survey of a representative sample of medical practitioners about key aspects of their willingness to disclose and communicate about incidents. By combining quantitative and qualitative methods I intended to complement my findings from both studies (Hammersley, 1992) to establish waht contributes to the maintance or rebuidlign of interpersonal trust after incidents.

3.2.2   The qualitative interview study

The dynamic model of trust that I introduced above, derived from literature research, suggested that a mismatch between expectation and actual outcome would lead to the erosion of trust. With an incident representing the mismatch between what a patient expected in their care and treatment and their perception of the outcome, I wanted to see whether there was empirical evidence supporting the assumed dynamic.

As outlined in Chapter 2, my understanding of an incident is broad in that I considered an incident to be any unexpected event in the treatment or care of a patient. Incidents may or may not be recognisable to the patient and medical practitioners. What accounts for an incident from a patient's perspective may be part of a normal treatment risk from the practitioner's point of view.

To determine situations that both the patient and the practitioner would perceive as an incident, I chose to look at patient complaints. A complaint about an incident was considered evidence that the incident was both experienced and defined as an issue by the patient and/or their family or carers. Through making a complaint, the relevant medical practitioner was also aware of the incident and the associated issues the patient had from their perspective.

Hence, the fact that there was a formal complaint meant that there was a shared understanding that there had been an incident and the practitioner had an understanding of the patient's perspective before offering their own perspective.

I chose to conduct semi-structured interviews to gain an understanding of the dynamic of trust in the patient-practitioner relationship and relevant factors from the participants' perspectives that influenced their relationship and trust levels. My review of relevant literature had revealed a gap insofar that I could not locate any empirical work inquiring into interpersonal trust in the patient-practitioner relationship after incidents. Given the absence of precedents, I considered a qualitative approach with its inherent flexibility to be more suitable than controlled studies or experimental test designs (Axelrod, 1984; Rotter, 1967) in exploring this area. As set out above, I also intended to minimise imposing my own preconceptions, which meant that I decided against using surveys with pre-defined scales that had been tested in routine medical encounters (Anderson & Dedrick, 1990; Kao, Green, Davis, et al., 1998; Kao, Green, Zaslavsky, et al., 1998; Thom, Ribisl, et al., 1999). A survey may not have fully captured the dynamic development over time and also had an inherent potential to (mis-)direct responses by imposing my own understanding of the phenomenon through the questions used in such a survey.

With reference to Thom (2001), I designed the semi-structured interview schedule to cover three broad categories – namely, communication, competence and care – in relation to which I developed mostly open-ended questions. I was mindful that trust may not be an established term of which people share a common understanding and which often is not even rationalised in a way that a person could respond to a question about who, when, how and why they trust (Fontana & Frey, 2000).

My approach to the interviews in a broad sense can be described as related to ethnography (Berg, 2009), as I shared the assumptions that as a researcher, I would be an active participant in the sense-making process of the participants (Holstein & Gubrium, 1995). Although for practical reasons I could not immerse myself and observe the incident and the patient practitioner relationship before, during and after the incident (Heyl, 2001), I was interested in how trust in the patient and practitioner's view had developed in the course of their relationship. Opting for semi-structured interviews, I gave participants the opportunity to describe freely their perceptions and priorities in regard to the incident while relating their experiences and emotions to the chronological timelines that would enable me to look at the dynamic developments in the relationship.

3.2.2.1 Practical implementation

Sample selection

The interviews were undertaken in New South Wales, Australia, with its unique legal and policy framework that in principle supports – and for practitioners working in the public system mandates – the disclosure of incidents to patients (NSW Health, 2007b). In addition, practitioners disclosing incidents and offering an apology were protected from their apology being considered an admission of liability in civil proceedings (*NSW Civil Liability Act 2002*, section 69). Thirdly, patients in NSW have the opportunity to make a complaint about a practitioner to the independent Health Care Complaints Commission which has the authority to investigate and prosecute practitioners with the possibility of disciplinary action being taken. As outlined above, often incidents may not be known either to the patient or the practitioner, and by making a complaint, there was a shared understanding that an incident had happened. Statistical data on complaints to the Commission is publically accessible and covers a range of different types of health service providers, regions, types of services and facilities.

Both medical practitioners and patients who had been involved in a complaint to the Commission, and thus an incident, were included in the sample.

The aim was to understand how both sides experienced incidents and whether and how perceptions overlapped or differed.

The analysis of the complaint data of the NSW Health Care Complaints Commission (HCCC 2013, p. 106) shows that complaints about medical practitioners are more common than complaints about any other type of health service provider. Practitioners working in general medicine and surgery attracted the most complaints. This mirrors the data compiled by the German expert assessor commissions and mediation bodies that also shows that general practice and surgery are the most commonly complained about areas in Germany (Bundesärztekammer, 2013b).

General practitioners and surgeons, in general, are different in the way they interact with their patients. The typical relationship between surgeons and their patient can be described as a limited period interaction relating to a specific, from a patient's point of view often serious, health problem for which surgery is required. While surgery may be routine for the trained surgeon, for the patient and their family, in most cases, it is an exceptional situation, commonly associated with high levels of anxiety, uncertainty and significant impact on the health status and life of the patient. The average patient's knowledge about surgical procedures can be considered less extensive than patients' knowledge about general practice, which also contributes to higher levels of uncertainty and a higher risk of misunderstanding and misalignment of expectation of patients and practitioners in surgery compared to general practice. In contrast, patients' interaction with general practitioners is much more common and therefore harbours less potential for uncertainty. Relationships between patients and general practitioners tend to be more frequent and long term compared to surgery and can cover a broad range of medical issues.

In Australia, compared to Germany, the distinction between general practice and surgery is clearer due to the requirement (*NSW Health Insurance Act 1973*, section 132A (2)) for all patients to be referred by another medical practitioner, usually the general practitioner, to a surgeon. In Australia, general practitioners usually act as a gatekeeper to the wider health system, except in emergencies. With specialists interacting with patients at a later stage of their health care journey, patients often have some knowledge and understanding about their symptoms and associated expectations. In contrast, German patients are free to choose their health practitioner and can consult specialists directly (Bundesministerium für Gesundheit, 2014c).

Initially, the study sample was designed to include both complaints that were resolved or handled directly between the medical practitioner and their patients and another group where the complaint was lodged with a third party, the NSW Health Care Complaints Commission. It was assumed that a successful resolution of the complaint at a local level may be associated with the relationship of trust between patient and provider being maintained or restored, whilst lodging a complaint with an independent third party – the Commission – could be an indication that the relationship between practitioner and patient had deteriorated to a point where trust could not be restored at all, or required the assistance of a third party. This assumption was reached from results of an earlier study of complaints to the Commission, in which only two of the 290 respondents stated that they would consult the doctor complained about again in future (Daniel, Burn, & Horarik, 1999). While one could assume that patients complain to the Health Care Complaints Commission about what they consider serious matters, while trying to resolve less serious issues directly with the provider, the Commission's complaint statistics (HCCC, 2013, p. 115) show that the vast majority of complaints the Commission deals with did not raise serious issues of public health and safety that warrant formal investigation under its legislation (*NSW Health Care Complaints Act 1993*, section 23).

Initially, the aim of the study was to explore the expectations and experiences of both patient and practitioner who were involved in the same complaint, with one group where the complaint was managed locally and another where it was made to the Commission.

Recruitment proceeded through the Health Care Complaints Commission, as well as for directly managed cases through the Royal Australian College of General Practitioners and the Royal Australasian College of Surgeons. The recruitment of participants started in July 2009. By November 2009, I had not been successful in obtaining the consent from both parties – the patient and the practitioner – in a single complaint that was made to the Commission. For practitioners involved in a complaint to the Commission, there were concerns that interviewing the patient might re-ignite the complaint. In cases where the patient was interested to participate, the relevant practitioner declined and vice versa.

There were no successful recruitments of practitioners though the Colleges. Acknowledging that complaints are a sensitive topic, of which most practitioners do not wish to be reminded, especially when they consider them resolved and the fact that there was no financial incentive to participate offered, may explain the lack of responses. After four months, due to the lack of sufficient responses, I had to adjust the initial design of the study in order to be able to proceed.

Revised sample

The revised sample broadened the eligibility criteria to include cases where one of the parties was willing to be interviewed. Although that meant that no direct comparison of the practitioner's and the patient's perception of the same case and their associated expectations would be possible, it was deemed sufficient to get a general understanding of the experiences and perceptions of practitioners and patients who were involved in complaints. A detailed journal of the recruitment of participants and the reasons for changes made to the sample and recruitment strategy is included in Appendix 3.

By concentrating on formal complaints to the Commission, the study excluded cases in which the patient might have been dissatisfied or their trust in the practitioner had deteriorated, but they did not lodge a complaint. The NSW

Population Health Survey indicates that almost one in ten adult patients (9.6%) was not satisfied with the service received at a public hospital (NSW Health, 2009, p. 99). Extrapolating this data to the total number of patients admitted to public hospitals in NSW that year (HCCC, 2009, p. 104) would mean that almost 150,000 patients were not satisfied with the service that was provided at a public hospital to them.

In addition, some incidents or errors may not be visible to the patient. The data of the Incident Information Management System (IIMS) reported by the NSW Health and the Clinical Excellence Commission (2008) indicate that in 2007 the public health facilities overseen by the NSW Department of Health recorded 111,625 incidents (p. 12), of which 16,133 (14.5%) (p. 38) were recorded as complaints. Although these numbers apply to all public health facilities, public hospitals represent the greatest part. Data of the Health Care Complaints Commission shows that in 2007-08, 763 complaints were made about public hospitals, which suggests that only a small number of patients who are dissatisfied with the service they received actually make a complaint to the Health Care Complaints Commission.

German data for 2009 states that 40,000 complaints are lodged every year, of which about a quarter are dealt with by the medical board's expert assessor commissions and mediation bodies (Gutachterkommissionen[8]) (Bundesärztekammer, 2010). This number appears small in the context of over 18 million patient services provided in hospitals alone in 2012 (Statistisches Bundesamt, 2014b), which does not take into consideration the significant number of patient services provided in the primary health care sector.

---

[8] Gutachterkommission für Fragen ärztlicher Haftpflicht der Landesärztekammer Baden-Württemberg; Gutachter- und Schlichtungsstelle bei der Landesärztekammer Hessen; Schlichtungsstelle für Arzthaftpflichtfragen der Norddeutschen Ärztekammern; Gutachterkommission für ärztliche Behandlungsfehler bei der Ärztekammer Nordrhein; Schlichtungsausschuss zur Begutachtung ärztlicher Behandlungen bei der Landesärztekammer Rheinland-Pfalz; Gutachterkommission für Fragen ärztlicher Haftpflicht bei der Ärztekammer des Saarlandes; Gutachterstelle für Arzthaftpflichtfragen der Sächsischen Landesärztekammer; Gutachterkommission für ärztliche Haftpflichtfragen bei der Ärztekammer Westfalen-Lippe; Gutachterstelle für Arzthaftpflichtfragen bei der Bayerischen Landesärztekammer (Bundesärztekammer, 2013a)

Privacy and risk considerations

Researching complaints is a very sensitive area. Concerns raised by the Human Research Ethics Committee of the University of Technology, Sydney, which reviewed the study design, related to measures protecting the privacy of the participants, as well as minimising any potential harm caused by 're-living' the experience.

As I was the sole person having access to consent forms and contact details of the participants, privacy issues were limited. Not being a medical practitioner also meant that I did not have any legal obligation to report certain conduct to relevant authorities should I become aware of it during the interviews.[9] On advice given by AVANT medical indemnity insurance, I was also considered exempt[10] from Freedom of Information legislation in Australia at the time of the interviews, which otherwise could have meant that patients would have been able to seek access to recordings or transcripts of interviews.

Some patients became distressed or emotional during the interviews. In these situations, I paused the interview. There was no case in which the interviewee wished to end the interview prematurely. Although participants had the opportunity to contact an independent conciliator to talk about their grief, none of the participants actually did. A potential risk was also that talking about the incident could re-ignite the patient's grief and may lead to the patient taking further action against the practitioner. This risk was higher with the initial

---

[9]   Since August 2008, medical practitioners in NSW, and since July 2010 all registered health practitioners have the legal obligation to report 'notifiable' conduct to the relevant authorities. Notifiable conduct includes where a practitioner has a reasonable belief that another registered practitioner practised the profession whilst affected by alcohol or drugs; engaged in sexual misconduct in connection with the practice of the practitioner's profession; placed the public at risk of substantial harm in the practitioner's practice of the profession because the practitioner has an impairment; placed the public at risk of harm because the practitioner has practised in a way that constitutes a significant departure from accepted professional standards (*Health Practitioner Regulation National Law (NSW)*, section 140).

[10]   The exemption was based on the reasoning that there would be public interest in publishing identifiable information that would override the protection of the privacy and confidentiality awarded to participants.

design of the study and was cited as a reason by some practitioners who declined to be interviewed, if the related patient would also be interviewed. With the amendment to the sample, the requirement to interview both sides in the same cases was removed and thus this concern was addressed.

In some cases during the interviews, I was asked for advice about steps to take against the other party, or I was asked my opinion or evaluation of the facts as presented to me. Partly, this might have been due to my disclosure that I worked for the Health Care Complaints Commission, although the research was conducted independently. In all these cases, participants accepted my response that it would be inappropriate for me to provide any advice or opinion.

Face-to-face interviews can include strong emotions and in rare cases aggressive language. Indeed, many participants displayed emotions and some aggression during the interview; however, it was never directed at me but at other parties involved in the incident and its aftermath. Letting participants vent their anger, or pausing the interview when they felt distressed, were successful strategies I employed to deal with such situations.

I also considered the potential risks to my own safety when visiting people in their homes, often in the evening or on the weekend. The initial phone contact gave me a reasonable perception of any potential risks and in one case, I decided not to proceed with the interview due to safety concerns after the initial phone contact. In other cases, I suggested meeting in a public place rather than in the home of the participant.

Ethics approval

The study was formally supported by the Royal Australian College of General Practitioners, NSW Research Branch; the NSW Health Care Complaints Commission; AVANT Medical Indemnity Insurance and the Royal Australasian College of Surgeons. Formal ethics approval was granted by the Human Research Ethics Committee of the University of Technology, Sydney in July 2009, as well as the ethics committee of the Royal Australasian College of Surgeons. Amendments to the original ethics application in relation to the sample, recruitment of participants and mode of interview were approved in December 2009 and July 2010, respectively.

Research question and assumptions

With the change in the design and scope of the interview study, the overall research question was modified to reflect the characteristic of the sample and the data I would have access to. Ultimately, the research question that guided my interviews with patients and practitioners was:

> *What is the relationship between the interpersonal trust in the doctor-patient relationship and communication in the context of health care incidents?*

I intended to explore any themes that would emerge from the interviews that were associated either with building or maintaining trust in the interpersonal relationship between patient and practitioner, or with the deterioration of trust between the parties. Accordingly, the following sub-questions guided my research:

- What themes emerged from the interviews that are associated with the building and maintaining of interpersonal trust?
- What themes emerged that were associated with the deterioration of interpersonal trust?
- What triggers a patient complaint?
- What emotions do patients and practitioners experience in relation to an incident / complaint?
- What role does an apology play after health care incidents?

With reference to the results of Thom (2001), I assumed that the emerging themes would broadly fall into the three categories of competence, communication and care. Further with reference to the dynamic trust model developed in Chapter 2, I assumed that a discrepancy between expectations and actual outcome would have a negative effect on the reported trust levels, while where expectations were met or exceeded by the action or outcome, it would have a positive effect on reported trust levels.

To explore the dynamic of trust or the development of trust during the patient-practitioner interaction, I attempted to capture changes in the relationship, trust levels and communication before, during and after the incident.

Data collection

I conducted semi-structured, explorative interviews with 22 patients[11] and 12 practitioners between March and December 2010.

Miles and Huberman (1984, p. 27) note that any 'researcher, no matter how unstructured or inductive, comes to fieldwork with some orienting ideas, foci and tools'. Accordingly, I used some guiding questions that broadly covered the areas of communication, care and competence that were identified as related to interpersonal trust with reference to Thom (2001). I encouraged interviewees to talk as freely as possible about their experience and later in the interview asked them any outstanding questions I had. I considered this appropriate given the explorative character of the interviews and in order to limit my own influence on the way the interviewee constructed their accounts of experiences, their perceptions and understanding of trust in their relationship with the practitioner. The study was trialled with two practitioners and two patients. No substantial issues were identified and these interviews were included in the final analysis.

Most interviews were conducted face-to-face. Some interviewees volunteered that they preferred to meet me to see whether they could trust me

---

[11] In one case, the interview was conducted with the patient's wife, as the patient did not recall most of the circumstances, and in another case, I interviewed both the patient and his wife together, again due to the patient having a very limited recall of the incident. In both cases, the complaint about the incident was made by the wife.

before sharing their experience. In nine cases, the interview was via telephone where this was the participant's preference, or where participants lived in remote areas.

All interviews were voice-recorded with prior permission, which allowed me to concentrate on the conversation and later to transcribe the conversation from the recording. The de-identified transcripts were provided to each participant to confirm their accuracy. Given that I conducted all the interviews, any interviewer related bias (Atkinson & Silverman, 1997) would apply to all of the interviews.

In the process of conducting the interviews, I became more confident in letting interviewees give their own account with very limited prompts or questions from my side, as I came to understand the importance of not only what was being said, but also how and in what order and priority. Letting interviewees describe their experience as freely as possible and not interrupting them especially at the beginning of interviews was also conducive to them sharing authentic emotions they associated with the experience they described.

The study was completed with a total of 34 interviews, including six interviews with surgeons, six interviews with general practitioners, and 22 interviews with patients, all of whom had been involved in a formal complaint to the NSW Health Care Complaints Commission. Of the patients, 10 made their complaint about a general practitioner, 12 about a surgeon. In the interviews, most medical practitioners referred to several cases where they had experienced a conflict with a patient and/or an official patient complaint. The duration of interviews ranged from 22 minutes to over two hours, with an average of approximately one hour per interview.

Table 3.1   *Participants by gender*

	Female	Male	Total
Surgeon	-	6	6
General practitioner	2	4	6
Patient of surgeon	8+1*	-	9
Patient of general practitioner	7+1*	5	13
Total	**19**	**15**	**34**

* *The interviewee was female, but spoke on behalf of her husband, the patient.*

All interviewed surgeons were male, which reflects the gender distribution in the professions according to the activity report of the Royal Australasian College of Surgeons (2013) that states that in 2012, 91.2% of all active fellows of the College in NSW were male (p. 36). According to a 2006 study by the Department of Health (2006), women represented 38% of general practitioners in NSW, which was reflected in the study where 33% of interviewed general practitioners were female.

The majority of interviewed patient were female (77.3%). In general, women account for more health service attendances than men (except for emergency department visits) according to the 2010 NSW Health Population Survey (NSW Health, 2011), although not to a comparable extent. Reasons for the high proportion of female participants may include that women more commonly lodge complaints, or were more willing to share their experience than men.

Motivation to participate

Exploring the participants' motivations to be interviewed about their experiences can have an impact on the interpretation of the data. Complaints are a difficult topic for both patients and practitioners, as in most cases they are associated with negative emotions. For patients, incidents may have had a significant impact on their health status as well as other areas of their lives, including their relationships, their financial situations and their ability to work. Similarly, for medical practitioners, incidents and complaints are challenging as they may feel that they made a mistake, or someone implies they did. There was no financial incentive to participate in the interviews. Considering the time pressure of practitioners in particular and the topic, only a small number of patients and practitioners were willing to be interviewed.

Indeed, most practitioners had unique reasons to participate, including that they had a personal connection to Germany and wanted to support a German researcher's work. Other participants were critical of the way the Health Care Complaints Commission had dealt with the complaint and saw the opportunity to voice their opinion as the research was distributed through the Commission and given that I had disclosed that I work for the Commission.

On a more general level, almost all patients who were interviewed stated that they wanted to share their experience to prevent others from having to go through something similar, and secondly, to be heard by practitioners. This suggests that despite a complaint being finalised, for a number of patients their issues remained unresolved.

3.2.2.2 Reflection on my role as a researcher

Disclosing my work for the Commission led to some participants viewing me as someone who knows the system and could therefore understand their experience and may be able to make their voice better heard. Being familiar with the complaint-handling system also allowed me to concentrate on people's perceptions of what had happened, rather than having to ask a lot of process-related questions.

I discussed with my supervisors and peers several times how to deal with situations where participants viewed me not as an independent researcher, but a Commission representative or as someone they can seek advice or feedback from. Despite stating that I could not offer advice or my opinion, during the period in which I undertook the interviews, I reflected on the attempts to use me as a feedback tool to the Commission and discussed how to deal with these situations with other researchers at the Centre for Health Communication at the University of Technology, Sydney. I have, on occasion, used my understanding about people's perceptions, gained through the interviews, in my professional role at the Commission to suggest ways the Commission can improve its processes. At no time did I disclose any detailed information from the research, but I have drawn on the information given to me as a researcher in a generalised way. Importantly, at no time did I influence the handling of individual complaints, but have used the information to advise on improvements of Commission processes, particularly relating to the way it interacts with the parties to a complaint.

3.2.2.3 Data analysis

Approach to data analysis

Given a constructivist approach guided the design of the interview study, it influenced the way I analysed the interview transcripts. Having considered a number of possible approaches to the analysis, including content analysis, grounded theory and phenomenography, ultimately, I chose thematic analysis as the most suitable method.

Initially, I considered content analysis (Gribch, 2007; Neuendorf, 2002), as I was most familiar with this type of analysis from prior empirical studies I had undertaken (Beitat, 2004). However, when starting to define a coding system, I found that the methodological rigidness of content analysis, which essentially is a quantitative tool, was not suitable for capturing the depth of the data in semi-structured interviews. Even with a refined coding system, results could be distorted with certain categories such as 'I did not understand' being coded quite often, but the coding would not capture how the lack of understanding impacted on the interviewee's perception of a situation or person. Although I might have been able to define a detailed coding system to capture such contextual information, I considered that this approach would be overly complex, particularly when searching for relations between categories and codes. Also, some interviews focused on a small number of themes that were most relevant to the interviewee, while others covered a wide spectrum of themes the interviewee associated with their experience. I considered that using content analysis in these circumstances carried the risk of the results misrepresenting the data (Vaismoradi, Turunen, & Bondas, 2013). A third reason for not using content analysis was that I considered myself an active partner in a dialogue where the interviewed patient and practitioner reflected upon their experiences, and as a result, the transcripts were not considered an 'objective' source of data to be analysed.

In the search for a more suitable method to analyse my interview data, I considered grounded theory (Cutcliffe, 2005; Glaser & Strauss, 1967; Gribch, 2007, pp. 70-83; Mills, Bonner, & Francis, 2006) and phenomenography (Entwistle, 1997; Marton, Dall'alba, & Beaty, 1993; Richardson, 1999) before settling on thematic analysis (Buetow, 2010) also referred to as narrative analysis (Grbich, 2007, pp. 216-228).

Phenomenography has its origins in educational research (Entwistle, 1997) and aims to describe the attitude a subject has towards a specific phenomenon. I empathised with the assumption of ethnography that every subject has a different perception of the same phenomenon and that it was important to try to describe these different perceptions considering the individual context (Marton et al., 1993, p. 283) in order to understand the phenomenon. However, my reading of the phenomenographic approach (Barnard, McCosker, & Gerber, 1999) was that I could only interpret the data (rather than merely describe it) if I could compare my own perceptions of a phenomenon with those of others. Not having been involved in the incident or the patient-practitioner relationship, I was unable to compare my own perceptions with those described by the interviewees and hence, a phenomenographic analysis would have been limited to the description of categories of how people related to trust or other phenomena.

Similarly, I empathised with a number of assumptions and techniques used in a grounded theory approach according to Strauss and Corbin (1994). In essence, using their approach, the researcher immerses oneself in data, and formulates categories, codes and codings using both deduction and induction. This means that categories and codes, used to formulate a theory that is grounded in the data, are constantly reviewed and adjusted depending on the material that presents itself to the researcher. The categorisation and re-categorisation continues until the researcher finds that new data does not change the developed categories and codes and so can be satisfied that the phenomenon is accurately described. As such the theory has been grounded in and discovered through the data. There are other approaches to grounded theory (for the classic approach see Glaser, 1998; for the constructivist approach see Bryant & Charmaz, 2007) that I will not describe in detail, as they were less relevant for my decision-making process. Given that I had designed the semi-structured interviews with some guiding questions, and had based the design on some broad preconceptions of the trust being related to communication, care and competence, I felt it would have been misleading to use a grounded theory approach that in essence requires no or minimal preconceptions towards the data.

Ultimately, I chose to use thematic analysis (Braun & Clarke, 2006; Buetow, 2010; Grbich, 2007) to analyse the narratives in a socio-cultural context that was provided through the interviews. This allowed me the flexibility of starting with a broad framework derived from my theoretical model to analyse the data while allowing new themes and unexpected patterns to emerge from the data. In contrast to grounded theory, it allowed me to combine a deductive with an inductive approach to the data without generalising my findings to inform a predictive theory. Thematic analysis allowed me to offer an interpretation of the themes that I discovered in the narratives, taking into consideration not only my own socio-cultural background and knowledge, but also those of the interviewees (Sandberg, 2005). As such this approach was less limited than the phenomenographic approach described above.

Implementing the analysis

As Berg (2009) describes it:

> The reflexive ethnographer does not merely report findings as facts but actively constructs interpretations of experiences in the field and then questions how these interpretations actually arose. (p. 198)

I related to Berg's view when analysing the interview transcripts. Through conducting the interviews, mostly face-to-face, and transcribing the recordings, I was already quite familiar with the material and some themes stood out immediately. I used the themes that stood out to form an initial classification system. Reading through all transcripts several times helped me to create the following broad categories for the coding of the transcripts:

- Relationship/interactions
- Communication
- Emotions
- Trust
- Health
- Timeline
- Incident
- Complaint
- Personal information

I used the software NVivo 9.2, which enabled me to code and cross-reference data and also allowed me to re-code the material when re-defining categories that emerged during the analysis. Starting with the broad coding system, I added codes while analysing interview by interview, restructured code hierarchies in the process and started to note preliminary themes and patterns emerging from the data either through repetition or something that was unexpected. Where new categories emerged, I returned to already coded transcript and re-coded relevant parts where they fell into new emerging categories. Although not coded in the transcripts, my observations during the interview helped in applying the most suitable codes to the transcript data.

All transcript contents were fully coded to capture unexpected themes. This meant coding all transcripts, mainly sentence by sentence, in several aspects, including the timeline (before the incident, after the incident, etc.), in relation to perceptions and narratives about the patient-practitioner interaction, communication, health, associated emotions and values. I constantly reviewed the coding structure to identify overlapping or related codes, some of which were merged to better distinguish different codes and categories. The process of coding the interview transcripts took eight months to complete.

Next, I started my analysis by looking for quantities in coded categories, as well as relations between particular codes, for example emotions of patients by timeline. I mainly used the matrix analysis tool included in the NVivo software. The results gave me an understanding of the most prevalent associations, which I then analysed in more detail by referring back to the underlying transcript passages. In parallel, I started to write about my initial findings and after several rounds of refining the themes that had emerged, most indeed broadly fitted the categories derived from the literature review – communication, competence and care.

I compared themes that emerged from the interviews to identify where practitioners' and patients' narratives overlapped or contrasted. To validate my findings, I used frequent data extracts illustrative of the themes I identified and also included contextual information, where relevant, as well as diverging views that I had found (Silverman, 2001, p. 69). I was cautious not to interpret my findings until the discussion in Chapter 4, to aid the reader's own interpretation.

Section 3.2 presents the results of the analysis of practitioner interviews, and Section 3.3 of the patient interviews. In Chapter 4 I will discuss the findings from both sections and place them in the context of relevant literature.

3.3   Medical Practitioners Survey

Initial findings from the interviews suggested that communication immediately after an incident was crucial for maintaining or building trust between patients and practitioners. While patients appeared to expect transparent and responsive communication in these situations, they described perceiving the practitioner withdrawing from the relationship or trying to avoid any interaction with them, both of which were in direct contrast to the patient's expectations (see also Iedema, Allen, Britton, Grbich, Piper, & et al., 2011). I built on these initial findings when deciding to conduct a quantitative survey that specifically aimed at ascertaining a better understanding of factors influencing the practitioner's willingness to communicate about incidents and prior experiences that may have had an impact on their attitudes.

From the literature review it appeared that although the typical patient-practitioner relationship is changing, commonly the practitioner remains the more active communicator in the relationship (Szasz & Hollander, 1956). This means that after an incident, patients most commonly would expect that it should be the practitioner who discloses the incident to them, rather than the patient prompting the disclosure through their questions. A review of the implementation of open disclosure – transparent communication after incidents – in Australia (Iedema, Mallock, et al., 2008b; Iedema, Mallock, Sorensen, Manias, Tuckett, & et al., 2008a; Iedema, Sorensen, et al., 2008) also showed that in practice, practitioners remain reluctant to disclose incidents to the patient.

Using an anonymous survey, I aimed to identify current attitudes of practitioners regarding the disclosure of incidents and perceived barriers to open communication about serious incidents in practice. With permission, I adapted a suitable survey instrument that initially had been developed by Gallagher, Waterman, et al. (2006) to inquire about the attitudes and experiences of practitioners in the United States of America and Canada. The adapted survey was undertaken both in Germany (in German) and Australia.

3.3.1 Research question and definitions

Returning to my overarching research question that guided the interview study, I was interested in What is the relationship between the interpersonal trust in the doctor-patient relationship and communication in the context of health care incidents? With the initial findings of the interview study suggesting that open and responsive communication was expected by patients to maintain their trust in the practitioner, I was further interested in the practitioner's perspective, what factors influenced their willingness to openly communicate with patients after incidents. In contrast to the interview study, the survey concentrates on 'errors' rather than incidents. Incidents in the patient's treatment and care may sometimes only be perceived as such by the patient, while the treating practitioner interprets the same situation as a routine part of the treatment with its inherent risks and possible side effects. Medical errors represented an incident type where I expected that practitioners and patients had a shared understanding of it as an incident.

Referring to medical errors, I followed the definition used by the World Health Organisation (2005, p. 8) which defined a medical error as '[t]he failure of a planned action to be completed as intended ... or the use of a wrong plan to achieve an aim ...'. Medical errors include serious errors, minor errors and near misses, which for the purpose of the survey were defined as follows:

- serious error – error that causes permanent injury or transient but potentially life threatening harm
- minor error – error that causes harm which is neither permanent nor life threatening

- near miss – an error that could have caused harm but did not, either by chance or timely intervention

According to the behavioural psychologist Kurt Lewin (1943), individual behaviour is the result of the current constellation of two types of forces: facilitating forces and limiting forces, both internally as well as in the person's environment. To achieve change, both the facilitating forces that support change and the limiting forces, or barriers, need to be identified. According to Lewin, change can only occur where barriers are removed first before employing 'facilitating forces'. I concur with Lewin's assumption and aimed to clearly identify current barriers to open communication about medical errors in practice, in order to discuss strategies to overcome these.

The research question for the survey was: *What are medical practitioners' experiences and attitudes about medical errors?* The survey specifically assumed that the following six areas are related to the overall willingness of a medical practitioner to communicate openly about medical errors and inquired about:

- the general attitude towards medical errors
- communication about medical errors with patients
- experience with medical errors
- dealing with medical errors
- communicating about medical errors with others
- receiving information about medical errors

The survey included a mix of questions including multiple choice questions using a 4-item Likert-scale ranging from *strongly disagree* to *strongly agree*; multiple choice questions with pre-defined response options, as well as questions inviting free comments from the practitioners. The survey instrument in English and German can be found in Appendices 5 and 6.

3.3.2   Sample

The sample for the survey was indented to reflect the sample of the qualitative interview study to allow discussion of results across the two studies; hence general practitioners, including practitioners working in general practice, and surgeons, were included in the sample. While there are slight differences between the German and Australian sample due to the different ways of specialisation among medical practitioners in the two countries, the selection was based on the similarity of the types of services practitioners provide, rather than position titles, to achieve the highest level of comparability between the German and Australian samples. Accordingly, the German sample includes a range of medical practitioners who do not identify themselves as general practitioners but as physicians[12] who despite being formally specialised mainly provide general community based primary health care services. For example, paediatricians were included in the German sample, as they provide a broad range and often generic type of service compared to their more specialist Australian peers. In Australia, general practitioners cover a broad range of comparable services provided by German paediatricians. Similarly, in the German sample, general physicians who visit patients at home were included, while in Australia, these services are typically provided by general practitioners.

In regard to the geographical boundaries of the sample, I replicated the limitations used for the interview study by concentrating on medical practitioners working in NSW, Australia and Saxony, one of the German Federal states, which I chose because the study was part of my PhD dissertation at the University of Leipzig, which is located in Saxony.

---

[12] Physicians in Australia have completed specialist training and are fellows of the Royal Australasian College of Physicians as opposed to general practitioners who underwent specialised training in general practice and are fellows of the Royal Australian College of General Practitioners. Physicians commonly further specialise in areas including oncology, paediatrics, internal medicine, haematology, cardiology, etc.

3.3.2.1 Recruitment of participants

For the German survey, I contacted the *Sächsische Ärztekammer* (Medical Board of Saxony) and the *Kassenärztliche Vereinigung Sachsen* (Association of Statutory Health Insurance Physicians), asking for their assistance in distributing the survey. The Association of Statutory Health Insurance Physicians eventually agreed to distribute the survey to its members who fell into the defined sample, namely *Allgemeinarzt* (general practitioner), *hausärztlich tätiger Internist* (physician working in general practice), *Kinder- und Jugendarzt* (medical practitioner specialising in paediatrics and adolescent medicine), as well as both general and specialised surgeons. Although practitioners who exclusively treat private patients were excluded from the German sample, their number is considered very small and not significant (Günterberg & Beer, 2010). Due to the structure of the German health system, the vast majority of practitioners in the primary health care sector have a registration with the Association of Statutory Health Insurance Physicians, as this is required to be able to receive reimbursement for services provided to patients who are insured with a statutory health insurance.

In December 2010, the Association of Statutory Health Insurance Physicians included information about the survey in its member magazine 'KVS Mitteilungen' (Kassenärztliche Vereinigung Sachsen, 2010). In addition, Dr Gunnar Dittrich from the association introduced the survey to the General Managers of the three regional branches of the association that are located in Chemnitz, Dresden and Leipzig. I then provided the printed survey, information on how to access the online version, and reply-paid envelopes to the three regional branches of the association who, in January 2011, distributed these materials by post to 3,211 medical practitioners who fell into the defined sample.

In relation to the Australian survey, I contacted the Medical Council of NSW, the Australian Health Practitioner Regulation Agency (AHPRA), as well as the professional Colleges to assist in the distribution of the survey to relevant practitioners. Both the Australian Health Practitioner Regulation Agency[13] and the Medical Council of NSW[14] declined my request. The Royal Australasian College of Surgeons declined to write to members directly[15], but agreed to include an invitation to participate in their weekly member publication – Fax Mentis – in September 2012. Similarly, the Royal Australian College of General Practitioners included an invitation to participate in the study in their September 2012 faculty update to 5,500 fellows in NSW. Both invitations included an incentive of $10 to be donated to a chosen charity for each response. Practitioners were able to nominate either Medicines Sans Frontiers or Save the Children, both of which were chosen because they provide medical services and have no religious affiliations.

Given the lack of a personalised invitation to participate, response numbers were very low. With permission from the Human Research Ethics Committee of the University of Technology, Sydney I then personally invited a small number of practitioners whom I knew, to participate. Given the poor response rate of the Australian survey, I discussed whether or not to include the results with my supervisors. Ultimately, the results are included to provide an anecdotal, although statistically not valid, comparison with the German results, and to indicate some aspects that may be relevant for future research.

---

[13] The reason for declining my request to assist in the distribution of the anonymous survey were included in a letter of 9 July 2012 that stated that the 'project presented a potential difficulty in that the involvement of AHPRA as the regulatory body may be seen as inviting practitioners to disclose information around medical errors and thus issues which may be associated with performance in a regulatory sense. In this context the committee decided that your project was not well aligned with the objectives of the National Law and the public interest.'

[14] The Council declined assistance citing that since July 2010, they are no longer responsible for the registration of medical practitioners and referred me to the Australian Health Practitioner Regulation Agency (AHPRA) or the professional Colleges.

[15] The College's reason given when declining my request was: 'Unlike many other countries, surgeons in Australia are required to participate in audits of morbidity and mortality – these audits cover many of the same issues that are discussed in your survey. It was felt that further surveying of our Fellows in relation to these sensitive issues would not be of benefit either to the Fellows or to the College.' (Personal email correspondence from the Royal Australasian College of Surgeons, received 5 September 2012)

3.3.3   Methodology

The survey that I used for the study was adapted from an instrument developed by Dr Thomas Gallagher, Waterman, et al. (2006 with Dr Gallagher's permission. The adaptation process included a review of terminology and some adjustments to fit in the Australian context. I shortened the original instrument, by excluding hypothetical examples of serious and minor errors. The adapted English survey was reviewed by Dr Peter Kandlbinder, Senior Lecturer at the Institute for Interactive Media and Learning, as well as Professor Roderick Iedema at the Centre for Health Communication, both from the University of Technology, Sydney. I then translated the English survey (Appendix 6) into German, my native language. The German survey (Appendix 5) was reviewed by Sandra Jenke, a psychologist specialising in market research; Sandra Mühlberg, a communications specialist, as well as Dr Gunnar Dittrich and Dr Jan Kaminsky from the Association of Statutory Health Insurance Physicians. Feedback mainly related to discussions around the most appropriate translation of terms used in the English version of the survey. For example, the term 'disclose' was initially translated as 'offenlegen', which can have a connotation of divulging secret information. After discussion, it was agreed to use the more general German term of 'mitteilen', which can also be translated into the English 'convey'.

3.3.3.1 Data collection

It was estimated that on average it took 15-20 minutes to complete the survey. Responses to the German survey were received both online and by reply-paid envelope between late January and May 2011. Responses to the Australian online survey were received between September and November 2012. There were no formal reminders sent, following the preferences expressed by the partners in the distribution of the survey.

3.3.3.2 Data analysis

Responses to the German paper-based survey were entered using unique codes for each question and response option, matching codes used in the online version of the survey. This allowed an easy merging of data from both sources. Results from the Australian online survey were analysed using the same methodology as was used for the German surveys.

I used Microsoft Excel 2007 to analyse the data. As part of the cleansing process, I had to exclude a small number of responses for logical reasons. For example, a respondent selected an answer for what type of action they had taken after their last medical error they were involved in, but had earlier responded that they had never been involved in any type of error. Due to the anonymous nature of the survey, I could not clarify any answers and therefore excluded illogical answers on a question-by-question basis, meaning that other responses from the same participant were still included in the analysis. The results of both the German and Australian surveys are summarised in Section 3.4 of this chapter.

3.3.4 Privacy and risk considerations

The survey was anonymous. Given the sensitive nature of the subject, it was crucial to offer the highest protection of privacy to participants. In the process of recruiting potential participants I had no access to any personal or contact data of the practitioners who received the invitation to participate in the survey, except for the last stage of the Australian survey, when I was allowed to contact a small number of medical practitioners that I personally knew to invite them to participate.

The postal responses to the German survey all went to a postal box that I had opened purely for this purpose. The online version of the survey was password protected and both the link and the password were included in the postal mail-out. The online survey was hosted on a password protected database run by the University of Technology, Sydney.

In the case of the Australian surveys, the approach of inviting potential participants through professional college publications was considered low risk by the Human Research Ethics Committee of the University of Technology, Sydney. In relation to the small number of practitioner that I approached personally, I made it clear that participation was voluntary and that I would not be able to identify who had responded to the survey.

Before presenting the results of the anonymous survey of medical practitioners about their experiences and attitudes with medical errors in Section 3.6 of this chapter, I summarise the themes that emerged from the explorative interviews with medical practitioners and patients in the following sections 3.4 and 3.5.

3.4   Themes emerging from practitioner interviews

The section starts with practitioners' views on why patient trust matters. It then continues to describe themes that were related to building and increasing trust, before contrasting these with themes that practitioners identified as destroying or decreasing patient trust.

In the third part of this section, I analyse how practitioners described dealing with a patient complaint and how they described their emotions associated with both the incident and the complaint. Lastly, I look specifically at the role of an apology and how it may or may not have influenced the relationship between the practitioner and their patient. The themes that emerged will be contrasted with the themes that emerged from patient interviews in the discussion Chapter 4.

The research question and underlying assumptions introduced in Section 3.2.2.1 were broken down in the following questions that guided my analysis of the interview data.

Why does trust matter? How do practitioners describe how trust builds and how it deteriorates? What triggers a complaint? What happens after a complaint to the trust and the relationship and how do interviewees reflect on their experience with a complaint in retrospect?

The results of the interviews with six surgeons and six general practitioners are presented first. Themes that relate to trust building and maintenance, as well as themes relating to the deterioration of trust, will be structured into three broad areas: communication, competence and care. The same structure of analysis will be used for the patient interviews and comparisons will be made throughout the analysis, but specifically in the following discussion in Chapter 4. The assumed link between expectations and actual outcome and their impact on the trust relationship will also be discussed in Chapter 4.

3.4.1   Why does it matter?

3.4.1.1 Practitioners feel more comfortable to treat patients who trust them

When asked whether practitioners believed that the patient had a certain amount of trust in them to see them, most agreed.

During the interviews, practitioners expressed the view that they needed to feel comfortable treating a patient and having the feeling that the patient trusts them. Where they have the impression that this is not the case, practitioners prefer to refer the patient to another practitioner or encourage them to see another practitioner for a second opinion, as the following statement illustrates:

So, my personal bias is towards forming a relation of mutual trust and will, if I don't sense that, choose, on occasions, not to operate on people, or not to intervene and encourage them to seek other opinions. (Surgeon 02)

Particularly among the interviewed surgeons, this was a point commonly made, with all of them expressly talking about encouraging the patient to seek a second opinion, if they felt that the patient had reservations or hesitated to proceed with surgery. This also reflects that these surgeons recognise that surgery is a highly emotional situation for a patient and they are usually very vulnerable and often anxious before the operation. To alleviate the uncertainty and anxiety as far as possible before surgery was considered elementary and beneficial not only for the outcome, but also the relationship between doctor and patient.

Practitioners conceded that when it comes to initial trust and first impressions, the doctor-patient relationship does not vary much from any other social interactions in so far that there is an immediate judgement of whether or not the other side is likeable and that does influence how the relationship evolves.

There are some women who I feel that I have an instant sort of rapport with them and/or their partners. I don't know how to put it into words .... It is just natural human interaction. With some people you click, with some you don't. And I have some women who have seen me for five or six years now and every time I see them I think very fondly of them; I will have almost a chat ... and I have to make sure that I do their medical aspects. But they ask how my kids are, they say 'I remember when I was operated before your son was born; he must be five years old now'. And I guess it has been a two-way path. (Surgeon 04)

Interestingly, despite describing that patient trust was beneficial to the relationship with the practitioner, it was not essential, in other words, practitioners spoke of their obligation to treat patients, independent of whether they liked them, or whether the patient trusted them. This is an interesting point when contrasted with patients who, at least in non-emergency situations, have the choice to continue the relationship with the practitioner despite a lack of trust. Often, they would end the relationship and walk away. In contrast, practitioners cannot just walk away from a patient; they acknowledge their professional responsibility to provide care to anyone who requires it.

There is an underlying conflict between the practitioner in their professional role and the practitioner as a private person. As a professional, they cannot walk away from a patient; however, the instinct to end the relationship is manifested through asking the patient to seek a second opinion or referring the patient where there is a complete breakdown in the relationship.

Another aspect of this theme is when practitioners mentioned the goodwill of the patient being helpful, but not essential for the treatment relationship. Patient goodwill may be useful to achieve cooperation and compliance, especially where recovery times are very long and not necessarily linear. But, where it is not given, it would not mean that the practitioner would deny treatment.

3.4.1.2 Patient trust enables practitioners to be proactive and holistic

Patient trust allows the doctor to explore wider health issues with the patient and to dig deeper than the symptoms the patient presents with. Some of the general practitioners interviewed described a dynamic whereby more delicate health issues are seldom volunteered by a new patient in their first consultation. Often it takes a number of consultations for the patient to open up to the practitioner.

> *Not usually in their first consultation; a little bit maybe in the second; but probably by the third consultation, if they felt that they could trust you they'd come back and then discuss it. (GP 05)*

This may include health issues such as depression, anxiety, stress factors impacting on general well-being.

3.4.1.3 Practitioners can be open and transparent despite uncertainties

Doctors feel that they can openly talk about being uncertain or having inadequate knowledge of a specific issue or problem with the patient when they feel that the patient trusts them.

> *If people come in and I don't know, then I am perfectly happy to say, 'look, I'm sorry; I really don't know anything about this, but I will find out about it. So come back and we'll discuss it when I know what I am talking about.' (GP 06)*

> *Interviewer: And do you feel that the patients find that acceptable?*

> *Yes. Yes. ... most of my patients are very, very long-term patients, so we have a very good trust. (GP 06)*

It should be noted that the practitioner's observation relates to long-term patients, and other practitioners mirrored this during the interviews. It was the recurring theme that practitioners talked about, having to earn the trust of the patient rather than having it from the outset.

3.4.1.4 Trust enables openness about mistakes and acceptance

The relationship between trust and errors is two-fold. On the one hand, where a patient trusts their practitioner, they may accept an error by the practitioner and even justify it without losing trust in the doctor. However, this scenario was mentioned usually in relation to long-term patients, or where there has been more than one interaction:

*with a patient you have seen a few times and you feel you have
got a relationship ... With those patients – and there is sort of a
reciprocal trust – [they think] 'he knows what he is doing; he has
done that before; this is what it is all about'. With those patients,
if I find I made a [mistake]: sometimes I put down the wrong dos-
age on the hypertensive drug – I put on the old one, instead of the
new one – the chemist says 'oh, what's going on with the doctor?'
And then the patient says 'ah, he was just so busy'. They go again.
But I still got the patient back. And I would mention 'I am sorry, I
put down the wrong thing'; and it is sort of dismissed and accepted by them. Now, these are patients where I have proved myself
to them. ... But having said that, you can't always count on that.
(GP 01)*

Practitioners appreciate patients' trust, as it can decrease the risk of conflicts after (minor) errors. On the other hand, where the patient's trust is obvious, the practitioner may be less stringent in their approach to the health problems, which in fact may even increase the risk of errors (Pehm, 2009).

3.4.1.5 Patients want one person to primarily deal with

Practitioners also spoke about the difficulty of building and maintaining patient
trust in the fragmented way health care is delivered today. Particularly in the
public health system, which does not allow for a choice of treating doctor and
often means that the patient will see several practitioners, including junior staff
members, it appears more difficult to maintain the interpersonal trust relationship, as the following quote acknowledges.

I mean if I were a patient I feel I want to trust my surgeon. And I think that is important to probably a lot of patients. One of the hardest things I have got to gently tell public patients is that although I might be there and I may or may not do some of the surgery, that in all likelihood I won't do all of it. But I will be there, if there is a problem, I will take over from the registrar who will do it. It is a training hospital and things like that. You definitely get a powerful sense that there is disappointment. (Surgeon 04)

Specifically with surgery, patients do not wish to expose themselves to any unnecessary risk. Being operated on by a junior person, even under supervision, is a difficult aspect of care in the public health system. The trust the patient places in the senior practitioner's competence and skill level does not transfer fully to junior staff being supervised. It is clearly a sign that trust is person specific. What I could not establish through the interviews was whether there is a difference in patient perception in cases where the registrar is involved in the interaction with the patient all the way alongside the senior practitioner. However, in the way health care delivery is structured, this would only be the case in a small number of treatment situations and usually connected to emergency situations, rather than elective situations.

3.4.1.6   Trust can impact on judgement

While a trusting relationship can enhance treatment and the way errors are dealt with, it may also have the unintended opposite effect of increasing the risk of errors being made.

Patients just seem to trust their doctors outright, out of hand – maybe for the wrong reasons, but they just do. (Surgeon 03)

With long-term patients, where there is a relationship of reciprocal trust, practitioners sometimes pay less attention to new and emerging information and instead rely on assumptions based on previous information about the patient. This may limit their diagnostic or treatment approaches and this can be to the detriment of the patient.

It is therefore important to be aware of this dynamic to remain stringent and thorough in the diagnosis, treatment and care of long-term patients.

3.4.1.7   Trust required to overcome information asymmetry

While some practitioners believed that trust is ideal, but not essential, in a doctor-patient relationship, others believed that there cannot be a treating relationship without trust. The following practitioner said that he would not proceed to operate on a patient without them trusting that their decision to proceed with the surgery was the right one, which implies trusting the surgeon's skills and competence.

> They [the patients] need to trust you 100%. … The patient coming from a lay position, they don't really know; you could tell them anything, how would they know? And if I sense that I haven't really explained to them, or … if they haven't really understood and are not sure, I suggest they get a second opinion. I say, … 'You can come back and see me again. … You need to trust that what you are doing is the correct thing. And if you are not happy that you are doing the right thing, you need to go away and think about it.'
> (Surgeon 03)

The statement shows that the practitioner acknowledges the information asymmetry in the patient-practitioner relationship and the need for the patient to make their own, informed decision to proceed.

3.4.1.8   Trust helpful in dealing with incidents

One surgeon offered that although it was not essential for the patient to like their practitioner before undergoing surgery, it was helpful to counter-balance unrealistic expectations in regard to the surgeon's competence. This is of particular relevance if the patient experiences unexpected treatment outcomes or complications.

> *People who have interventions sometimes don't mind what the demeanour of the person is provided that the technical outcome is good, perfect. Nevertheless, those people seeking perfection in technical outcome will often magnify perceptions of failure and problems in the make-up of the surgeon, if there is a flawed outcome. (Surgeon 02)*

3.4.1.9 Summary: Trust, why does it matter?

From a practitioner's point of view, patient trust was important and helpful, but it is not essential for a treating relationship. Where practitioners, particularly general practitioners, described patient trust, it usually related to long-term patients. It implied that practitioners view trust as something that develops over time and something they have to earn. As I will show below, this contrasts with the patients' perspective which mostly mentioned trust as being essential from the outset, even if it may grow over time.

Another aspect of the practitioners' perspective is that trust was seen as enabling open communication both in routine situations, as well as after errors had occurred.

3.4.2   First impressions

To understand the way practitioners perceived the relationship with their patients, I looked at how they described their first impression of the patient. My assumption was that the first impression would shape the practitioner's expectations of how the relationship will evolve and would influence their communication with and behaviour towards the patient.

As the following statement exemplifies, the effect of the first impression of a patient is comparable to the effect of a first impression of other people outside the doctor-patient relationship:

> *[W]e do that instantly with everyone in any situation. When people come through the door, you know. I don't know. It is not a gut feeling; it's aura; whatever it is, you know immediately [whether] this is going to be a successful, positive relationship or it's not. (GP 06)*

The practitioner acknowledges that first impressions are an element in any social interaction, independent of the role – as a private person or as a practitioner. Referring to it as a gut feeling indicates that it is often not rationalised, but remains on an emotive or sub-conscious level. Nevertheless, it appears to influence the relationship and the way practitioners behave. As the following statements will show, the practitioners interviewed reported becoming careful when the first impression was inconsistent; however, the way they modified their behaviour differed. It included spending more time with the patient and attempting to communicate and explain better, seeking a second opinion or ceasing the relationship altogether.

When forming a first impression, the practitioner may not solely rely on directly observable information, such as the patient's behaviour and appearance, their voice and tone, but also on contextual information, such as knowing the medical history and drawing assumptions from it.

For example, a patient saw a surgeon and the knowledge that the patient had seen several other surgeons before, none of whom had operated on the patient, made the surgeon suspicious, despite the friendly behaviour the patient displayed during the actual first consultation.

I mean the penny dropped immediately that there is something peculiar about this bloke. He had seen three orthopaedic surgeons; none of them had offered to do his operation; you know immediately that something is strange. But he was pleasant to me. The guy had a hip replacement. [I] did a long good consultation with him, half an hour [to] 45 minutes to explain how I did it; what are the complications – all the usual stuff. He was happy. (Surgeon 01)

The example highlights that a first impression might be formed even before the practitioner sees and interacts with the patient the first time, solely by developing a picture about the patient based on the information they read about them. Expecting a difficult patient, the Surgeon 01 cited above modified their behaviour and spent extra time on the consultation and was extra careful.

In another case, the inconsistency between the patient's appearance and the verbal information about their symptoms in the first consultation made the practitioner suspicious.

She was not genuine in what she was presenting. She was trying to con me. ... people don't present like that when they are suicidal. They look sort of untidy; they don't present neat, perfect, immaculately dressed. The whole thing just didn't click as being genuine. (GP04)

In the above statement, the practitioner felt that the patient was trying to con him, indicating that their relationship would start with dishonesty. The inconsistency between the information provided by the patient and the information the practitioner collects though observation or other sources often leads to suspicion and the practitioner changing their normal behaviour and becoming more careful. Where a relationship starts out on this basis, it becomes difficult to establish trust.

> *My view was that he was drug-seeking for opiates. So again, there are a couple of patients who against the background of intravenous drug use, particularly opiates, it is difficult to form a relationship of trust [with]. And more often I might err on the side of not supporting intervention, or medication, or choose to try to find a way that the person is seeking the opinion of another clinician. (Surgeon 02)*

As the statement shows, where the practitioner is unable to trust the patient and their motives to seek treatment, he prefers to either not treat or get a second opinion. The practitioner conceded that where this is not possible, the obligation to provide treatment to a patient in need would override the feeling of discomfort – it is part of the professional self-perception.

> *Well, she fitted into that category of being a person with whom it was difficult to establish a relationship of trust, but again, I don't regard her as particularly unusual. She is just one where you have to go the extra yard to get the trust and even with a base of trust, as I say formed over a couple of years, people like her still find criticism, find fault and demonstrate a degree of lack of insight …. (Surgeon 02)*

The following practitioner excluded the possibility of having any future relationship with the patient based on her first impression of the patient as being demanding, aggressive and non-negotiable.

> *She [the patient] was so aggressive. One: 'You've kept me waiting. YOU kept me waiting'. Two: 'I have decided that you will be my general practitioner', it was no bargaining; no middle ground. And I said to her, – she was a diabetic obviously out of control – 'don't you have an endocrinologist or diabetologist that you could see?'*
>
> *[She responded], 'oh, I don't want to see those doctors. They only want to see me for my money.'*

And I said, 'no, that's not true.' I said, 'most doctors who are specialists have worked hard. What they charge is what they are worth'.

She responded, 'no, no, it's money.'

I thought: great. (GP06)

The characteristics displayed by the patient led the practitioner to believe that this patient would be very demanding, would not listen to her suggestions or explanations and would therefore make it difficult to build a relationship or have effective communication with.

In summary, where the first impression is that of a difficult patient, most practitioners became more aware and careful in their interaction. The majority spoke about attempting to continue the relationship, with certain safeguards, due to their professional responsibility.

As we will see from the analysis of patients' interviews, their first impression also influenced their expectation of the practitioner and their own behaviour. Being aware of this bi-directional dynamic is a first step towards understanding certain patient behaviours and being able to respond early and appropriately.

During the interviews, two of the surgeons explicitly reflected on the patient's most likely first impression in order to better understand the patient's behaviour. They distinguished emergency from routine, elective situations.

Well, the difference is that in trauma the first time you see a patient is after he has been traumatised. Whereas a patient I operate a joint on, I build up a rapport before [I] start. So you know each other. With a guy who was hit by a car, you don't say, 'please come back next week'. You have got to put him together tonight. ... It's a different situation between trauma and elective, because the timeframe is different. (Surgeon 06)

The opportunity to build rapport or trust is very limited in emergency situations. While a negative first impression in elective situations would usually lead to the patient not returning, and seeking treatment somewhere else, in emergency situations, the first impression will shape the patient's interpretation of future interactions and outcomes.

> *In emergency situations where they generally don't exercise their choice, that's where those little things that were said or not said, or even the way you examined the patient ... You hear people say 'oh he picked up my leg and dropped it again'. And you think – you may know the person involved and you can't imagine them doing that – the patient perceived it as rough. Examining the leg that was perhaps injured you've got to be so gentle. And if they perceive that you are very gentle, they relax. But if you are a bit rough, they think 'this guy is a butcher'. And if the operation doesn't go well 'I knew it; he is a butcher; he picked my leg up and he dropped it; he doesn't care'. That first impression will colour everything that happens after the operation. (Surgeon 05)*

In summary, the interviews included evidence that practitioners' first impressions of patients shape their perception and subsequent behaviour. In the next step, I look at perceptions and behaviours in three core areas relevant for trust building and trust decreasing – communication, competence and care.

3.4.3   Trust building elements – the practitioner's view

When developing the semi-structured interviews, the questions were intended to explore three areas that I saw as central to trust: communication, competence and care or relationship. The interviews with practitioners included themes in all three of these areas and I will present emerging topics and issues following this structure. I should note though that the relationship between these areas and trust was often not expressly described, but implied. For example, practitioners were talking about communication aspects that enhanced their relationship with the patient, which I interpreted as being representative of a relationship of trust. Although this was not necessarily explicitly suggested by the practitioner, it reflects the often unconscious nature of the phenomenon. Trust may be displayed in action, communication and behaviour without being explicitly named as such. To ease navigation, I will use the following symbols.

3.4.3.1 Communication

The relationship between communication and trust was the most prominent theme in the practitioner interviews. Analysing communication-related themes also reveals the explicit and often implicit expectations of both patients and

↑ Communication

Competence

Care

practitioners. Practitioners commonly referred to the expectations patients have and whether or not they were able to fulfil those expectations.

Communication relates to the 'what' – the factual exchange of information – or the 'how' – the manner or way in which the information is given.

Understanding what is wrong

Practitioners who reflected on patient expectations often at the same time reflected on their own persona or behaviour – what kind of doctor they are and what they offer to their patients.

The following statement highlights two expectations patients seem to have of their doctor. Firstly, patients expect a clear explanation for the problems they are experiencing; they want to understand what is wrong with them. This expectation is often explicit or obvious.

Commonly, there is a second, often implicit, expectation that patients want to understand how the practitioner came to their conclusion. To meet the second expectation, a practitioner must adequately communicate their line of thought and information they considered relevant for their diagnosis or conclusion.

> *Most patients expect something. What I believe they expect from*
> *me is to come to some sort of diagnosis and conclusion about*
> *what they were coming in with. Even if it's wrong – because diag-*
> *nosis is based on probability of 1, 2 and 3 – even if it's wrong,*
> *most patients are quite happy that they walk out with a diagnosis,*
> *with a provisional diagnosis and an explanation as to why I actual-*
> *ly did that; [why] I came to that conclusion. (GP 01)*

The patient expectation is that the practitioner can provide information that will fill their knowledge gap about what is wrong with them. Sometimes, the patient may already have the right information and knowledge and is seeking re-assurance.

Honesty and transparency

Where practitioners claimed that they had a good relationship with their (often long-term) patient, they described behaviour that was not only open, honest and transparent, but also aware of the responsibility of care they have.

The following example shows that the practitioner felt comfortable to acknowledge to the patient that they did not know something.

> *If people come in and I don't know, then I am perfectly happy to*
> *say, 'look, I'm sorry; I really don't know anything about this, but I*
> *will find out about it. So come back and we'll discuss it when I*
> *know what I am talking about.'*
>
> *Interviewer: And do you feel that patients find that acceptable?*
>
> *Yes. Yes … most of my patients are very, very long-term patients,*
> *so we have a very good trust. (GP 06)*

What this statement reveals is not only that the practitioner was comfort-able with being open about their limitations when they feel they have a trusting relationship with the patient. It also reveals that they acknowledge that the patient has come to them for an answer: the practitioner apologises before asking the patient to return. Another underlying expectation is that the patient expects the practitioner to offer help and a solution, even in a situation where they are unable to do so, immediately. The practitioner says that she will find out and the patient should come back.

Identifying and responding to expectations

The following statement reveals that practitioners are aware that different patients have different expectations, even if they may present with the same health conditions. The way this particular practitioner addresses this challenge is to take time in the first consultation, where expectations can be explored and addressed and future expectations are formed.

> *I take the attitude that all patients are different and you have to account for their different personalities and whatever. But I give people lengthy consultations, you know, I explain all the terms to understand; I don't rush things, answer questions. I mean the only thing you could complain about my practice is the waiting time. I often go overtime. My secretary does half an hour for new patients and 15 minutes for follow-up, and often I go 45 minutes to an hour with a new patient, because they have questions and I sit there and answer them. I never rush them. (Surgeon 01)*

Another practitioner spoke of the assistance of his secretary in identifying specific issues patients may have and that needed to be addressed in the con-sultation.

If someone, for example, might have rung up half a dozen times with questions, she might mention that; or if they have changed their appointment five times. If there is something like that she might mention it. And she is quite a good ... people person; she reads people very well and she is good in soothing them down as well. That helps a lot. (Surgeon 05)

This is an important point for practitioners to use other sources of information to establish the patient's obvious and underlying expectations, rather than solely relying on the presentation during the consultation. In addition, referring to the patient's phone calls to the secretary also shows that the practitioner has listened and acknowledges the uniqueness of the patient rather than having the same approach to every patient. The patient feels heard and respected, which is beneficial to building a trustful relationship.

Patients are often not sufficiently skilled and/or prepared to articulate all relevant questions in the limited time of a consultation. Having an indication about what their priorities might be at the start of the consultation can shape the communication and address many more of the patient's needs, proactively rather than reactively.

Consistency in information and communication

A recurring theme in the practitioner interviews was the importance of and challenges related to the consistency of information the patient receives. I distinguish two types of consistency: horizontal and vertical, both being equally important. Horizontal consistency refers to the same or similar information coming from different sources. Vertical consistency refers to the same or similar information by the same source over time.

Consistency in information contributes to patient trust, but at the same time is one of the most challenging aims to achieve. Firstly, practitioners often do not fully know which information sources the patient uses and how the patient evaluates the information from these different sources. Secondly, information given to the patient may change over time as new facts, such as test results, emerge and make previous assumptions obsolete. It is the nature of medicine that it is art as much as science – a perspective that practitioners understand, but patients do not always appreciate.

When becoming aware of inconsistency in the information the patient receives, it is important to address and explain to the patient the actual or most likely reasons for that mismatch, so they can understand and form a coherent opinion to move forward and underpin their future decision-making.

A common example is where practitioner opinions differ about the diagnosis or treatment approach. A practitioner describes:

> *People don't like that [inconsistency]. But if you spend a little bit of time with them, they can understand that there can be differences of opinion and that there could have been more than one path that could have been a reasonable one to adopt. Because the other thing is that often later on, we got information that wasn't apparent to the doctor at the time. Like my man that had the stroke – later on, we knew what was happening, but not at the time, you 've got to put yourself in the shoes of the doctor that made the decision at the time with whatever information they had. People have to think about that. (Surgeon 05)*

Vertical inconsistencies, if unaddressed, may also have an impact on the patient's perception of a practitioner's competence and skill level. As the statement suggests, more information becomes available and, with hindsight, may have led to a different decision taken earlier in the treatment of a patient. The practitioner points out that it is important to discuss both what was known and what was not known at the time.

In summary, from a practitioners' point of view, the main elements in relation to communicating with patients that assist in the patient trusting the practitioner are that the practitioner is perceived to be honest, transparent in their decision-making, responsive to the patient's needs and consistent in both their communication with the patient and their family over time as well as consistent in what is said and what is done. The next area of factors that support patient trust from a practitioner's perspective is competence.

3.4.3.2 Competence

Competence was the second theme that appeared to be important to trust building and maintenance from a practitioner's point of view. Competence in my understanding captures a range of topics, including reputation, technical skills, professional judgement and behaviour, as well as treatment outcomes.

↑ Communication

Competence

Care

Reputation

Trust in a person without prior interaction is often built upon reputation. This does not only include the practitioner's reputation, but also the reputation of the person who recommended or mentioned the practitioner, the reputation of an information source, or the reputation of the hospital they work at.

Asked about what they thought was most important for a patient's decision to see them, the following practitioner statement exemplifies the role reputation commands.

I think that you come ... well recommended either by the GP or from friends or someone else who has seen me. That I have some experience. And I don't know, maybe where I operate. I operate at [a hospital] and a lot of people say that they are very relieved, because [this] hospital has a very good reputation as being a very good hospital – rightly or wrongly, but nevertheless, that's our [reputation]. And I think that is one of the reasons people quite often come to [this hospital]. They want to be sure and they want that you come highly recommended; got some experience (Surgeon 03)

The quote points to the link between reputation and trust. A good reputation is a vehicle to interpret the factual information a person has in a positive way. For example, the patient may know the size and services of a hospital, but they cannot evaluate whether or not it is good or bad. Reputation plays a significant role in helping in that evaluation and as such assisting in the patient's decision-making. Believing in the reputation displays trust and as a result lowers the anxiety about making the wrong decision.

It is important to note both the importance and limitations of reputation. Reputation may bring people through the door, but the first consultation or interaction between patient and practitioner is crucial in testing the 'belief' that was based on the reputation, against reality.

When someone comes to the rooms with arthritis for example, [he or she] has the chance to ask their friends 'this painful hip, should I go and see this [doctor]? Is he a good surgeon?' They go to their GP asking 'is this doctor a good surgeon?' so by the time that they walk in here, they already feel they made a choice to see someone that they can trust. And if the interview goes well; the operation goes well, everybody is all smiles. And even if something doesn't go well, they can kind of accept that it's part of life. (Surgeon 05)

If the practitioner behaves as expected in the first consultation, the initial trust is confirmed and strengthened. If the initial expectation the patient had of the practitioner is not confirmed in the first consultation, usually, the patient will not return.

Technical skills

Most practitioners named technical skills and being competent in what they do as the most fundamental prerequisites for a patient trusting them.

> *I felt that anything that I tackled I was competent at. I was doing tonsillectomies, I was doing circumcisions – things people want you to do well and trusted you with. (GP 05)*

Avoiding serious mistakes

Most practitioners explicitly talked about the importance of avoiding mistakes to maintain patient trust. Although this may sound simple, a closer inspection revealed that often there is a discrepancy in the perception of patients and practitioners about the severity or seriousness of an error.

While for practitioners a serious error often equates to a serious mistake in judgement and knowledge, patients attributed the seriousness of an error more commonly to the outcome and the impact it had on their lives.

Judgement

The distinction between technical competence and judgement and their importance was highlighted in the following practitioner statement:

> *First of all, he has got to know what he is doing – that's number one. It's far better from my perspective that a surgeon knows what he is doing; that he operates for the right indications rather than that he should be warm and cuddly and fussy and doing operations for the wrong indication on the wrong patients, even if he does them well. … [T]he judgement when to go in is even more important than the technical skills. The judgement is important. (Surgeon 06)*

The practitioner refers to the lack of professional knowledge that would enable patients to judge the practitioner's actions objectively. This also refers to the situation where patients unknowingly or naively place their trust into a practitioner who does not have their best interest at heart. The practitioner may do so because they are a good communicator. However, although short-term trust may be built in this manner, long-term, it is a risky strategy as it assumes that the patient primarily or solely relies on information given to them by that particular practitioner. Such a situation may be more common in the field of surgery, where interaction between patient and surgeon usually is a one-off, rather than in an ongoing relationship.

The importance of physical examination

Where the patient's ailment is of a physical nature, they often expect a physical examination to be part of the consultation. This is a crucial point, as more commonly today, diagnosis is being based on the verbal information given by the patients in connection with the practitioner's observations and information from referral letters and test results. Although practitioners may view the physical examination as not necessary, if they have other more relevant information at hand to make their judgement, for the patient, physically looking at the problem is often still an important element of the consultation.

One practitioner described it as follows:

> *[M]ost patients are quite happy that they walk out with a diagnosis, with a provisional diagnosis and an explanation as to why I actually did that; [why] I came to that conclusion; and I actually have done something to them that helps to reinforce their perception that I actually have done something. The physical examination is very important. (GP 01)*

Overall, practitioners were well aware of how the reputation regarding a practitioner's competence plays a role in the patient's decision-making, particularly at the beginning of the relationship. Once the patient is seeing a practitioner, practitioners described the importance of an adequate examination, i.e. physical examinations for physical problems, technical skills, professional judgement and not making serious errors that have a great negative impact on the patient's life.

After having identified the communication and competence related factors that practitioners view as underpinning trust, the last area I look at is care.

3.4.3.3 Care

The third area of trust building elements is what I like to refer to as care: it includes concepts such as empathy, relating to the patient, respecting the patient, seeing and treating the patent holistically as a person rather than a condition.

Communication

Competence

Care

Being comprehensive and proactive

Some of the general practitioners interviewed mentioned that it was important to their patients that the practitioner proactively offers services that may be beneficial to them, rather than responding only to the conditions or issues as the patient presents them. I identified three aspects of this theme: being comprehensive, accessible and proactive.

For example, one general practitioner described his approach in the following words:

> *I was trying to be a one-stop shop and to be as comprehensive as I could in the one visit. Trying to solve as many problems as possible in the one visit. And a lot of them did appreciate that, because it is very hard to get back to a doctor, once they have seen one. They feel that they want more, but they didn't know how to get it. (GP 05)*

Referring to the statement that patients would like to ask their doctor certain things, but do not know how to, implies that the practitioner acknowledges that communication during consultations can often be asymmetric and as a result not all of the patient's needs will be met if the patient did not actively communicate them. This may be a reflection of the power asymmetry between patients and practitioners and how it manifests in the patient-doctor communication.

Another practitioner described their strategy to address this issue:

The other trait I have is always at the end of the consultation to ask, 'is there anything else you want to talk about?', because that often opens up avenues for them to talk. (GP 02)

It seems a simple way of encouraging the patient to be open with the practitioner about their needs. However, it also requires the practitioner to listen and take the time to respond, should a patient make use of the offer to share other information about issues and ailments with the practitioner. It would be counter-productive to encourage the patient to open up and then rush through a response, or in the worst case not responding at all. Being mindful of the practical balance a practitioner has to achieve, this area can be challenging.

For a practitioner to be proactive in the care they provide often requires some knowledge about the patient, their background and history to make assumptions about what potential problems there might be. Having proven yourself to the patient before may help to encourage them to open up about other issues they do not feel comfortable talking about.

[Y]ou eventually get to know them and there is always something you can help them with. And once you proved your technical standards with them, you can then tackle the harder issues with them. (GP 01)

One person, long-term

I referred above to the structural challenges for building trust by the way health care in public hospitals is organised. General practitioners also talked about the impact of structural changes to general practice over the past decades with higher rates of specialisation, a focus on effectively resolving the problem the patient presents with, more services being provided in medical centres with multiple staff, higher staff turnover, and more common part-time working arrangements, all of which have made it more difficult to establish and maintain trust. This need not be seen in the context of the old model of the trusted sole practitioner who was anchored in the local community and made it easier for the patient to relate to one person and building a relationship over time. Certainly bigger practices did exist in the past and sole practitioners do today. But the proportions have shifted and often sole practitioners cannot afford to offer their services to their patients without charging an additional fee, so, often patients who would like to have personal attention are required to pay more for their health care.

> And that's why I find this so tragic the way modern medicine is going. The old-fashioned GP has gone. I mean I used to go and see patients in their homes; have visits – they've gone. You just know from the day they are born almost – from the day the relationship is established that it is going to build. (GP 06)

Roles and expectations

Not only has the structure of health care delivery changed, making it often more challenging to build and maintain trust. Practitioners also commented on the shift in patient attitudes that influence the relationship and trust.

The older Australians – and I am talking about the people who grew up during the Great Depression – they have a totally different attitude to what I call the post-Whitlam years, the ones that grew up thinking that life owes them a living. The older people are appreciative of what you do for them. The younger [ones] make demands and they expect you to [fulfil] them. And they cannot understand, if you say that's not a good idea, because they demand it. It is their right to have it. (Surgeon 06)

According to this practitioner – who holds a view shared by other practitioners during the interviews – overall patients have become more aware of their rights and appear more vocal and assertive in pursuing their expectations. This generational shift becomes more prominent as the 40-55 year old age group that is referred to is moving into an age bracket where they require more frequent health care services. Notably, in the interviews with practitioners who themselves were older than 60 years, this opinion was voiced, while younger practitioners between the age of 30 and 55 were more accepting of the 'demands' of the patients, accepting them as the patient's rights and it was just a matter to find a way to properly respond to them.

Overall, the interviews appeared to reflect a generational shift from a traditional model of patient-practitioner interaction, with an active practitioner and a mainly passive patient, towards a model that is much more equal in the patient-practitioner relationship and open for patient involvement in their own care. This shift is also reflected more broadly in the policy area, with a noticeable shift towards patient-centred care and empowering patients to take responsibility for their health care.

Relating this theme back to the two points I made above in relation to providing comprehensive, long-term, personal care, this was more commonly raised by older practitioners, who appear to feel a greater obligation towards the patient, may be based on their perception that the patient is more passive. This is contrasted with younger practitioners less often voicing issues with the way modern medicine is structured, implying that they were more accepting of the idea of the patient who is more active and involved in their own health care, taking the onus off the practitioner to a certain extent. As one surgeon described it, it is a matter for the practitioner to get a feeling of how actively their patient wants to be involved and respond with appropriate level of care:

> *There are some women who I feel that I have an instant sort of rapport with them and/or their partners. I don't know how to put it into words, but ... I think sometimes, they might offer some humour back, or they ask questions – intelligent questions – that show that they are interested in their condition beyond the fact that they have cancer, that they think a surgeon can provide answers to and I think they appreciate that. Some women don't want to have the technical details, they think I could make the judgement; and some women really want to be led by the hand – do this, this and this. And I try to do so for those women where I perceive that. It is just natural human interaction. With some people you click, with some you don't. (Surgeon 04)*

The last sentence also reflects the attitude that a practitioner cannot be there for all of their patients to the same extent. As one practitioner said during the interview, 'there is a practitioner for every patient and there is a patient for every practitioner', referring to the fact that a good patient-practitioner relationship cannot be purely based on the skills and expertise the practitioner offers, but includes the important aspect of whether or not the personalities of patient and practitioner align.

Empathy

Although the above suggests that sympathy for the patient plays an important role in good patient-doctor relationships, it was not presented as an essential element by practitioners. The difference between empathy and sympathy[16] and the fundamental nature of the former was notable throughout the interviews.

> *I hope I haven't kept them waiting too long. People said some-times that the rooms are fairly calming, because it is not too big or busy, because often people are a bit tense when they are going to see a surgeon. You can imagine that: 'he is going to tell me that I need an operation and there is going to be pain; it is going to cost money and I'd rather not be here'. When they arrive and [my sec-retary] is really nice to them and it seems calm and you can see that generally they relax. (Surgeon 05)*

The same practitioner then continued to describe the importance of listening to the patient and that it is a sign of respect towards the patient to let them speak about the things they feel are important in connection with their care. The practitioner gave the patients the opportunity to talk about what is most important to them.

> *[W]hen they start to talk and go on and on and on about the most extraneous of things, I think it is important to sit back and listen for a while, because then again the person will relax. If you are cutting in saying 'I don't need to know that; I just want to know about the knee' then they are going to think 'but I haven't' told him all the things I wanted to tell him about; my auntie's knee and things like that. They are important to them; you have got to let them get it off their chest. (Surgeon 05)*

The practitioner further suggested that empathy helps in understanding the reasons for patient behaviour and thus may make it easier to accept and deal with challenging patient behaviour.

---

[16] The understanding of empathy and sympathy follows the Oxford Dictionary, which defines empathy as 'the ability to understand and share the feelings of another', while sympathy is defined as 'feelings of pity and sorrow for some-one else's misfortune' (Oxford Dictionary, 2014).

You have to understand the trauma they are going through and have to understand that they will be irrational; they will be hostile; there won't be trust particularly in the trauma situation. They don't know you from a bar of soap. You have this vision of yourself, but to them you are just some figure at the end of the bed in theatre gear. There is no trust until you've earned their trust. And you earn that in all the little things you do, I find. I try to teach the registrars 'be very careful what you say to people. Never make offhand comments, certainly no rude, or cheeky, or disrespectful comments'. Not that many of them would, but it is amazing what people remember. (Surgeon 05)

Finally, the practitioner described their strategy to show empathy, particularly in trauma situations.

Show them that you will help them through that episode and give them a little bit of an idea what's in store for them. I usually try to be not too pessimistic; a bit of advice on how long the recovery is likely to be just so that they can start adjusting to that. Make them realise that you are interested and competent and [will] look after them so that they can relax. I always try to ring up a relative too. It only takes a minute, but people really appreciate that, because when someone is in surgery, often the family are at home and they don't know what's going on. (Surgeon 05)

Analysing the above statement, the practitioner describes a range of steps in interacting with a patient, including the following:

- showing the patient that the doctor will be there
- informing them about treatment and possible outcomes
- being positive
- shaping realistic expectations about long-term recovery
- showing interest in the patient
- showing competence
- assuring that the practitioner will look after them

- informing the family or next of kin

Notably, only the second point relates to the obligation of a practitioner to communicate the treatment, while all the other points are non-essential for the treatment, but appear important in caring for the patient. Some of the points – being there, being competent and being interested in the patient – are not commonly expressly communicated by the practitioner; often they are con-veyed to the patient by the practitioner's behaviour and action, which in return is open to interpretation by the patient.

Connecting on a personal level

Another theme practitioners referred to during the interviews was the im-portance of connecting with patients on a personal level, which was usually considered beneficial in building trust. What became clear in the ways practi-tioners described such personal connections was that they happen naturally and voluntarily, rather than being pursued by the practitioner.

> *With some people you click, with some you don't. And I have some women who have seen me for five or six years now and every time I see them I think very fondly of them. I will have almost a chat [with them] and I have to make sure that I do their medical as-pects. But they ask how my kids are. They say 'I remember when I was operated [on] before your son was born; he must be five years old now'. And I guess it has been a two-way path. (Surgeon 04)*

What is important to note is that the personal connection appears much more symmetric than communication about care and treatment where, regard-less of how well informed the patient is, their role is one of a more or less pas-sive recipient of treatment. The information exchange about personal aspects of the patient's and practitioner's lives lets them interact on a much more equal level. This might explain why connecting on a personal level is beneficial to trust building, as it equalises the power asymmetry between the patient and the practitioner and allows the patient to be more active in sharing information.

Permitting that personal connection when offered by the patient is an important element in building a good relationship with them.

> *When I get the old war veterans in their 80s or 90s, ¾ of the consultation is often [about] when they were out fishing last, what they catch and how the golf is going, that sort of stuff. They just want to sit down and talk to someone. I could do a consultation about their hip or knee in two minutes. But, they just want to sit down and have a yarn about things. And I have patients that regularly bring me fish that they have caught. I am sure a lot of doctors do that, a lot of doctors get that. And they are probably the ones that don't get sued – doctors whose patients like them and bring them gifts and all that sort of stuff. (Surgeon 01)*

What the above statement alludes to is the link between being able to connect to the practitioner on a personal level, patient satisfaction and the decreased risk of a complaint being made. As another general practitioner summarises it, patients stay with practitioners they feel comfortable with.

> *And then they think, 'well, I feel comfortable with you; I'll come back'. (GP 06)*

The statement can be read to also imply the opposite – that patients do not return to practitioners they do not feel comfortable with, unless they have to for other reasons, such as a lack of alternatives. If so, the decision of a patient to be treated by a practitioner is rarely solely based on their satisfaction with the competence and technical skills, but is often underpinned by their satisfaction with the personal interaction they have with the practitioner.

Overall, care related elements that support trust from a practitioners' perspective can be summarised as viewing the patient not only as a patient, but as a person. That means respecting the patient's preferences when it comes to treatment approaches, respecting their background, being empathetic with their situation beyond their health condition, connecting with them on a personal level by sharing experiences both the practitioner and patient can relate to; being accessible to the patient; and thinking proactively what would be the best for the patient from the patient's point of view.

3.4.3.4　Summary: Trust building elements – communication, competence and care

The interviewed practitioners were asked to reflect on the main elements they believe build and maintain patient trust. Usually, practitioners described a mix of communication, care and competence. There was a difference between general practitioners and surgeons insofar as surgeons emphasised skill and technical competence, while general practitioners usually first referred to caring for the patient and being a good communicator. However, overall practitioners believed that all three elements contribute to building and maintaining trust, particularly long-term.

After having looked at elements that support a trustful relationship between practitioners and patients from the practitioner's point of view. I now turn my focus to the elements that were considered as destructive to trust, the relationship and often related to triggering the complaint the practitioner had experienced.

3.4.4 Trust decreasing factors and complaint triggers – communication, competence and care

When analysing what practitioners believed decreases the patients' trust in them or other practitioners, I found it useful to cluster the emerging themes into the same areas: communication, competence and care, which also enabled me to contrast themes in those three areas in regard to whether they enable or destroy trust.

Before I continue my analysis, I would like to make a few observations. In the interviews, practitioners talked much more generally about what they believed builds or maintains trust, while the decrease of patient trust was more commonly talked about in relation to a specific patient complaint. The reference to a specific complaint could be the result of the study design that only selected practitioners and patients who went through a complaint experience rather than being able to select both positive and negative experiences. On the other hand though, it could be interpreted as a sign that practitioners in general think of their interaction with patients as positive and supportive in developing trust, while complaints are considered isolated, singular events and are compartmentalised as such by the practitioner.

Based on the dynamics of the trust model that I introduced above, my assumption was that a mismatch between the patient's expectation and the actual behaviour or outcome results in a decrease of their trust level. If the mismatch continues, trust levels decline to the point where there is no trust or even mistrust. I will explicitly refer to underlying expectations that are related to the themes that emerged from the interviews in the following analysis.

Most of the following examples from the interviews refer to a specific patient complaint; some are generalised statements by practitioners.

3.4.4.1 Communication

Lack of information, inadequate information, making sense

Communication

Competence

↓ Care

Lack of information or inadequate information was cited commonly as a suspected trigger for the patient's complaint. Particularly, where there was a serious outcome, such as the death of a patient, the lack of proper explanation, or inconsistency in the information given to the patient's family, appear to have played a role in the patient's or their family's decision to lodge a complaint.

> *[T]he boy died. I sat down with the mother and I said 'nobody knew why he died'. I talked to her, but obviously they needed [to blame someone] – and I can understand when your son dies it is a terrible thing. But it was very badly handled. ... And the other trigger, I suspect, was that the next door neighbour was a GP and he knew nothing about what was going on and made some very unguarded comments to [the patient's family], which they picked up on. (Surgeon 06)*

Underlying this statement is the family's expectation to know and understand exactly why their son died, who was involved in his treatment and care and whether there were any mistakes made. Where there is no clear explanation, people will attempt to make sense with the limited information and experiences they have. The need to find a cause for what happened in order to be able to understand is very common, as the analysis of the patient interviews will also show.

Where there is inadequate information, patients attempt to make sense of the situation with the information they have and that can result in completely different interpretations of the situation, as the next example shows.

I can see, from his perspective, what he is trying to link together to make a case. He basically said that he thought I was caught out. He couldn't believe that a specialist of my standing could be caught out by this sort of situation. And the bits of information he was throwing together: my assistant is a lady who is a breast physician ... – he then transcribed her speciality that she was a specialist surgeon and I was caught out and called her in, a specialist surgeon to help me out with this difficult operation. ... She is [in fact] my regular assistant who helped me operate on the other eight woman on that day. She was just the person who was there on the day. (Surgeon 04)

Differing opinion and actions of others

Another trigger for complaints that was more commonly mentioned by patients, but also reflected upon by practitioners, was the opinion of respected or trusted others that had led to the patient eventually making the complaint, as the following statement illustrates.

And somehow they got talking and she told [the Member of Parliament] and [they] sided with her and said, 'that's not good enough. He is just getting too old and he shouldn't be doing things like that'. (GP 05)

It suggests that although the patient may have considered making a complaint, it was the opinion of the trusted or respected other person that made the difference and resulted in action.

Other practitioners may be involved, for example, a previous treating doctor may have contributed to different expectations the patient had:

[Patients] comment, like 'my usual GP does this; my usual GP does that; he never said this'. (GP 03)

Notably, the way practitioners would manage differing opinions of other practitioners is more cautious than the way they would manage different opinions by other people.

> *I think you've got to try to preserve people's trust in their original doctor. Particularly, if it is someone you know and you know that they are conscientious. I mean, you have got to be honest about the result they have got and the patient can make their own judgement. And they might say 'I am still not happy with it', and I understand and accept that. You should never say that guy is an idiot, because it is this sort of work where people have different opinions. (Surgeon 05)*

The practitioner making the above statement implies that there appears to be a professional ethic not to go against fellow practitioners in front of a patient in the interest of preserving the trust in that practitioner, but also more broadly the trust in the profession, which was also mirrored in the following statement:

> *... You have to smile, grin and bear it. We all have our different opinions. ... You can't professionally bag your colleague, especially your boss. ... You just can't say bad things about your colleagues. ... We realise that we don't know everything and sometimes, what patients say may not actually be facts. There could just be a misunderstanding. (GP 03)*

So where there is a difference in professional opinion, practitioners noted that they would try to manage that very carefully with the patient and would try to stress the imperfections of medicine that are not necessarily based on a lack of skill or judgement. It was not absolutely clear from the interview data whether this implied professional ethic would only apply to the patients of immediate colleagues, or any patients. The following statement seems to broaden it to any peer, not limit it to immediate colleagues.

> *If someone had an operation somewhere and there is a definite*
> *problem that has to be done, then you have to say 'look this actu-*
> *ally is the problem; this piece has to be taken out and put in again*
> *in at a different angle'. You have to be honest about that. But I*
> *would even then try to explain to the patient how [difficult] it is*
> *putting those components in and how we are all human and it is*
> *not possible to replicate the exact same alignment every time, de-*
> *spite the best of techniques we have; and trying to make them re-*
> *alise that it is that type of work and we have those sorts of issues.*
> *(Surgeon 05)*

Overall, the communication related themes that practitioners considered contributed to the decline of patient trust and often were a factor that triggered a patient's complaint were lack of information, inadequate information or inconsistency in information, specifically where the inconsistency was across different practitioners. I will now look at competence related themes that practitioners spoke about during the interviews.

3.4.4.2 Competence

Communication

Competence

↓ **Care**

When practitioners reflected on what they believed to be the trigger for the patient's complaint they commonly cited as a possible reason that the actual outcome of the treatment did not meet the patient's expectations. Expectations about treatment outcomes are commonly linked to the perceived competence of a practitioner and in return where the treatment outcome does not meet the patient's expectation, this may have a negative impact on the patient's view of a practitioner's competence.

Complications and side effects

Patient may form their expectation based on information they select from all the information given to them during the process of obtaining informed consent. In the following example, the interviewed practitioner made sense of the patient's complaint by referring to a similar dynamic, whereby despite being informed of the risk of having an impaired capacity to have an erection after prostate surgery, the patient did not expect that it actually could happen to him and became angry because the side effects had a great impact on his life.

> It must have had a very big impact on his lifestyle and when he had been told about it earlier, he probably had thought, 'oh well, it won't happen to me. They'll look after me.' And when it happened, I just think he was really upset. I presume that was all. He just couldn't accept it … There is nothing else I could have said to him; there were no other tricks; there was no other treatment. He just had to accept it and he could never accept it. (Surgeon 03)

It can be difficult to work through such situations where the practitioner cannot offer the patient an alternative treatment or any further action they could take. The patient may perceive the lack of alternatives as lack of care and ignorance on the part of the practitioner. Patients can get frustrated and angry as a result.

Perceived lack of competence

Patient perceptions are important to analyse to understand the patient's behaviour and opinions. Particularly interesting are situations where the patient's perception and the facts as understood by the practitioner differ widely.

We often give women a lot of choice in breast cancer. You can do it either this, this, this, or this way. And how I deal with this problem is that I say 'I tell you of the options and if in the end you can make a decision, that's great. If you can't, I can tell you what I would do if you were my mum, my sister, or whoever depending on what their age is.' But this lady, I told her all the options and I think her perception was 'he doesn't know what he is doing! He asks me to make a decision. How should I know? I came to him for advice!' And by the time I got around saying 'if you were my sister, I would suggest you had this', I had lost her. And I just sensed it somehow. And I asked her whether she had made a decision, and she said 'no, that's fine; I'll let you know'. And she walked out of there and I knew that she wasn't going to let me know and that was fine. (Surgeon 04)

The above statement illustrates the differences in patient expectation of their practitioners and how it shapes their perception, assumptions and generalisations about them. The way the practitioner communicated was not responsive to the style the patient was used to or expected. A second observation is that the patient did not test her perceptions, but made up her mind and did not return to the practitioner. This illustrates the influence that communication, which is not specific to the patient's expectations, can have on patient choices and decision-making.

Wrong diagnosis

Inadequate information and unmet expectations can be influenced by differing assumptions of what the role and responsibility of a practitioner is, particularly where they are not regular patients. As the following example illustrates, incomplete communication can have a serious impact on patient outcome.

She mentioned the diarrhoea, but she came to me for a skin condi-
tion. And she was going to another doctor, so I didn't investigate
it very much, because I thought she was coming to me for her skin
and was going to another doctor for her diarrhoea. Anyway, even-
tually, it turned out that she had cancer of the colon; or cancer of
the bowel. (GP 05)

From a practitioner's point of view, it appears that the treatment result
takes precedence over other factors. Where there is a positive treatment outcome, patients may overlook inadequate information, rudeness or ignorance of
their wishes. In contrast, where there is no trust, even minor technical flaws can
be interpreted as much more serious by the patient.

People who have interventions sometimes don't mind what the
demeanour of the person is provided that the technical outcome is
good, perfect. Nevertheless, those people seeking perfection in
technical outcome will often magnify perceptions of failure and
problems in the make-up of the surgeon, if there is a flawed out-
come. So, my personal bias is towards forming a relation of mutu-
al trust and I will, if I don't sense that, choose, on occasion, not to
operate on people, or not to intervene, and encourage them to
seek other opinions. (Surgeon 02)

Challenging the common perception of practitioners that treatment outcomes take precedence over expectations regarding other aspects of the patient's care, some practitioners also spoke about examples where despite a
good treatment outcome, patients complained because their expectations regarding the overall care were not met. Sometimes, these factors may not be
under the control of the relevant practitioner, but from the patient's point of
view, they are considered the primary carer and therefore responsible, or at
least accountable.

> *I got a lady last week who complained about my registrar, alt-*
> *hough she is very happy with her physical outcome, she com-*
> *plained about her perception of the level of care in the hospital. ...*
> *I apologised broadly for the system. I told her that I would follow-*
> *up with the relevant doctor. I tried to steer the conversation as*
> *much as I could towards the positive: The good pathology, which I*
> *have no control over, but the fact that under the circumstances it*
> *is a really good result. And her cosmetic result was exceptional*
> *under the circumstances. (Surgeon 04)*

Patients may see their practitioners being accountable for their overall care experience. Interestingly, the statement above shows that the practitioner seems to accept being a representative of the system when he apologises for issues the patient had experienced that he had no control over.

Making a point about inadequate safety and quality

Practitioners also offered as one possible explanation why patients complain that they want their dissatisfaction to be heard and their practitioner to know that it is important to them. This implies that the patient had the perception that the practitioner did not take the incident seriously or did not care.

A general practitioner who out of courtesy had removed a corn from an elderly patient's foot so that she did not need consult and pay for a podiatrist, slightly cut into the skin. The patient made a formal complaint:

> *She wanted me to be aware and that it was probably not trivial.*
> *She didn't consider it trivial. And she considered it outside my*
> *competence to be doing corns on the feet of a patient and [that] I*
> *had no special qualification [to do so]. There were other people*
> *who could do that sort of thing. They may do it better. ... Her sug-*
> *gestion was that I should not offer that type of service. (GP 05)*

This example also highlights the difference in perception about the seriousness or severity of an incident. While the cut in the skin might have been painful, the doctor did not consider it in any way posing a risk to the patient. For the patient, however, it was serious enough to bring to the attention of a regulatory body, the Health Care Complaints Commission, with the aim of stopping the doctor from providing this service not only to her but to anyone else, implying the doctor posed a risk to her and to his other patients.

Questioning practitioners' actions

In the following case, the negative perception of the patient was primed by her fear of infections, which was unknown to the doctor and hence not specifically addressed during the consultation despite the practitioner quickly becoming suspicious.

> *I said to her what I would like her to do … I pulled out the packet and opened it and pulled the speculum out by the handle. Now, I did not have at that point gloves on. However, by this time, she was already asking questions: Is it sterile? Is it this? Is it that? And I cottoned on quite quickly that this patient was quite obsessive about what was going on. … Now, she maintains I didn't wear gloves. Now, there is no way I am going to do a pap smear and put my hands rather my fingers in anyone without gloves on. But she maintains I didn't do that and she didn't see me wash my hands. … She maintains that I didn't wash my hands at any point in front of her, which I know very well, I did. I do know I wore my gloves. … I was not really surprised [by her complaint], because I'd already picked up there was going to be a problem …. (GP 06)*

The practitioner uses the word 'obsessive' which implies that the patient's behaviour was unusual or out of the ordinary, which implicitly defends the practitioner's side of the story by suggesting that the patient was not acting rationally.

Differing expectation about the level of care

One practitioner reflected explicitly on the gap between patient expectations and achievable outcomes, suggesting that some patients' expectations may be unrealistic and could never be met.

> *I actually think there is a small but significant minority of public patients who have chosen, or for whatever reasons are, public patients who, in my judgement, have expectations of the level of care far beyond what is the norm and probably beyond what would be [possible] ... no one would be able to meet them, whether they are [in the] public system or private sector. They are expecting perfection and medicine really doesn't achieve that. (Surgeon 04)*

The statement implies that a complaint is more likely where expectations differ about what level of care and treatment is possible or realistic in the given circumstances. The finding underpins the importance of expectation management.

Overall, from the practitioners' point of view the main factors that contributed to a deterioration of patient trust and eventually triggered a complaint included patients experiencing a wrong diagnosis or (often unexpected) poor treatment outcome, patients questioning the practitioner's competence, or feeling that their suffering is not taken seriously. Importantly, it is the patient's perception of the practitioner's competence and quality of care, which may differ from the practitioner's or other people's perceptions.

3.4.4.3 Care

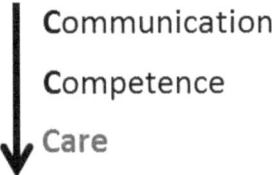

Communication

Competence

Care

During the interview, most practitioners referred to care-related inadequacies that they believed had triggered or contributed to a patient complaint. Often care-related themes were interlinked with communication and competence factors, but I have chosen to present them separately in the analysis. Some of the statements may have been included above in relation to a different aspect.

Delays

In the interviews with patients, lack of punctuality came up as a regular theme. Patients' interpretation of this varied from some perceiving it as a sign of the practitioner's lack of respect for them, others referred to delays as a sign that the doctor did not take it as seriously as it deserved to be, while still others derived an opinion about the practitioner being disorganised and therefore lacking in competence from the fact that there were these delays.

Practitioners also mentioned delays as a contributing factor to patient complaints during their interviews.

> *The other was a woman who'd objected to the fact that she was the first scheduled patient for the morning – a clinical review at 8.30am – and I appeared at about 9.15am having been involved with a patient who needed intensive care management and other interventions within the hospital. And she objected to that 45 minute wait as the first patient for the day. Nevertheless, her complaint to the Health Care Complaints Commission then required a formal response from me. (Surgeon 02)*

The above statement illustrates the differing perception about priorities: while the practitioner's priority was to provide emergency assistance, the patient's priority clearly was her own operation. Considering that the patient may have been very anxious about her operation, it would have made the delay even more difficult to deal with. It is unclear in that example whether or not the patient had been informed of the delay early on and was told the reasons, or whether that was only done at the time the surgeon finally attended on her, or was not explained to her at all.

Another case mentioned by one of the practitioners related to the delay in a non-life threatening treatment of a child with a common cold that lead to the parents lodging a formal complaint.

> [A] child had a cold that I treated. I sent the child to our nurse to have oxygen and ventolin by nebulizer. And I think the nurse was delayed and the people got impatient and took the child to the hospital. And then they wrote to the Medical Board too and complained that the treatment was inadequate. (GP 05)

The difference in the perception of priorities may have contributed to the patient complaint in the above example. Overall, practitioners viewed delays or issues with punctuality as not a serious issue that justifies patient complaints in their opinion. Often delays were seen as a contributing factor, but rarely the only reason a patient makes a complaint.

Feeling rushed and unresponsive

One practitioner summarised the patient complaint:

> And she thought that she didn't like the way I treated her in the room: that I didn't give her enough time and I didn't listen to her and I rushed her through and I didn't give her enough attention. (Surgeon 03)

The lack of time, attention and understanding triggered a complaint, despite no treatment being provided and the practitioner perceiving the consultation at the time not as an incident.

Unbefitting consultation style

Notably, one general practitioner said that she suspected the reason for the patient making a complaint was two-fold: unmet expectations combined with unmet demands. The patient used to see a different practitioner at the same practice who had a very different consultation style, in a sense more conversational and having a chat rather than focussing purely on the treatment and health problems of the patient. Hence, when this patient saw the new general practitioner, her straight-forward style focussing on the symptoms and treatment did not meet the patient's expectation based upon prior experience with the other practitioner. In addition, the patient then requested antibiotics, which apparently were prescribed to him in the past for a similar condition. This practitioner refused the request based on her clinical judgement, which then led to a discussion about her reasons, wherein the patient constantly questioned the validity of the practitioner's reasoning.

> *I don't think that this person is challenging so long as they get the demanded medicine. ... I spent 20 minutes – I didn't charge him a long consultation. He challenged whatever I said. When I explained it further, he questioned me further. He was trying to catch me out. And eventually I gave him the script, which he virtually came in for and then he actually, before he left, said, 'is there someone I can complain to? ...*

> *I think a couple of things triggered him. First the patient's expectations were not met. I know the consultation style of his usual doctor, which is having a nice chat, giving him the script, usually quite on time and then a chat about sport or the weather.*

> *This time, the reason why I asked him a few question was just to gauge the level of knowledge. Sometimes, I deal with doctors and nurses and I start explaining things and they look at me and say 'I am in the medical profession; you don't have to tell me this.'*

And he felt challenged by me asking him to explain what he already knew, or didn't know. (GP 03)

The example illustrates how prior interaction with practitioners, particularly where they work at the same practice, shape patient expectations.

Being charged for unsatisfactory service

One practitioner specifically mentioned that the two complaints she [GP 03] had received were both where the patient was charged for the service, rather than bulk-billed[17]. The same practitioner spoke about situations where she did not meet patient demands and expectations, but instead of giving in, apologised and did not charge, with none of these resulting in a complaint.

This suggests that where an additional payment for medical services is requested, patient expectations about the quality of service and treatment may be higher than where there is no charge to the patient. However, a patient may also be willing to (co-)pay for their health care expecting to gain faster access to medical services or preferential treatment, rather than having an expectation about a higher level of care or treatment.

Lack of responsibility

Finally, I would like to highlight one other situation some practitioners experienced in relation to patient complaints. It appeared that where something unexpected happened, especially when it had a great impact on the patient's life, patients looked for causation. In the absence of a clear cause, they then tend to look for someone who may be responsible and accountable.

---

[17]   Bulk-billed in the Australian system means that the practitioner accepts the Medicare rebate as full payment and there are no further costs for the patient. Medicare is the basic health insurance that covers treatment for Australian citizens and permanent residents.

[S]he was going to have a breast reduction and she had a mam-
mogram which was negative. And she went to the plastic surgeon.
And then, she was waiting for her reduction and she had a lump in
her breast. And she maintains she'd come to see him and he had
said, 'don't worry about it; the plastic surgeon will sort it out for
you'. But, he wasn't found [guilty]; there was no complaint found
against him either, because there was no record of her ever hav-
ing attended our surgery between her mammogram and seeing
the plastic surgeon. So where she got that from, I don't know. (GP
06)

This example shows how the recall of verbal information a practitioner gives to a patient during a consultation may be unreliable and in the absence of another 'logical' explanation for the situation, the patient may attribute blame directly to the practitioner.

The snowball effect

In understanding what triggered a patient to make a complaint, it was suggested that the practitioner has to consider a variety of potential factors and their relationship to understand how the patient has perceived a situation. Often not knowing all the factors or addressing them only partially will not resolve the complaints. Notably, this practitioner also highlighted that once a question or negative perception arises in the patient's mind the subsequent actions are interpreted to fit that initial perception.

The other thing that I found when there is a complaint and some-thing doesn't work well, it is usually a coincidence of a number of factors. It is not usually the one thing that has gone wrong, people don't get too worried, if one thing goes wrong. But if multiple things seem to have gone wrong, that's when they get worried. You can see [that]. And once they get worried, they start looking at everything and they start remembering things. You can see them building a case in their mind that the people looking after them are incompetent. And it can sort of snowball from there. You have to try to understand what it is that triggered the process. (Surgeon 05)

The statement summarises the finding that often it is a combination of different unmet patient expectations that triggers a complaint. It appears from the way practitioners talked about it, that they believed that competence-related issues had a higher possibility of leading to a patient complaint. Contrasting this perception with statistical data from the Health Care Complaints Commission shows that complaints to the Commission about communication issues are often not related to treatment outcomes (Kable et al., 2014).

Overall, the care-related themes that were associated with the loss of trust by practitioners almost perfectly contrasted the care-related themes that were considered to enhance trust. Not respecting the patient as a person, being indifferent and unresponsive to the patient's needs and expectations were mentioned by practitioners as contributing to the patient losing trust. Often, a combination of multiple communication, competence and care-related aspects that decreased trust eventually led to the patient thinking of making a complaint.

3.4.4.4 Summary: Elements that decrease trust

It appears from the practitioners' accounts that trust is lost through lack of or poor communication, the patient suffering from unexpected complications or treatment outcomes, or the perceived lack of respect and care afforded to the patient. Those are not only factors that may decrease the patient's level of trust in the practitioner, but may at the same time trigger a formal complaint. In the next section I analyse the response of practitioners as to how they would deal with complaints or have dealt with them in the past.

3.4.5   Dealing with a complaint

The strategies practitioners described having taken in response to a complaint varied from trying to understand the patient's perspective to ceasing the relationship they had with the patient altogether, with the latter more commonly mentioned as the method of choice.

3.4.5.1 Complaints as the end of doctor-patient relationship

A belief shared by some of the interviewed practitioners was that if a patient does not trust them, they would simply choose not to return, if possible.

> *And if you don't live up to their expectations, they go. They don't stay. (GP 06)*

It appears that a complaint may not always be an indication of a loss of trust, as practitioners on rare occasions reported patients returning after making a complaint. Interestingly, one point that was not raised by a single practitioner, but came out in the analysis of patient interviews, suggested that there are situations where a patient is forced to return to the practitioner given the reluctance of other practitioners to accept them as a patient where there was an obvious complication or error suffered. The patient's perception was that other practitioners did not want to touch them as they were afraid of being implicated in the incident or error.

3.4.5.2 Impact on treating relationship

Asked whether practitioners would continue to treat a patient who had made a complaint against them previously, the responses were mixed. Some declined outright to see the patient again, citing a breakdown in their relationship, whilst others thought there was an ethical and professional obligation to treat a patient the best they can, independent of a complaint.

> *[The patient] would be seen on her own merits. Now, we have made repeated attempts for [the patient] to come back to the rooms; all of those letters, requests have gone unanswered. And that is not unusual once somebody has lost trust. Nevertheless, as I said, unless you are a doctor, you won't understand, you can't fully appreciate the ability to change gears and do that, but that is the reality of what we have to do day after day after day. There is no paradox in that, but it is part of the highest level of ethical practice and again part of the desired attributes in the doctor. (Surgeon 02)*

The statement implies that there is a specific moral code that only applies to doctors which requires them to act in the patient's best interest regardless of their own emotions, thoughts and opinions they hold of the patient. It is an extension of the Hippocratic Oath in conflict situations. The practitioner reiterated this position later in the interview.

> *Every step of the way from my first encounter with her, she is a woman whose default is to complain. That makes interactions difficult but not as a carer; you can't avoid the obligation to provide care and you work within it. (Surgeon 02)*

The ethical obligation to cooperate and provide treatment despite any negative patient behaviour or complaint appears to be unique to the treatment relationship and in the opinion of this practitioner would extend to situations where there is no trust left between the parties.

This has got nothing to do with trust. If you once, as I said, inflated a matter to the level of an agency [the Health Care Complaints Commission] like this, you have lost all trust. And whichever the parties, the appellant or the defendant in a matter, there is complete lack of trust. (Surgeon 02)

3.4.5.3 Identifying and addressing differing expectations

In response to the question what he would do when getting a complaint, one surgeon noted the need to collect the facts and identify the patient's perceptions first, which may well differ significantly from the recollection the practitioner has.

I suppose the first thing is, you want to get the facts and trying to understand what they are unhappy about, because as I said, it could be something quite unexpected. As a surgeon you would think this, but it could be something completely different, like someone was rude to them in the ward, or someone said something that is upsetting them. It could be something like that. So you need to gather that information and gather your own recollections of the patient so that you can try to understand the context. (Surgeon 05)

The practitioner not only talks about certain facts or what happened, but how something was perceived. In the last part of the statement, the practitioner refers to trying to ascertain the patient's perception of the situation, but also to the need to recollect the practitioner's initial perception of the patient to make sense of what the patient needs. This links the first impression a practitioner had to interpreting incident situations and determining appropriate action.

In summary, the cultural predisposition of practitioners is to cease a treating relationship where the patient has made a complaint. Some practitioners override this predisposition with a professional obligation to provide further treatment, but nevertheless, the relationship had changed, mostly towards the negative. In the next section, I look more closely at the emotions practitioners reported in relation to an incident and in relation to a complaint.

So far, I have analysed what practitioners believe makes trust important in a relationship with patients, what role first impressions play, what factors enhance and what factors diminish trust. I have also looked at how practitioners described dealing with a patient's complaint and the impact it had on their relationship with the patient.

In the next section, I focus on emotions that practitioners described in association with the incident and the complaint.

3.4.6   Emotions

When talking about a specific incident, practitioners focussed on describing patient emotions. In contrast, when talking about the patient's complaint, practitioners more commonly reported their own emotions.

Practitioners did not describe many emotions – positive or negative – in regard to the patients before the incident. Immediately after the incident, emotional descriptions focused on feelings displayed by patients. Most commonly, practitioners perceived the patient to feel any of the following:

1. Dissatisfaction and disappointment
2. Distress and upset
3. Anger, antagonism
4. Acceptance
5. Fear and anxiety
6. Blame

Notably, only one neutral emotion – acceptance – is included in this list by frequency of otherwise negative emotions patients were believed to have had regarding the incident.

Once a complaint was lodged, practitioners did describe their own emotions. An explanation may be that incidents and dealing with difficult patients are accepted as part of the job and there appears to be a professional ethic to deal with them. However, once an incident triggers a complaint, it is lifted onto a different level. Complaints are not considered a routine part of the practitioner's job. The complaint process is often foreign to a practitioner and practitioners tend to have a more emotional response to a formal complaint to a third party. The fact that a complaint was made to a body like the Health Care Complaints Commission has also lifted the conflict stemming from the incident from an interpersonal conflict to a more complex, more formal, and potentially more serious level.

Finding someone to blame was not only an emotion attributed to patients, but also to complaint-handling authorities. One surgeon described his experience of a hearing before the (former) NSW Medical Board. The complaint related to the death of a trauma patient who had died after being referred from Intensive Care, despite the practitioner's protests that this would be inappropriate given the patient's condition. Still, the practitioner felt accountable – not responsible – for the death, as he was the head of the department in which the patient died.

> *There were many doctors looking after this guy ... when he was shut out of the intensive care unit, he was put into the orthopaedic ward. Even though I did not want him there, I did take him.*
>
> *So we were looking after him, but he died for reasons not quite clear; but he died. The point was that it went to [a coronial] inquest – which it should have – but then they tried to find someone to blame, so the doctor who is the head of the bed is always to blame. (Surgeon 06)*

The surgeon accepts accountability by supporting that there should be an inquest as the reasons for the patient passing away were not fully clear. He also expressed in the interview that reviews are important to learn from, but in his opinion, are often only being misused to blame someone without having a proper look at systemic failures and issues that led or contributed to the incident. In this case, the surgeon felt blamed as he was the only provider that was being held accountable. Asked whether he was aware whether there had been an internal investigation by the hospital, he responded:

> *I have no idea. If it was, nobody had come back to me ...*

He then offered the following causation:

> *[T]he administration's job is to protect itself. The first function of any administration is to look after itself. So when they are doing an in-depth investigation into what was going on, the first principle is to find somebody else to blame; so they like purity. ... I was set-up as the fall guy. Undoubtedly, this is what they needed and my name was the head of the [department]. (Surgeon 06)*

He then describes his experience of the complaint process, as part of which he was requested to attend a hearing before the former NSW Medical Board. It reflects the feeling of antagonism he perceived and his frustration with the process.

> *When I went to see the Medical Board – ... you can take a lawyer, but the lawyer can't say anything – well, I took the lawyer along. At least, I have an expert witness who could listen to what was going on. And I sat an hour with them and I gave them a couple of barrels. You know, this wasn't on and it is a disgrace. They looked a bit stunned. I was angry as hell about it. ... the system was deeply flawed. It was a deeply unpleasant part of my life for a while and I feel very sorry about this boy. (Surgeon 06)*

The last part displays three emotions: dissatisfaction with the complaint system, personal upset at having to go through the process without any positive outcomes and relating it back to the actual incident – a young man died – which was a sad event, from which, in the practitioner's opinion, nothing was learned or led to improvements.

Another important aspect of the interviews was the residual emotions practitioners had about the incident and complaint and whether it may have had an impact on their expectations and behaviour in general.

Practitioners described the impact the incident and complaint had on them professionally and personally. In some cases the incident had resulted in a more relaxed approach to similar situations. In others, it resulted in the practitioner becoming more defensive in their professional judgement, or a complete loss of confidence in the complaint system, or fear of the patient.

3.4.6.1 Acceptance and resilience

Some practitioners noted that they had become more accepting of the fact that patients have a right to complain and that it is not necessarily an attack on them as a person. One surgeon said that he used to worry a lot, but now after having had a few minor complaints, is much more able to compartmentalise and leave work without taking the professional concerns into his private life.

> *Look, I don't [worry] much now, I just compartmentalise. I used to worry a lot and things, but now when I go home I switch off. I could almost forget that I have a patient in hospital until the next time I think, oh, I better do a ward round. But before that I was worrying …. (Surgeon 04)*

One practitioner reflected that in relation to the patient who made a complaint about her, she would not have changed anything she did during the actual consultation, but may have been more proactive in responding to the actual complaint. Asked whether she would have changed anything, she responded:

> *No, no, because I knew that that woman had a huge personality problem. I only pray for the person who took her on. And I still feel sorry for her. She was her own worst enemy, but I was very pleased not to see her, all the same. And as I say, this patient doesn't come to the practice anymore anyway. So I don't have to confront her in any sense. But, if I'd been aware, should I have rung her up? Yes. The answer is yes. Maybe , if I'd been a bit more sensitive to the fact that she was going to complain, I might have rung her up and said, 'look, I'm sorry this has happened. Can we talk about it?' But I was too busy and didn't think [of it] anymore. (GP 06)*

It is clear that the above practitioner blamed the patient for the incident and the complaint. Although she said that perhaps she should have called and apologised, she did not consider it essential and necessary.

One surgeon spoke about the benefits of a complaint system for not only the patient but also as a feedback and learning tool for the practitioner.

> *I think the system is quite good. Everybody thinks that it is rotten to get complaints, but in a way it does make you examine your own practice and the way things work at the hospital and often something good comes out of it.... And if you didn't get the odd complaint you wouldn't realise what path of destruction you might be leaving. Unless someone stands up ... you may not think and stop [about] what might have been said or done. ... By and large when someone makes a complaint, you can see that they are reasonable people, but a few things have gone wrong and ... often what they say is that they don't want this to happen to someone else. So they want the system, or whoever is responsible to take notice: ... they are trying to help the system by making a complaint. So we shouldn't get too upset about it. (Surgeon 05)*

What the above statement implies is also that complaints are a tool to ex-amine practice and that in some circumstances, it may be a more effective way than the existing peer review system. This practitioner views complaints as a normal part of professional life, rather than an upsetting exception to professional life. However, this was an opinion shared among a minority of interviewed practitioners.

One general practitioner reflected on his complaint experience and offered advice to other practitioners, to always apologise to the patient, whether or not their complaint is well-founded. He said:

> *Always apologise, even if you are right, because of the perception of the patient, the patient doesn't know what is right or wrong. The patient only feels the hurt, the fear and the wrong, even if they are wrong. The best way to explain it is: we can see; they are blind. A seeing man does not blame the blind man for walking into them. (GP 01)*

Although this statement may reflect a conciliatory attitude of the practitioner in the sense that he speaks of offering an apology to respond to patient dissatisfaction, it also reflects a patronising patient-practitioner relationship, with the practitioner having all the knowledge and understanding and the patient being the passive and powerless recipient of information and treatment. The practitioner also does not distinguish between different types of apologies that might range from showing empathy to asking for forgiveness for an error that occurred. I will analyse the role of an apology in complaints, from the practitioner's perspective, separately.

3.4.6.2 Changes to professional practice

While practitioners were reported above as being more careful in treating and interacting with people where they felt there was a lack of trust and/or a complaint, the caution appeared to remain with them in their working life after they had experienced a patient complaint. Some spoke about their more defensive approach to treatment.

I think I have to accept that if someone like that can make a com-
plaint like that then society in general will have to accept that
they are getting a lot more scans and things done on them, so
that we are not subject to that kind of allegation. (Surgeon 05)

The practitioner not only speaks about his reaction and changes to practice after a particular complaint, but placed it into a broader context of the way modern medicine becomes more complex, cautious, technical and as a result costly.

Other practitioners spoke about a changing patient-practitioner relationship in general, with the number of patient complaints increasing and potentially the outcome for the practitioner being more serious, which in their view contributed to a cultural change towards more cautious and resource intense medicine.

It's an awareness that you need to be a lot more defensive; that
you can't afford to say to someone with chest pain, 'look, I'm sure
it's not cardiac; don't worry, I am sure it is not.' You've got to say,
chest pain is cardiac until proven otherwise, so let's investigate.
Whereas 30 years ago, I would say, 'look, I am sure this is not your
heart. You are 35 years old; it is most unlikely'. But now, you've
got to go looking; you have got to check the cholesterol [level];
you have got to make sure they don't smoke. You have got to be
much, much more defensive. (GP 06)

The above statement is an example of what is referred to in the literature as 'practising defensive medicine'. This means that there is a greater responsibility on the practitioner to provide evidence for their diagnosis and treatment. It also means that there are increased risks of over-diagnosing and over-treating, which can lead to increases in health care costs through the greater use of diagnostic tools and tests, but also increases patient anxiety.

3.4.6.3   Fear of patient and the system

Two of the more extreme reactions to a patient complaint that practitioners described were fear of the patient and fear of the complaint-handling system. I like to start with the first – fear of a patient – that was described by a surgeon who had dealt with a patient who did not accept that he had experienced recognised side effects from an operation. The patient did not want to accept any explanation for his physical condition, either by the surgeon, or by the Health Care Complaints Commission that after assessing the complaint did not take any action. According to the surgeon, the patient had displayed angry and violent behaviour on several occasions and had threatened the surgeon and staff of the hospital.

> *[H]e is just a very aggressive man. And I really fear that he would come and do something, some injury to my staff or to my family. … My wife knew, … she met him when he turned up. And my secretary certainly was aware. In fact, what I had said to the hospital when he came back recently was that when he came back to my office, I would ring the police. They all knew. So I certainly made it very clear to all my staff that if he came back that I would call the police. (Surgeon 03)*

The surgeon did add that he fears that the patient would coincidentally see him or his family on the street, as they were living close by. Managing the situation and the fear was no longer only a part of the surgeon's professional life at the hospital, but also in his private life.

The second fear described by practitioners in the interviews was the fear of the complaint-handling system and the fear of being unjustly accused of wrongdoing.

You see, if you are a lawyer, you think like a lawyer and it is a job. You appear for the plaintiff or you appear for the defendant, it's your job – nothing personal. But for the doctor, it is very personal, because it is a blow to his self-esteem, to be accused of something and he doesn't feel that he has done anything wrong. And within the profession, there have been some real terrible upsets through judgements which are medically totally crap, but judgements have been made in favour of the plaintiff. And it causes great angst in the profession, because people feel, this isn't justice. It's the law performing, but it isn't justice. (Surgeon 06)

The statement implies that being a medical practitioner is not just a profession, but the basis of their identity. Secondly, the statement infers that wrong decisions are being made by the legal system on occasion. It displays a lack of understanding of how the complaint-handling and legal systems work, and suspicion of its outcomes. The lack of understanding of the complaint-system is also evident in the following statement that implies that there are no alternative dispute resolution mechanisms available to practitioners to deal with patient complaints, which is contrary to the facts.

People should be able to discuss their anxieties, tensions and problems in a non-adversarial set-up. … It is not really happening at the moment. Some people may go to a mentor and say such and such and such, but a lot of people [practitioners] just clam up and get morose and that's it, they carry on. (Surgeon 06)

In summary, the impacts of incidents on practitioners that were described were overwhelmingly negative. It appears that a lack of understanding and mistrust of the complaint-handling system and an adversarial attitude towards patients during the complaint process contribute to this negative attitude.

The open disclosure policy, which existed at the time of the interviews, was not mentioned a single time by any of the practitioners.

3.4.6.4 Emotions and trust

In the analysis, I correlated the emotions practitioners described with their description of factors and the effect of decreasing trust. Most commonly related to the decrease of trust were the following:

- being careful
- feeling not understood by the patient
- unhelpful, unsupportive, unresponsive
- worried

This order remained unchanged when taking into account emotions correlated with experiencing a manifest perception of mistrust or distrust towards the patient.

In contrast, practitioners associated positive emotions with trust building factors and the effect of patient trust. Most commonly, they were the following:

- being helpful, supportive, responsive
- accepting
- feeling happy

While the emotions associated with trust decreasing factors were mainly experienced by the practitioner, the emotions described in relation to trust increasing factors and patient trust were more commonly the patient's emotions. This supports the themes that emerged earlier in the analysis.

Lastly, I turn to the role of apologies practitioners described during the interviews. I did not prompt practitioners to talk about apologies, as I wished to see whether they mentioned them and what importance they assigned to them as a possible trust restoring measure when talking about incidents and their relationship with patients.

3.4.7   Role of an apology

My hypothesis was that where the practitioner offered an apology, no formal complaint would be made. Given that the sample for the interview study only included incidents that had actually triggered a complaint, I looked more broadly into the role an apology had in the practitioner's view.

In general, two areas can be distinguished and will be analysed separately: (1) practitioners speaking about the lack of an apology, and the reasons and circumstances for this, and (2) practitioners speaking about an apology, and their intention in making it and the outcome. How practitioners talked about apologies revealed some of their underlying attitudes and expectations.

3.4.7.1 Lack of apology

Examples of practitioners' reported reasons for not offering an apology were that:

- they had no chance to apologise as they were not aware that there was a problem;
- their indemnity insurer advised them not to apologise as it could be used against them; and
- they should have apologised, but were too busy.

Where practitioners spoke about their lack of apology to the patient, it usually related to a situation after an incident had occurred. All of the above statements imply that, in principle, the practitioner was willing to apologise, but there were circumstances that prevented them from doing so.

Some practitioners also spoke about the lack of an apology they had expected from the patient. For example, the patient did not apologise for swearing at the practitioner, which had prompted the doctor to ask the patient to leave; or the patient did not apologise for coming to a consultation without bringing along relevant information, including test results. The lack of an apology by the patient usually related to a situation before the incident. The way these situations were described by the practitioner implied that the patient was partially to blame for the complaint and the escalation of a situation, as their own behaviour had triggered the deterioration of the relationship or situation.

3.4.7.2 Apologies

Where practitioners made an apology, different functions of such an apology can be distinguished. One function of an apology was the acknowledgement of the patient's or their family's grief, for example, where a patient had passed away. Sometimes, the apology was coupled with an explanation of what had happened and why. This is the closest version of an apology described by practitioners that correlates to the open disclosure concept. But the function of the apology can be two-fold: either the apology is an acknowledgment of an error and a sign of taking responsibility, or it could serve to calm the patient down to then be able to defend the action, or both.

On a different level, a practitioner apologised on behalf of the system for the disappointing experience the patient had had and proceeded to steer the conversation towards the positive results of the actual treatment. Here, the practitioner made himself accountable for the system he is part of, but did not take personal responsibility.

There was one practitioner who spoke about apologising to a patient, saying 'sorry, there is nothing more I can do' to end the conversation.

Overall, practitioners reported that patients often reacted to an apology by calming down, dismissing or accepting the issue and being able to move beyond emotions and listen to the information and explanations given.

Interestingly, two practitioners mentioned that they had apologised to staff or another practitioner for sending a difficult or rude patient to them.

Here, the apology served to maintain a positive relationship with colleagues or staff.

Overall, apologies and apologising to the patient were only minor themes in the interviews, which might be a reflection of the level of importance practitioners assign to it. Where there was an apology, it was often instrumental in achieving a desired outcome or behaviour.

3.4.8   Summary: Trust, the practitioner's perspective

The analysis of interviews with general practitioners and surgeons about their experience with patient complaints showed that most believed that the patient's trust is beneficial for the relationship in routine situations, but also has a positive impact on the relationship after incidents. While trust makes relating to the patient easier, most practitioners would treat a patient who does not trust them – viewing it as their professional obligation. However, most would be very careful in their interaction with the patient and some would encourage the patient to see another practitioner or seek a second opinion.

The analysis distinguished three areas that contribute to building trust, or in contrast, to diminishing trust – communication, competence and care. Practitioners said that if they are able to work out the patient's priorities it helps them to respond appropriately and build a relationship. However, various doctors also said that an initial liking of the patient, a feeling of connectedness, helps in establishing the rapport that is needed to build a trusting relationship. Most practitioners believed if they displayed technical competence, it would most likely outweigh any issues with communication and care the patient might have. In other words, practitioners believed that a high level of competence would outweigh other behaviour that may be deemed problematic by patients.

In the opinion of practitioners, reputation, patient choice and first impressions play an integral part in establishing trust in a practitioner. They believe that a patient comes with pre-conceptions to the first consultation and that the first impression will either support this pre-conception, or make them doubt their initial choice. In other words, patients come with an initial level of trust that is being tested during the first consultation.

Practitioners agreed that, given the opportunity, most patients would not wish to see a doctor again whom they do not trust or have lost trust in.

In summary, practitioners viewed trust in the doctor-patient relationship as two-directional. Patients come with preconceptions and expectations, while practitioners have certain communication styles, manners and specialised skills. It seems that the better the match between patient expectation and practitioner skill and personality, the easier the practitioner feels it is to establish and build trust.

I now turn to how patients described their relationship with practitioners before and after incidents and when they made a complaint. I will use a similar analytical cluster as I used for practitioners to assist in comparing practitioners' and patients' views about dynamics of trust in relation to incidents.

3.5   Themes emerging from patient interviews

This section summarises and illustrates the themes that emerged in patient interviews in relation to trust. The section starts with the patient's perspective on why trust matters in the relationship between patients and practitioners. It continues with an analysis of the first impressions a patient had of a practitioner and the emotions related to the patient's experience. Following from this I present an in-depth analysis of the emerging themes relating to trust building and the loss of trust. Similar to the structure used when analysing themes from a practitioner's point of view, I distinguish communication, care and competence related themes.

The section then moves on to why patients decided to make a complaint and what the outcome of the complaint was. Lastly, I look at the role of apologies and how patients with the benefit of having reflected upon their experiences describe their ideal doctor. The results will be contrasted with the themes that emerged for the interviews with practitioners in the later discussion.

The research question and sub-questions that were introduced in Section 3.2.2.1 were used both for the analysis of the practitioner and patient interviews and were broken down in the following questions that guided my analysis of the interview data: Why does trust matter? How do patients describe that trust is built or diminished? What triggers a complaint? What happens after a complaint to the trust and the relationship and how do patients reflect on their experience with making a complaint in retrospect?

I interviewed 22 patients. In one case, the wife of the patient responded, as her husband had almost no recollection of the events. In another case, I interviewed both the patient and his wife, as the patient, due to his condition at the time of the incident and thereafter, could not recall many of the events.

3.5.1   Trust – why does it matter?

Practitioners mentioned a range of reasons why, from their perspective, patients' trust in them as clinicians mattered, mirroring findings in the literature (Krupat et al., 2001; Lee & Lin, 2009; Macintosh, 2007; Trachtenberg et al., 2005). The practitioners mostly spoke about the benefits of patient trust in general terms rather than with reference to specific cases.

In contrast, few patients spoke directly about why trust mattered to them, but inferred it in statements they made in relation to the particular experience they had. Notably, patients spoke about trust rarely when describing their relationship with the practitioner before the incident. This might underpin the assumption that trust is not consciously on their mind and is implicit in their decision-making until the point in time when it is challenged through an incident that signifies a mismatch between what the patient expected and what actually happened. Patient expectations may be influenced by what the practitioner promised or was hoping to achieve with the proposed treatment or care, but expectations may also be influenced by other sources of information and how the patient selects and interprets information both from the practitioner and other sources.

3.5.1.1 Patients who trust give benefit of the doubt

Trusting their practitioner appeared to matter for some patients when something unexpected happened in their care or treatment. This was often immediately after an incident, when patients were unsure about what had happened, and why, and at the same time talked about what they thought possible explanations and reasons could be. Where patients trusted their practitioner, they believed that there must be a reason for the incident. Trust in these situations often led them to suspend judgement and give the practitioner an opportunity to provide an explanation.

For example, one patient who underwent breast reduction surgery had insisted on a particular size of her breasts post-surgery. Her surgeon had assured her several times before the surgery that she would achieve the wanted outcome. The woman went into the surgery with the expectation that her wish had been fully understood and been confirmed by the surgeon.

> *The next day when I woke up … it felt very, very strange … The question did come to me [that] it feels really, really flat. This feels really flat. But I was still in the zone of trusting the surgeon and thinking, 'well, maybe tissues settle; maybe fat deposits; maybe there is a specific bra that she wanted me to wear and by putting that on in a couple of days that would help form the shape.' So I was suspending my disbelief about the process, because I think, ultimately, I was still trusting the surgeon. (Patient 13)*

The example shows that although the patient had doubts about the outcome of the surgery, because she trusted her surgeon, she assumed that there must be an explanation for the result and reserved her judgement at that stage.

In summary, when patients spoke about why trust mattered to them it primarily related to the particular incident or situation. Immediately after the incident is a critical point in the patient-doctor relationship, as it is the moment in which trust is usually being questioned and the patient tries to rationalise why they should continue to trust the practitioner. As seen below, it is also the moment in which patients very commonly feel uncertain and anxious and begin to question their trust in a practitioner, depending on the practitioner's behaviour and actions.

3.5.2   Decision to see practitioner

As part of the interviews I asked patients how they found or decided to see a particular practitioner. The most common response, with nine patients stating this, was that the patient's general practitioner had referred them. Given that most patients also reported a high level of initial trust in the practitioner they were referred to, the trust the patient had in the judgement of their general practitioner may have contributed to the initial high level of trust in the practitioner they were referred to.

Five patients said that other people, including family members, friends, other patients, and in one case their dentist, had recommended the practitioner to them. Only three patients said that they did their own research, mostly via the internet, to find a practitioner. Notably, in all cases it had been a fall-back option to do their own research when either there were no available appointments with the initially referred to practitioner, or their waiting list was too long. In one case, the patient was so dissatisfied with the treatment and care she had received from specialists in her area, she looked for someone outside her region, as she suspected that most specialists in her region knew each other and of her case and as a result would not be willing to help her.

Overall, it appears that patients primarily relied on their general practitioner, followed by other trusted persons, to recommend a practitioner to them.

An interesting side theme emerged in relation to some of the patients who also sought treatment from alternative health providers. It appeared that these patients were more active in their decision-making and did their own research before seeing an alternative health practitioner rather than relying on the recommendation of other people or providers. In the following statement, the patient contrasts how differently she makes a decision to see a conventional medical practitioner compared to an alternative health practitioner.

> *[With] the conservative treatment, I generally don't look before-hand and I go and get the referral or see someone and that's that. On the kind of more alternative side, ... that's where I really want expertise. I want people who are the best of the best; who know what they are doing .... And then I research it, and I talk to people. ... What reputation have they got? Would people recommend [them]? I guess if I was not to do that, my confidence level wouldn't be so high. (Patient 05)*

Other deciding factors in the patient's decision to see a particular practitioner were image and reputation, as well as convenience and financial considerations. Where the problem for which the patient sought help was minor or routine, a small number of patients reported that despite not fully trusting a practitioner's competence or not feeling cared for, they consulted that practitioner, because their practice was conveniently located, or because there were no additional expenses. The following statement describes this scenario and the patient's reasoning:

She is enough to have a basic knowledge as long as I keep my eyes and ears open. I guess, this probably seems a bit strange why to keep going – she is close by and also she isn't an expensive GP, the clinic isn't expensive. It used to be bulk-billed when I used to go with my daughter, so I didn't pay a cent. (Patient 05)

The patient implies that her relationship with this particular practitioner is different to most other relationships patients have with practitioners, implying that ultimately it is the practitioner who is responsible for the quality of treatment. Here, it is the patient who feels in control, but who also takes responsibility for the quality of the health service provided. This particular patient is medically trained although not working as a health practitioner and this may explain the confidence in being able to evaluate the competence of a practitioner.

The following quote comes from a patient who also has an in-depth medical understanding and knowledge although not being a health practitioner, and who described their relationship with their general practitioner along similar lines:

We have got this very crook GP in [our area] that we go to and he is pretty well useless. He has the worst bedside manners you could imagine and I actually use him. ... He bulk-bills. I know all my ailments. ... And I will go and say things like this to him: 'look, I need an x-ray; ... I need to get my cholesterol checked; I need a blood test'. And I tell him. He is not at all interested in anything about us. ... but we use him. We still use him occasionally to bulk-bill. (Patient 06)

When I asked both these patients whether they trusted these practitioners, both rated them low on the trust scale that I used during the interviews. This suggests that a lower level of trust in the practitioner had been mitigated by the patient having a greater sense of control over the relationship and its outcomes.

Where patients researched on their own which practitioner they should see, all used the internet as the main source of information. For all patients, the image and reputation conveyed over the internet played a role in their decision-making. One patient summarised how she looks for information and evaluates it.

The websites can really vary. They can look really poor and the person is very good, and the other way around. Still it is as with any business; if the website looks good you do think 'well, this person is probably quite organised; they know their stuff'. So, it definitely plays a role. Most important is what I can find out there. So it can look great and make them look as if they are fantastic and that their reputation is awesome, but if all I see are clichéd lines and a bit of background of the clinic or things like that, then that doesn't really help me very much in making my [decision]. (Patient 05)

The patient continues to describe how she evaluates information the practitioner has no control over, for example blogs, forums or websites of other organisations or publications.

I look at what types of positive things have been said and what types of negative things. ... partly what I am looking at is [is] this person pioneering? Is this person someone who really wants to keep up with everything that's going on; that is really passionate about 'I really want to crack these cases?' ... (Patient 05)

Notably, a negative opinion about a practitioner did not automatically mean that the patient perceived the practitioner negatively, if it is in a context of differing opinions and there may be valuable arguments supporting the practitioner's side. Where the overall perception is that of an innovative and passionate practitioner, the patient may still decide to consult this practitioner. That same patient also clarified what information indicates a competent and trustworthy practitioner to her:

> *Again, if I see a few different sources with their name on it, …*
> *there might be a conference in America … or it might be an article*
> *they have written, a published article [in a medical journal] or just*
> *magazine style, I see that favourably. Seeing them doing things in*
> *different places; seeing them mentioned by other practitioners as*
> *well, although that in itself isn't the most important. (Patient 05)*

Similar to the patient relying on their general practitioner making a judgement as to the competence of a practitioner, this patient relied on peer opinion to assist her decision-making. The difference is that the peer opinion is in the form of presentations at professional conferences, or peer reviewed publications in medical journals.

Overall, the majority of patients were relatively passive in their decision-making about seeing a particular practitioner. Many relied on the professional judgement of other health practitioners regarding the competence and skills of a particular doctor they had not seen before.

3.5.3   First impressions

First impressions are often based on a mix of factors, and can influence the patient's decision making, which often is not rationalised at the time.

> *I think that you know straight away when you meet someone*
> *whether he is going to be good or not really good. I think it is*
> *straight away that you have that feeling. (Patient 08)*

First impressions appeared to matter in shaping the trust levels patients had when they first met the practitioner they later complained about. However, as the interviews took place at the end of the complaint process, the first impression as described by the patients appeared sometimes coloured by the later experiences the patient had in an attempt to make the first impression fit in with the rest of the patient's journey.

In general, where patients described a positive first impression, they also reported a high level of trust in the practitioner. In contrast, where patients had had a bad first impression of the practitioner, they reported a low level of trust at their initial encounter with the practitioner.

3.5.3.1 Negative first impression

Of the patients who reported a negative first impression, all described the practitioner as not being able or willing to help them with their health problem. Their expectation to see the practitioner for help had not been met and had an immediate impact on their perception of the practitioner, as the following example demonstrates:

> *[H]is first comment was, 'ah, sleeping problems are very hard to deal with. [It is] very hard to fix those problems.' … I [had] never met him before. I didn't have a warm and friendly feeling. … I simply went to see this guy without any expectations apart from getting a letter of referral …. (Patient 14)*

The practitioner's comment that her condition was difficult to deal with was interpreted by the patient as the practitioner not being willing to help her. Patients perceived practitioners who dismissed their health problem as being rude, cold, uncaring, disrespectful or incompetent.

> *I've seen him and tried to show my right arm, which is broken and he didn't even look. He was very rude … He was just looking at me like I am a kind of bikie guy or criminal, because I have long hair; a couple of tattoos and I look like a bikie …. (Patient 15)*

The statement shows that this patient tried to make sense of the perceived dismissive behaviour of the practitioner by implying that he was prejudged on the basis of his appearance.

One patient described their negative first impression being shaped by the lack of communication from the doctor.

I just gave him the letter and he got me up on the chair with my knees up so that he could check the back of my leg, or feet, or whatever he was doing. He didn't say very much at all. ... [H]e didn't actually say anything [about complications] to me. He was talking into his recording thing. [He was] mainly talking to that instead of talking to me. ... I thought he was quite rude. Another patient that I know that was in hospital with me, she thought that he was quite rude, too, when she had seen him. And she had complications after the operation as well. (Patient 20)

The patient did not receive the information they wanted, but apparently did not ask the practitioner during the consultation. The lack of direct communication with the patient was made worse by the practitioner dictating his findings into the recording machine, presumably using medical terminology that could not be fully understood by the patient. In short, the patient felt that the practitioner was disrespectful and made her feel like an object. Notably, the patient spoke about their impression with another patient and felt confirmed in her opinion. The patient inferred that the poor communication was linked to a poor treatment outcome experienced by the other patient, which again validated her own experience.

3.5.3.2 Positive first impression

The vast majority of patients reported having a positive first impression of their practitioner. This coincides with the vast majority having a high level of trust initially in their practitioner. Patients referred to different aspects of their interaction with the practitioner that contributed to their impression.

One patient described their practitioner as being:

Very professional, very easy to talk to. I was very pleased with his attitude in those days. (Patient 11)

It seems a mixture of perceived expertise and responsive communication contributed to the patient's good first impression.

The way the first impression was retrospectively described during the interviews was often coloured by reflecting on the whole experience. For example, the patient feeling initially assured by the practitioner's confidence and expertise after the incident, the patient reinterpreted their first impression of the practitioner as the practitioner being 'overly confident'. On several occasions, patients looked back to an earlier interaction and in hindsight offered an alternative interpretation of what had happened that was more in line with the final outcome.

> *Overly confident, very, very, very confident, overly confident, because I spoke to him about getting a second and third opinion and he insisted not to see anybody; that he was the god of head and neck. … At that point, I felt [that he was] 100% trustworthy, because basically he said that he was the god of this. I didn't think to question it any further. … And my doctor – my GP – … goes: 'don't worry, you will be in great hands'. (Patient 07)*

In the above example, the surgeon's display of confidence translated directly into their trustworthiness as perceived by the patient. The patient acknowledges that their impression was influenced by both their own lack of knowledge in the area as well as the positive comment from their general practitioner. Another patient described her first encounter with a surgeon along similar lines:

> *[M]y GP had referred me to [the surgeon], and after discussion, he paraded this wonderful hip in front of me – … 'and you get 30 years out of it'. … and I thought: '30 years – this is going to be great'. … I thought he was a god …. Confident. He said 'these hips are new, look at my design on the wall, I have all these awards. This would be the hip for you.' I trust a doctor. My GP has never let me down. (Patient 02)*

Both patients mention the role their general practitioner's opinion played in shaping their first impression. Both patients said that they trusted their general practitioner or their judgement and that this contributed to the patient perceiving the specialist they were referred to as trustworthy. Both statements also imply that the expertise and technical skills were the most important factors for the patient to trust their practitioner after the first encounter.

Some patients mentioned seeking information about the practitioner on the internet before their first consultation. Again, the perception of professional expertise appeared to be the most important aspect of how they interpreted the information they found.

> *[E]specially, I looked on the internet at his profile, when he did his study and for how long. (Patient 19)*

Patients named the place and field of study and training as a factor in assessing a practitioner's expertise, but also mentioned the influence of where the practitioner works, their patient base, academic publications, communication style and caring attitude. One patient said about their first impression:

> *It was very positive. In the city that I live in … usually the specialists have offices and waiting rooms in small old houses. His was a modern, white building – large, with his name across in very modern words – his name and 'surgeon'. I walked in and it was a beautifully appointed, positive image of great success. His demeanour was very gentle, very caring. I had to wait three and a half hours in the waiting room to see him, but when I did get in to see him he didn't rush; he apologised for me waiting and explained about the operation. (Patient 04)*

The patient was impressed by the professional and modern appearance of the practitioner's practice, which conferred the image of the surgeon as being professional and modern. The long wait was not perceived as negative given that the patient felt that the practitioner took time during her consultation to explain the treatment and to respond to her questions. Some patients appeared to be willing to overlook or accept less positive aspects about their consultation, if they felt that overall the practitioner responded to them and their needs. Particularly, a caring attitude of the practitioner together with perceived professionalism had a positive influence on the patient's first impression.

> *He seems to be very nice. He seems to be very thorough. He is an elderly man. I was quite impressed with him …. He said, 'I want you to go and have a blood test, and let's see whether you need that.' He seemed to be quite professional.*
> *(Patient 18)*

The practitioner's explanation to await the outcome of the test before reaching a conclusion about the treatment and whether it was necessary was perceived as professional by the patient.

In summary, patients' first impressions appeared to matter in their evaluation of the practitioner's expertise and were linked to the level of trust patients reported at the first encounter. Patients described perceived expertise, professional surroundings, good communication skills and a caring attitude as contributing factors to feeling confident in the practitioner and believing that the practitioner was trustworthy.

Before I continue to look more closely at the three areas – communication, competence and care – and how they contribute to the establishment or re-building of patients' trust in their practitioner, or are linked to the decrease and loss of trust, I would like to examine the emotions patients associated with their experience in general, and in relation to trust in particular.

3.5.4   Emotions

When coding the transcripts of the patient interviews I classified explicit and implicit expression of emotions. In total, I distinguished 94 different emotions, of which 85 categories were coded in patient interviews at least once. When correlating the chronology of the patients' experiences with all emotions, over-all patients described or expressed emotions most commonly when talking about the period immediately after the incident to the end of the relationship with the practitioner or the end of the complaint.

3.5.4.1 Emotions – ungrouped

Using all categories of emotions, overall the most common emotions patients described in order of their frequency were:

1. being dissatisfied and disappointed;
2. feeling not understood by the practitioner;
3. perceiving the practitioner as being unhelpful, unresponsive, or un-supportive; and
4. being distressed and upset.

Contrasting this with what practitioners believed patients had felt shows that practitioners also placed the patient feeling disappointed and dissatisfied at the top of their list, but perceived patients to be more commonly angry and antagonistic and blaming the practitioner than patients actually expressed during the interviews.

3.5.4.2 Emotions by timeline

Emotions that patients described were most common in relation to the period after the incident, but before the complaint was made. Often this coincided with the patient fully becoming aware that there has been an incident and trying to come to terms with it. In this period, patients commonly tried to seek information or tried to make the practitioner or someone aware that they believe something had gone wrong. During this period, the most common emotions patients referred to were:

1. perceiving the practitioner as being unhelpful, unresponsive, or un-supportive;

2. feeling not understood by the practitioner;
3. feeling abandoned; and
4. experiencing pain.

These results mirror the themes that emerged as complaint triggers, which I will discuss below in this chapter. The result also shows that for those patients who experienced physical pain after the incident, it influenced their perception of the practitioner and situation.

In contrast, patients' emotions of disappointment and dissatisfaction most commonly related to the time where the relationship with the practitioner ended, which may have been at the time they lodged a complaint or at the end of the complaint process. This may be an indication that the lack of support and the lack of responsiveness to the patient's needs after the incident turned into disappointment.

3.5.4.3 Grouping related emotions

In a second round of analysis, I grouped related emotions and a slightly different picture emerged. The most common groups of emotions expressed by the 22 patients overall and the number of codings related to them are shown in Table 3.2.

Table 3.2   *Most common emotions coded in patient interviews*
              overall (grouped)

Merged categories of emotions*	No. of codings
unhelpful, unsupportive, unresponsive & not understood	173
doubt & surprise, unexpected & not confident & uncertainty, risky & fear, anxiety	118
concerned & worried & critical	111
dissatisfied, disappointed	86
distressed-upset	78
Pain	76
aggressive & confrontational & angry, antagonistic	71
absent & isolated, alone & abandoned	69
annoyed & frustrated	66
happy & satisfied & grateful	65
understanding, empathetic & helpful, supportive, responsive	61
other emotions	652
Total	**1,626**

'&' indicates the merging of different categories of emotions.

Notably, when merging the category of 'unhelpful, unsupportive, unre-sponsive' with the category of 'not understood', it becomes the group of emo-tions that patients most commonly referred to in the interviews – I will refer to it as 'unresponsiveness'. The second most common group of emotions I sum-marised under 'uncertainty' – it contains the categories of 'surprise, unex-pected, uncertainty, risk, fear, anxiety, doubt, not being confident'. This group of emotions was closely followed by a group I refer to as 'concerned' which includes 'being concerned, worried or critical'.

In summary, many patients after the incident felt left alone, uncertain and concerned. It appears that a high level of trust at that point in time could be instrumental in mitigating these emotions. Therefore, I looked separately at the correlations between emotions and trust, which I summarise in the next section.

3.5.4.4 Patient trust and emotions

I was interested in emotions patients associated with certain dynamics of trust. Therefore, I correlated the emotions coded in patient interviews with the coding for trust categories. Most commonly, patients associated trust decreasing factors and the effects of decreasing trust with emotions of:

- perceiving the practitioner to be dishonest;
- being angry or antagonistic towards the practitioner; and
- being distressed, or upset.

Where patients referred to a residual feeing of distrusting the practitioner, in addition to the emotions above, they commonly blamed the practitioner.

In contrast, patients most commonly associated trust increasing factors and the effects of trust with the emotions of:

- being happy;
- being satisfied; and
- perceiving the practitioner to be helpful, supportive, and responsive.

In the next step, I will examine whether these results correspond to themes that emerged from the patient interviews in relation to both trust building and the decrease of trust in their practitioner.

3.5.5 Trust building elements – the patient's view

In this section, I look at factors relating to communication, competence and care that patients associated with the trustworthiness of a practitioner. Patients referred both to their experience with the particular practitioner they complained about, as well as to experiences with other practitioners.

3.5.5.1 Communication

Communication, as care, is an area on the interaction with practitioners that patients can directly evaluate, which differs from forming an opinion about the competence of a practitioner. The criteria for what is considered good communication do not differ much from interactions with people in other areas of the patient's life.

↑
Communication
Competence
Care

Explaining

The most commonly mentioned quality of the practitioner communication that was positively noted by patients was giving explanations. Patients want to understand. They want to understand their diagnosis, the treatment and more importantly, when something goes wrong, they want to understand the reasons. In the following statement, the patient contrasts how they experienced the communication about the incident they had with their general practitioner on the one hand and with the specialist on the other.

> *My GP, he is wonderful. He would just go into everything with me. He will even go into the internet with me and show me examples – he went into the internet and explained everything to me, explained what had happened to me. And he spent a long time doing that, even though he sees up to 70 people a day! And this guy, this surgeon, was seeing me as if he didn't have to bother, because he did look after himself and he didn't want to be sued. (Patient 04)*

The lack of explanation from the surgeon, under whose care the incident happened, was interpreted negatively by the patient, while the detailed explanation the general practitioner offered was directly linked to a positive perception of the practitioner.

Several patients described practitioners who spend time explaining to the patient the reasons for their diagnosis or treatment advice as caring.

> *I am happy with him. He is an Asian doctor and he is so, so caring. It doesn't matter how long he spends with you and he just describes everything. So [I am] very happy there. (Patient 11)*

Offering explanations was not only perceived as caring, but was explicitly linked with the patient being satisfied with the practitioner. One patient said that the reason she would rate her trust in her practitioner as high as 9 out of 10 was due to the practitioner answering her questions and offering explanations tailored to the patient's circumstances.

> *I put her there, because she answered my questions. ... She came across as really negotiable. We were talking quite specifically about the way my body is. (Patient 13)*

Assurance

Another communication-related aspect that emerged as a theme in the patient interviews was how verbal communication is supported by other means, for example brochures, or the internet. One patient noted that brochures on the practitioner's desk about his area of expertise, together with the verbal explanation and assurances given by the practitioner, made her feel very secure and confident.

> *One thing that also gave me a very positive, secure feeling was that he had a pile of papers that had the digestive system printed [on them]. And he explained where he would make incisions. And then he said that there is one problem; there is one difficulty with this operation: that there could be a nick in one of the other organs. 'But that won't happen, because I am doing it.', was exactly what he said.*
> *(Patient 04)*

The practitioner backed up his verbal information to the patient with written material from a different source, indicating consistency beyond the practitioner's personal and professional opinion. In this case, when the practitioner mentioned possible complications, but at the same time assured the patient that it would not happen under his care, it was perceived by the patient as a sign of a high level of competence.

Honesty and transparency

In general, patients greatly valued a practitioner's honesty.

> *[W]hen you asked a question [he] doesn't hesitate to give you the most honest answer, because he knows the truth. … He is one in a million, he tells the truth. (Patient 02)*

Even where this meant that practitioners were honest about limitations in their expertise, this was viewed positively overall.

> *But this guy was a fantastic guy. … he was great, because, if he didn't know something, he went on to say 'I will look it up'. And I think people just want honesty, that's all they want. (Patient 06)*

However, if the practitioner was honest about the limits in their skill or knowledge, there was a related small decrease in the reported level of trust.

> *Probably about 7, because he said that not a lot of people know about haemacromatosis and he was actually looking it up; reading about it. And he said that he wasn't 100% sure about it. That might be a bit of a worry. But he said, 'well, we'll get your iron tested and blood.' So on the first visit, I found him very thoughtful and very professional. (Patient 18)*

Where the treatment outcome eventually was positive, patients interpreted the openness about limitations as carefulness and evaluated it positively. There were no examples in the interviews where a practitioner openly discussed limits in their expertise at the outset and the patient later suffered a poor outcome. However, it may be possible that in such cases the patient might in retrospect perceive the earlier disclosure of the practitioner as a warning sign of the poor outcome they eventually suffered. However, this theme was not present in the interviews.

A number of patients mentioned that they wished the practitioner would have been honest with them about the incident and just told them what had happened. This point will be revisited below when I look at aspects of communication that contributed to the decrease and loss of patient trust.

3.5.5.2 Competence

Competence and the feeling that the practitioner is able to help the patient with their health problem were closely associated with patient trust and confidence. When patients perceived the practitioner to be competent, they ignored or accepted flaws in the practitioner's communication and care.

Communication
Competence
Care

> *I wouldn't even care too much if their bedside manner wasn't good provided they were up to date and they had a decent knowledge. I am pretty accepting of a lot of things. (Patient 06)*

Asked what first comes to their mind when asked what makes a patient trust a doctor, one patient responded:

That they have adequately researched their decision. So if they say 'you have xyz', that they can say 'because that test result was that; and in your medical history you had that, because of..., and therefore I think you have got that'. Trust – I think that I can see that they are active members of the medical world in various forms, not just, for example, only with pharmaceutical companies. That they are out there; that they are schooling themselves; keeping up with things; they go to the right places; and actually the third thing is broad knowledge, ... if I notice that a doctor is able to talk on this topic, but also on that topic, and that is related to that, then my trust definitely goes up a lot, because I think 'oh, here is someone who is switched on.' (Patient 05)

The answer reveals several areas that the patient names as indicators of the competence of a practitioner. A trustworthy practitioner according to this patient supports their diagnosis and treatment proposal with evidence and is able to explain their reasoning to the patient. In addition, practitioners who are active and independent members of the medical profession, who stay up to date with progress in their field and who are able to consider and treat the patient and their condition holistically, were perceived as competent and trustworthy.

Reputation

When patients evaluate the competence of a practitioner, the opinion of other practitioners is a common source of information to them. As described above in the section on first impressions, the opinion of a patient's trusted and often long-term general practitioner plays an important role when patients form an opinion about the competence of another practitioner. Similarly, when seeking information from other sources, such as the internet, patients appear to value a good reputation of a practitioner among their peers.

[If] I see a few different sources with their name on it, ... there might be a conference in America and they might have been there; or ... a published article [in a medical journal] or just magazine style, I see that favourably. Seeing them doing things in different places; seeing them mentioned by other practitioners as well, although that in itself isn't the most important. (Patient 05)

The statement suggests that although professional standing and a good reputation among peers is an important indication of a practitioner's competence for patients, it may not be the only source of information patients use to form an opinion.

Overall, it is difficult for patients to directly evaluate the competence of a practitioner at the beginning of the relationship. Patients rely on other sources to form an opinion, foremost including the opinion of other practitioners, other patients, or information found in public sources, including the internet.

An aspect that patients found easier to directly evaluate is care, which I will look at next.

3.5.5.3 Care

Being empathetic and concerned for the patient's well-being

Communication

Competence

Care

Most patients volunteered during the interview that it is important to them to be treated by a caring practitioner. There were differences in what patients considered expressions of care, but overall, it was seen as an essential part of the patient-practitioner relationship.

One patient described why he perceived a practitioner as caring:

[H]e was very good. He told me; he touched me. Sometimes, you go to the doctors and the doctors don't even want to know you. What do you have?' – 'A cough.' – 'Ok, just take this.' And that's it. But I was concerned, because the pain was hurtful. And he was concerned as well, because he said [that] he touched a lump. So he sent me to have all these things [tested]. (Patient 08)

The patient compares his perception in this case with other experiences where he felt his health concerns were not taken seriously by the practitioner. The practitioner referred to here was considered caring because he showed an interest, he acknowledged the patient's concern and responded to it by investigating the possible reasons for the pain the patient experienced. The same patient later in the interview spoke about his current general practitioner in whom he had the highest level of trust, by explaining:

He goes that extra mile for you. If you need something extra to be checked up, it is not 'just sign here and go', no, he would do it. If you need him at home, he'd come. He works Sundays! So he is always there when you need him. (Patient 08)

The statement shows the link between care and trust. The last sentence in particular sums up what patients expect of a caring practitioner – they are there when you need them and look after their patients. This particular patient reiterated this point several times throughout the interview:

I go to the doctor thinking that he is going to try to fix me. ... I want to have tests done. I am not the one that should tell him that. He should tell me, 'look, we are going to do this, that and that.' Then I'll probably feel comfortable with the doctor, because he is interested. He is interested in my health. Not someone who says to me, 'no, there is nothing wrong with you.' (Patient 08)

The statement illustrates that the patient not only expected the practitioner to respond to their needs, but also to be proactive, empathetic and feel responsible for them. When he first consulted this particular general practitioner, the practitioner said:

> *'yes, I will look after you. Don't worry about it'.*

> *So he fixes everything. He fixes it with the specialist and everything I have to do, I go and see him. He has got all my records and everything. (Patient 08)*

The patient noted that the practitioner's caring attitude was re-assuring and that he no longer questioned whether he had received the right advice or whether he should see another specialist, as he felt that this practitioner felt responsible and used their professional judgement in the patient's best interest.

Respecting the patient

The following description of a caring practitioner combines several elements of the reason the patient perceived their practitioner to be caring. The practitioner took time, listened, was interested and was open to alternatives, all of which showed respect for the patient.

> *We are very impressed with her. She cares; she does hour appointments when she first meets you; she doesn't rush you; she genuinely cares; she is open to listen to the alternatives and the medicines I was on – well, the so called natural products I was on. She immediately looked it up on the internet. She said 'look, I am interested in that too.' She checked it; she read it. That's the sort of person you want: someone who doesn't look like they are after the money even if they might be, they shouldn't be showing it – not to a patient. (Patient 06)*

Friendliness was another aspect of showing respect to a patient:

> [A] friendly face and a smile doesn't hurt. I like to smile; I like to
> laugh; I like to do jokes and I like to see a doctor [with] a bit [of a]
> smiley face. ... That is important, yes. It is not a big deal to give a
> smile. (Patient 15)

Connecting on a personal level, long term

When practitioners related to their patients beyond the immediate health problem, some perceived this as a sign that the practitioner cared about them:

> [S]he had known me for years, from when my kids were babies.
> {She] has seen me as a human being. (Patient 07)

The comment that the patient felt treated as a human being, as opposed to solely as a patient whose immediate health problem needed to be addressed in a consultation, suggests a wider connection between the practitioner and patient beyond their medical problems. In this case, the practitioner had listened to the patient telling them about the incident and the impact it had on the patient and her family. Although not involved in the patient care at the time of the incident, the practitioner had re-assured the patient that what she had experienced was not right and that she would support her should she consider making a complaint. The patient later expressed the view that she trusted the practitioner, partly because she was interested in her as a person.

3.5.5.4 Summary: Trust building elements – communication, competence and care

Overall, patients described elements in their relationship with the practitioners associated with developing and maintaining trust in the practitioner that relate to communication, competence and care. In contrast to the practitioners' interviews, where competence related aspects were most commonly referred to, patients more often spoke about communication and care-related aspects.

These areas are easier to evaluate directly for patients and the standards expected of practitioners in regard to communication and care are comparable to other professional services or interactions.

Overall, the patient interviews included less evidence of trust enhancing themes, but more relating to the decrease and loss of trust. This may be the result of the sample consisting of only patients that ultimately made a formal complaint about the practitioner, indicating a loss in trust.

The following section summarises aspects of communication, competence and care that patients associated with the loss of trust.

3.5.6   Trust decreasing factors – communication, competence and care

3.5.6.1 Communication

While patients emphasised good communication skills in building trust and rapport with a
practitioner, communication related issues also
played a great part when patients talked about
the deterioration of their relationship with the
practitioner and the associated loss of trust.

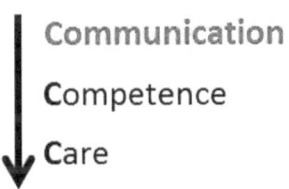

Communication

Competence

Care

Lack of communication

A common theme among patients was the lack of communication with the practitioner immediately after the incident. This may indicate that patients expected the practitioner to proactively approach them when there was a problem. One patient commented on the practitioner's lack of communication after the incident, saying:

> *I wouldn't have lost confidence in him. Because, like I said, initially*
> *he was very, very good. He took an interest; seemed to take an in-*
> *terest in me. (Patient 01)*

The majority of patients I interviewed described having no or very limited contact with the doctor after the incident. Commonly patients said that the practitioner avoided seeing them, ceased communicating or became defensive towards them. Patients on the other hand expressed feeling let down, confused and sometimes abandoned by their practitioner immediately after the incident. Referring to that point in time, only few patients expressed anger. Where patients reported becoming angry, this developed later and was mainly due to the behaviour of the practitioner rather than the actual incident.

Inadequate communication

Patients not only described a lack of communication and the practitioner withdrawing from their care after incidents, but also situations in general, not related to incidents, where the practitioner's inadequate communication with the patient was associated with a loss in confidence and patient trust. One patient said:

> *If that doctor speaks less English than you and you try to explain*
> *what your problem is, and he is trying to [understand], or ... is*
> *looking at the computer – not listening to you; because if you are*
> *talking to someone, you [should be] listening to this person. But*
> *sometimes you talk to the doctor and the doctor is [distracted]*
> *just there, typing or he is not even aware that you are talking to*
> *him. (Patient 08)*

Inadequate communication made some patients feel not understood, not respected or taken seriously and had a notable impact on the patient's trust and confidence levels.

Wrong information

Patients viewed more seriously situations where they felt the practitioner had misled them. In contrast to inadequate communication described above, which may have been unintentional, giving wrong information was perceived as a deliberate act. Dishonesty was strongly associated with a loss of trust and a deterioration of the relationship with the practitioner.

> *[W]hen you query it and then again you are given the wrong information, I mean maybe he should have said, '[perhaps] take half a tablet, in case one is too strong'. But instead he said, 'no, no, just take [one tablet].' He was 100% sure. (Patient 14)*

In the example above, the wrong information was queried by the patient but confirmed as correct by the practitioner several times. When it eventually turned out to be wrong, the patient completely lost trust in the competence of that particular practitioner. Similarly, a patient who underwent breast reduction was devastated after the end result of her operation was considerably different from what she had expected despite the surgeon assuring her several times before the operation she would achieve a particular size.

> *So, I was a small C cup [size] and that was pretty devastating. ... I was a C cup [size], exactly what I didn't want – having expressed that to this surgeon; having said 'will you make me a DD [size]?', she had said 'yes'. (Patient 13)*

Patients may reserve judgement about a practitioner until they have confirmed through other sources that they were given the wrong information.

> *He was conflicting himself while he was talking; he was giving me conflicting information. He was insensitive and matter of fact, but he was giving facts that were incorrect. So I was confused. I didn't have an opinion yet. (Patient 17)*

The moment patients became aware that they were given the wrong information was commonly associated with a feeling of shock and disbelief.

> *That's what he said 'inflammation after the operation. It is just inflammation after the operation; your mouth will go back [to being] fine within two weeks.' That was his exact words. … Well two weeks [later]; I went back. He was gone. … [T]he intern goes, '… your nerve has been damaged, cut, damaged'. And I went 'what?'* (Patient 07)

Denial and defensiveness

Closely associated with patients perceiving their practitioner to be misleading or dishonest were the descriptions of situations where the practitioner denied taking responsibility for the incident. As the following quote illustrates, a practitioner expressly denied any wrongdoing and that became the trigger for the patient to make a complaint to the Health Care Complaints Commission.

> *He denied it all. He went on saying, 'she must have mis-heard; I would never have said that; no way would I offend her.' But I have a witness; my husband was there. He was sitting right next to me. [He also said], 'I am very up-skilled in that area and she is not an expert.' I know what I was told; I know what I heard. But at the end of the day, he just denied it. … And because he refused to respond, I had to take it to a body that would listen. And he just denied it all.* (Patient 17)

In the above statement, the practitioner not only denied having given the wrong information to the patient, but in attempting to defend his actions, insulted the patient when referring to her lack of knowledge in that area. The practitioner's blanket denial together with a defensive attitude became the trigger for the patient to lodge a complaint.

The next example is related in that the practitioner denied any wrongdoing and in defending himself by blaming the patient for being overactive after a hip-replacement surgery and thus causing problems with the recovery. However, the practitioner – here referred to as Dr One – did not clearly inform the patient which movements and exercises could adversely impact on her recovery and cause her hip to become loose. The patient eventually consulted another surgeon and subsequently underwent replacement hip surgery. She compared her experience:

> I wasn't allowed to do 30 laps in the pool with the margron hips in. This is my question to the Health Care Complaints Commission: why under Dr Two and with these new hips can I swim 10km, if I wanted to, yet I am manic and overactive with the margrons after 30 laps and a 10 minute walk. Why? What's the difference?

> Patient's husband: Dr One wouldn't give us an answer … so [the patient] would always live in fear [at] what had caused the hips coming loose. At least when we saw the new doctor, he told us straight away …. (Patient 02)

The quote illustrates again that the patient alleged that the first surgeon not only denied any responsibility for the issues she had, but insulted her by referring to her as manic.

Overall, where patients reported a lack of or inadequate communication after an incident, or where they believed the practitioner had deliberately lied to them, or displayed a defensive attitude, it had a significant negative impact on their trust levels.

3.5.6.2 Competence

Patients commonly associated poor treatment outcomes with their perception that the practitioner lacked competence by implying or expressly stating that it was the practitioner's fault that the incident occurred.

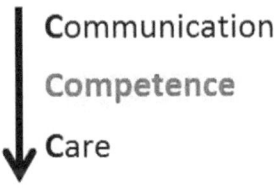

Communication

Competence

Care

Perceived lack of competence

Some patients who underwent surgery and suffered poor outcomes or side effects referred to the practitioner as a 'butcher', implying roughness and lacking the skills required by a medical practitioner. One patient said:

> The fourth [risk] might have been the scarring. He did mention that, but I didn't know that it would be so ugly and bad scarring, because I have seen other people's scars – this is a butcher's job. I had a butcher on my neck, not a surgeon.
> (Patient 07)

Comparing what had happened with the experiences of other patients in similar situations, or with their own experience in the past, was a common mechanism patients used to evaluate the competence of the practitioner. The following two statements from the same patient illustrate this:

> I suffered so much pain, I wrote a letter to Dr A. I said, 'this is your diagnosis; this is the hospital's diagnosis. And you told me I'll be all right in two days and they said it is broken.' (Patient 15)

The patient compares the diagnosis by the practitioner with the diagnosis subsequently made at hospital. Later the same patient underpinned his view of the practitioner lacking competence by comparing his consultation with this doctor to similar consultations he had with other doctors in the past.

> I saw several doctors. I had about eight bike crashes … and I saw several doctors…. But this doctor was so unusual. You can tell, he doesn't care about the patient, because he didn't look at my x-rays. (Patient 15)

For the patient, the fact that the doctor did not properly examine the x-rays subsequently led to the wrong diagnosis. The patient perceived this as a lack of care, but also a lack of competence in dealing with the condition.

While often the impact of perceived lack of competence on trust was only implied, a number of patients directly expressed the view that the reason they no longer trusted the doctor was the perceived lack of skill or competence.

> *I don't trust her anymore because I feel that her training in modern technologies is not there anymore. (Patient 03)*

Even with safeguards in place, patients may not trust a practitioner where they believe that there are issues with the practitioner's competence, as the following statement illustrates:

> *I found out that he is actually still practising, but he has to have a supervisor standing right next to him all the time, which would scare the hell out of me, if I had to go into surgery and someone who has been practising here for 20 years and then suddenly has to have a supervisor. I would be scared as hell to have him operating on me to be quite honest. (Patient 12)*

This viewpoint is particularly relevant when determining appropriate measures to ensure public health and safety, while allowing practitioners to practise, in some cases subject to conditions.

Bad reputation

Where practitioners have gone through disciplinary proceedings and the outcomes are public, patients can access this information in NSW on the internet[18] and often it is reported by the local media.

---

[18]   Decisions are published on the websites of the Health Care Complaints Commission (http://www.hccc.nsw.gov.au), the Australasian Legal Information Institute (AUSTLII, http://www.austlii.edu.au), the Medical Council of New South Wales (http://www.mcnsw.org.au/), or of NSW Caselaw (http://www.caselaw.nsw.gov.au/).

> *I got a phone call from the physio and she had seen it in the local*
> *paper, and I went, 'what happened?' ... And she told me that [Dr*
> *A] had been struck off, since August this year, he is not allowed to*
> *practise and he had to go back and be completely retrained. That*
> *was on the front page of the paper. (Patient 12)*

However, only a small number of complaints will be prosecuted before a disciplinary body with the decisions being made public. In other cases, and more commonly, a practitioner may be judged informally by word of mouth and rumours and this can have a profound influence on the perception of patients.

> *Yes, word gets around. And as I said, people started talking, 'oh*
> *yes, I had trouble with [the doctor], too'. So he has a [bad] reputa-*
> *tion up here, ... if I had known that, I would not have gone to see*
> *him. Or I would have gone to [another city] or something like that*
> *to see another doctor. (Patient 12)*

Overall, the perceived or proven lack of competence or inappropriate conduct is a major factor in patients losing trust in a practitioner. The perception of incompetence may lead to people talking with others, subsequently, resulting in a negative reputation of the practitioner. In other cases, hearing of the negative reputation caused the patient to re-interpret their experience with a practitioner. Almost all patients reported talking about their negative experience with other people. This included family members, other practitioners, or in some instances, patients approached the media, or used the internet to discuss their experience.

3.5.6.3 Care

Communication

Competence

A caring practitioner was very important to patients to build trust. In contrast, where patients perceived that the practitioner did not care about them, they reported lower levels of trust.

Care

Patients expressed their understanding of a caring practitioner by describing different elements: mainly empathy, being responsive and understanding, and respecting the patient as a person with their own unique experiences and backgrounds. In contrast, lack of care was associated with a lack of empathy, lack of responsiveness and understanding, and the feeling of being a case rather than a person and human being.

Lack of empathy

A small number of patients reported that they did not have a personal connection with the practitioner and perceived them as being cold. While some considered this part of professional behaviour and did not mind, others stated that they did not wish to return to a practitioner who was cold towards them despite having a positive opinion about their skills and competence.

> *I went to see the head and neck specialist and I went three times and [he] is very cold. I think that he is a good doctor, because he has his wall full of things in America, in France, in England, but I found him very cold … But he diagnosed that I have cancer, so it is not that I don't trust him, but because he is working in conjunction with the oncologist that I trust, so I don't mind if he is a bit cold. … If I had to go to see him on his own, I would change; I would go to someone else. (Patient 08)*

The patient said that he did not trust the 'cold' practitioner by himself, but only saw this practitioner because he trusted his oncologist's judgement. This is an example of trust being built through recommendations by trusted others that appear to override the lack of direct connection between patient and practitioner.

Dismissing the patient's fears

Patient fears in health care settings are common. It is a foreign environment to most and often they feel vulnerable and a lack of control over what happens to them when seeking medical assistance. Particularly in hospital settings, patients can feel confused and at times anxious. Ignoring or dismissing these fears, particularly when they are voiced, had a negative impact on the patient's confidence in a practitioner.

> *She had no business being a doctor. ... I am not very good with needles. And she got the needle and jammed it into my hand like this. So hard, my hand just burst with blood, and she tried to get the needle out and my whole hand got sucked up ... Nobody was caring about me – the patient .... (Patient 07)*

In the above statement, the patient generalised her experience with this particular practitioner to say that 'nobody' was caring about her. The practitioner became a representative of the health system. The singular experience had an impact in a much broader context.

Overall, a number of patients commented that the lack of care was magnified through them being treated as a medical problem, rather than a person. Practitioner behaviour that was perceived as indifferent, dismissive or disrespectful contributed to the patient's loss of trust in a practitioner.

3.5.6.4 Summary: Elements that decrease trust

All patients described some elements of communication, competence and care they were disappointed with and that resulted in their loss of trust in the practitioner. Patients placed different emphasis on these aspects; for some the perceived lack of competence was the main reason they lost trust, while for others it was dishonest communication, and for others still it was the lack of care. However, in most cases, a combination of these factors contributed to the loss in trust.

3.5.7 Effects of distrust

Where a bad experience had resulted in the patient not only losing trust in a practitioner, but actually distrusting the practitioner, this had a significant effect on their ability to interact with that practitioner, be it in the form of accepting further treatment, or in being willing to speak with and listen to a practitioner after an incident. There was a notable difference between patients reporting low levels of trust or no trust, and a patient stating that they distrusted a practitioner, the latter being associated with more intense emotions.

In the following example, the patient, whose facial nerve was accidentally severed during surgery, compared the experience of being asked to return to the surgeon to manage the complications with being asked to return to the perpetrator of domestic violence. She implied that victims of domestic violence receive more support to safeguard them against further violence than patients in her situation.

> *Now, had he been my partner and done that to me, the police would have arrested him and charged him and put an AVO (apprehended violence order) on him. Why should I be forced to go to the person [who has] perpetrated and done this to me? A perpetrator of violence! This is violent what he had done. There is an element of violence in all of this. Why would I want to go back and see someone who damaged me so badly? Who would? I mean, if someone came up and slapped you and hurt you and you were then forced to go back and see them, how would you feel? Would you or anybody else be comfortable with that? No. Sorry, someone that hurts me, I don't want to see them. (Patient 07)*

The patient's words reflect her belief that the medical error was violence against her, which in turn implies that it had been deliberate. She also clearly states that she would not return to the practitioner whom she no longer trusts. As I will illustrate below in this chapter, the vast majority of patients who had lost trust in their practitioner would not return to the practitioner.

While I have outlined both factors associated with building trust as well as with decreasing patient trust, it becomes clear that the fact that an incident happened and patient trust after the incident dropped did not automatically trigger the patient's complaint. In the following section, I look at the patient's reported motivation to make a complaint.

3.5.8   Making a complaint

A mismatch between what patients expected of the communication, competence or care of the practitioner and the actual behaviour or outcome they experienced was commonly associated with a reported decrease in the level of trust patients had in their practitioner. Immediately after the incident, most patients did not consider making a complaint, but tried to understand what had happened and why. Often it was the practitioner's lack of explanation, or withdrawal, that became the actual trigger for the complaint.

In one of the interviews, the patient recalled her communication with the practitioner after the incident like a dialogue. The incident was that her facial nerve had accidentally been severed during surgery. The recalled dialogue shows how the relationship between patient and practitioner deteriorated during their meeting and illustrates that the reason for the patient making her complaint was not the incident, but how she was treated by the practitioner afterwards.

> So anyway, 2 ½ months [later], ... we got hold of [the surgeon]. ... Everybody was [angry], because there were no answers ... and I was left like a mess. I was left torn apart. I was left looking like a monster. My friends weren't used to it; my family wasn't used to it and nobody was getting used to it – especially me.
>
> We were sitting; he was talking, and the question that I had asked him, which [my old GP] had told me to ask, 'who had actually done the surgery? Did the intern touch me at all?'
>
> He said, no, he'd just done some cutting from the outside, which explains the mess of this scar. And he goes, 'anything else?'

And I ask, 'what happened to my nerve?'

'It got damaged.'

And then [my friend] jumped in: 'Exactly what happened to her nerve? What did you do to her face? What did you do?'

And he looked at her and said, 'all right, I cut the nerve.'

And she goes, 'you cut the nerve. Why did you cut her nerve?'

He goes, 'I severed the nerve.'

And she goes, 'why?'

He goes, 'I accidentally cut the wrong nerve.'

And I went ...ah ... I was like ...ah ... I was in the twilight zone by this point. ... I think at the time ... – I felt relieved on one hand to know what was the problem, and I was angry on the other had that such a great king of surgery had stuffed [it] up. How did he do this?

My next question to him after this was, 'how did you stuff this up?' I was looking for excuses. 'Weren't you wearing special doctor's binoculars during surgery?'

'No.', he said, 'I don't need them.'

That's when I looked at him. He was cocky enough to say that to me. And I looked at him, 'you didn't wear your binoculars, yet you are working with people's veins, nerves – people's nerves! And you are not wearing binoculars?'

'No.'

I said, 'look, I am about 38. You are about 55-60 or something and you have confidence in your eyes like that? I wouldn't have this confidence in my eyes.'

'Because you are not a doctor!'

'I don't need to be a doctor. What does [being] a doctor mean? You just get a higher salary, that's all. I am not seeing any doctor in here; I am seeing a lot of butchering.'

And he looked at me.

I said to him, 'tell me specifically, what you have cut; how much damage have you done? I want to know. It is my neck.'

And he looked at me.

And I said, 'it is my right; it is my body. You tell me!'

He didn't want to say.

And [my friend] was going, 'you tell her!'

He went 'right', and then he explained it ….

I just went back, 'how did you make this mistake and you didn't tell me? How could you not tell me that you had done this? Don't I have a right?'

'You are a public patient. You don't have a right.'

That's what he said. You are a public patient; you don't have a right. I was amazed at that point. I thought, 'right, so I just should kill myself now and get it over with?'

'Well, you are not young', he said.

And I said, 'oh, ok, anything more? I just go and kill myself and make you happy now?'

'I don't care what you do', he said.

'I just get a gun and shoot myself and then it is over and done with, because I am just a public patient!'

The nurse comes in and she goes, 'you need some water; are you all right?' she goes, 'I heard what he's said'.

'I am fine'.

I got up with what little bit of self-respect, decency, pride I had left. I walked out of this office and I never came back. I went straight and made the complaint to the Commission. What other avenues did I have? I didn't have any. (Patient 07)

The example illustrates the defensiveness and passiveness of the surgeon in providing an explanation of the incident in direct contrast to the forceful questioning by the patient and her support persons. After the surgeon eventually admitted his mistake, without apologising, the situation deteriorated to an emotional and almost aggressive exchange and ended with a complete breakdown of the relationship. Only at that point did the patient mention making a complaint because she felt there was no other avenue left to her.

In general, I observed in the interviews that people did not make a complaint easily; they felt that they had a genuine reason and grievance that needed to be known to a neutral authority. The act of making a written complaint often made them feel that their experience was relevant.

I now summarise the themes that emerged in the interviews relating to why patients made their complaint.

3.5.8.1 Making the practitioner take notice

From many of the interviews with patients it became clear that making a complaint gave the patient back some control and power in their relationship with the practitioner, whereas after an incident they often felt hurt and powerless. The complaint was seen as an avenue to make the practitioner take note.

> *[T]he main thing was like shaking him awake a bit: 'hello, this*
> *might not be something that people appreciate'. And if he is doing*
> *it, he could be doing it a bit being unaware; he could be doing it*
> *quite consciously. If he is doing it consciously, at least there is*
> *someone – there is a commission – that looks into things. I was*
> *assuming that it would make him sit up and take notice. … I want-*
> *ed him to say 'look, I am really sorry for the way I treated you'. If*
> *he had a reason – great – if he didn't have a reason – fine. … I*
> *made the complaint to protect other people in the future. That's*
> *the only reason I did it. (Patient 05)*

The patient at the time of making the complaint considered that the practitioner may not be aware of their behaviour or that there was a problem, which left the opportunity for the practitioner to recognise a problem and rectify it in future.

Another recurring theme in the patient interviews was that patients not only wanted that the practitioner be made aware that there was a problem, but also that they understood what impact it had on the patient's life. The following statement from a patient and his wife illustrates their wish to explain to the practitioners involved in the incident how they perceived it, how they felt and what impact it had on their lives:

> *We would have liked to sit down with him. … I certainly would like*
> *to sit down with all of them and have a chat with them and let*
> *them walk in our shoes. And let them have a day in my shoes; see*
> *how they think. It would be good. …*

> *I think the best possible outcome that could ever come from this is*
> *if one day they might ask you, 'what is it that you feel … so that I*
> *know for next time.' I think that that would be worth more than*
> *anything, because it would vindicate; you would feel quite vindi-*
> *cated that they actually believe that there was something that*
> *they … that something went wrong and that something was*
> *wrong and that they would learn [from it]. (Patient 22[19])*

Patients did not only wish to understand what had happened to them and why from a medical point of view, but they also wanted the practitioner to understand how they experienced it and what the impact was on their life in general. Being physically or psychologically hurt by the practitioner (and often unacknowledged) was the most common reason patients gave for making a complaint.

> *When I first complained to the health complaints commission, I*
> *rang up and said that I suffer so much I have to complain to them.*
> *(Patient 09)*

Unresolved incidents can have a significant impact on the patient's well-being, as the following statement illustrates:

> *I was upset … and I just thought one day, I ring Beyond Blue[20],*
> *someone to talk to. I just felt so upset about it. And they then gave*
> *me the name of the doctor and also gave me the name of the*
> *health care complaints commission, if I felt I needed to make a*
> *complaint. And I didn't make one straight away. It took a while to*
> *reach the decision to ring the health complaints commission and*
> *that was very stressful for me to do that. (Patient 18)*

The patient needed to feel well enough and strong enough to make a complaint. This was echoed by another patient and his wife who said that while

---

[19] *The statement originates from a joint interview with both the patient and his wife.
[20] 'Beyond Blue' is a telephone service in Australia for people seeking support for depression or anxiety.

her husband was suffering from the aftermath of the incident, she had neither the time nor the energy to even think of making a complaint. Only when her husband was well into his recovery, over a year after the incident, did she complain with the help and encouragement from another practitioner.

A number of patients said that they made the complaint so that other patients could be spared a similar experience in the future.

> *I had hoped to achieve that nobody else would risk their lives with this surgeon. I had hoped that in some way it could be registered that this man had damaged me and tried to hide it. (Patient 04)*

Similarly, a patient noted that their decision was prompted by both wanting a personal apology and also wanting to protect other patients:

> *Everyone confirmed that I should do something about it. … basically, I wanted an apology myself – in writing or verbally, I didn't care. I wanted him to say 'look, I am really sorry for the way I treated you'. … I made the complaint to protect other people in the future. That's the only reason I did it. (Patient 06)*

3.5.8.2   Unresponsiveness to patient directly raising concerns

Some patients had raised their concerns initially with the practitioner or the manager of the practice or hospital where the incident happened. In all of these cases, they either did not receive a response to their concerns at all, or, where they did get a response, it did not address their questions, or they were directly referred to the Health Care Complaints Commission.

The following example illustrates this common scenario. A patient returned to her GP's practice after having undergone emergency brain surgery for an undiagnosed tumour and mentioned it to the receptionist to let the practitioner know what had happened. The practitioner saw the patient in the waiting room but did not talk to her at all. The patient described this moment.

I felt disappointed. I thought we had a friendship there. I respect her profession and I know her as supportive emotionally, but at the time – no comment. I immediately realised, she is protecting herself, because in our industry [child care] as well, you don't say sorry, because that is an admission that you did something wrong. I respect that as well. (Patient 03)

Despite drawing the analogy to her work place, stating that she understands the reluctance of the practitioner to apologise as it could be perceived as an admission of liability, the patient decided to make a complaint afterwards to receive answers to her questions.

'Why didn't you [the GP] send [me for tests]? You're a GP. You are trained for this industry. Why? How many times I went and had headaches. Ok, you've seen my scan in 2007. Didn't it occur in your mind that maybe something [was wrong] and send me for another scan?' (Patient 03)

When asked what she wanted to achieve by making a complaint, the patient said:

[I]mprove the training, because there are so many brain tumour cases now. They should really go back to the basics, checking your reflexes – it wasn't done on me when I saw her. … And another thing is, I was so frustrated that I became an expense. (Patient 03)

It appears that if the practitioner had provided an explanation, had assured the patient that she would update her knowledge on diagnosing brain tumours and had offered to bulk-bill her for future consultations that were required to deal with the consequences of the incident, the patient may not have made a complaint.

The lack of acknowledgement of the patient's concerns was a common theme during interviews. One patient, who initially wrote a letter to the practitioner, directly quoted from this:

'I would like you to respond to my letter. You know my phone number and you know my address, email everything. I just need [an] explanation and I believe I deserve it. Otherwise, I have to go to the health complaints department,' and he knew it. He actually didn't care about the health care complaint commission. He didn't care. I was waiting for that [response] for three or four days from him, but he didn't. Then I ... got ... a HCCC complaint form. (Patient 15)

The practitioner neither acknowledged nor responded to the initial complaint, which then triggered the patient making a complaint to the Health Care Complaints Commission. At that point, he declined the offer of a trained mediator assisting him to try and resolve the issues with the practitioner and getting the information he was seeking. The patient felt that the Commission had not taken his complaint seriously enough by referring him to a voluntary resolution process when the practitioner had declined to engage with him earlier.

3.5.8.3   Others encourage patient making complaint

A number of patients reported that they were encouraged or in some cases even requested by other health practitioners to make a complaint. Practitioners involved in the ongoing treatment, or general practitioners who had referred the patient to see a specialist initially, most commonly encouraged the patient to make a complaint.

In the following example, the patient was asked by her physiotherapist who treated her during the recovery from her operation to make a complaint.

> *[The physiotherapist] pushed, because she had that many people complain about [the doctor], but nobody is doing anything about it. She really pushed me, 'you have to do something. If no one is taking a stand, nothing is going to happen', because he stuffed up a lot of surgeries up here. ... He has caused a lot of problems up here. I heard if from a lot of people, because I have been on crutches for 12 months and people just talk .... (Patient 12)*

The patient had considered making a complaint, but was further encouraged by her physiotherapist and hearing about the experience of other patients.

The confirmation from someone within the health field that what a patient experienced was not alright was an important factor in their decision to eventually make a complaint.

> *I probably would not have had the strength to complain, would my GP not have encouraged me and [the capital city doctor]. Both men were my doctors as well and knew all the history of my blood tests and CT scans and what I had been going through. (Patient 04)*

In some instances, other health practitioners were more active in actually requesting that the patient make a complaint.

> *[The] the vascular surgeon] said to me ... 'this never should have happened. ... And he ... said, 'I want you to take this further. I want you to take this to the media', which we didn't, but I did put a complaint in to the Commission. ...*

> *[W]e were advised so by two other doctors ... and my GP ... said, 'it shouldn't be that people get away with it. It is not going to bring [the husband's] leg back, but it might make them all aware that the [local hospital] [has problems], because there had been so many complaints about this [local hospital], it is unreal.' So that's why we lodged the complaint. (Patient 16)*

The example shows that there are instances of informal knowledge about issues in the hospital among local health practitioners. Encouraging patients to make a complaint was an avenue for the practitioners to raise their own concerns, but do so indirectly.

Not only other health practitioners encouraged patients to make a complaint, family members, friends or lawyers were also mentioned in some of the interviews.

> *My family; my friends, they said, 'you weren't like this before the operation. If I was you, I would see somebody about it.' And then I was told by a solicitor to lodge a complaint [with] the complaints commission. (Patient 20)*

However, some patients made the complaint despite a lack of support from their family, showing the importance it had for them to be heard and acknowledged.

> *All the family is up against what I am doing, because [they think that] you don't sue a friend, but sweetie, I've been hurt. Boy, have I been hurt. (Patient 10)*

The emotional impact the incident had on the patient's life was so great that it outweighed the lack of support from his family.

3.5.8.4 Seeking accountability

Another theme that emerged from the interviews was that patients wanted the practitioner or someone to be accountable and take responsibility for what had happened. The terms of accountability and responsibility may be used with different meanings.[21]

Patients sought accountability for what had happened, and the lack of accountability was a recurring theme in the patient interviews.

> *[H]e should have said to me "I should tell you that [the hip replacement] is showing a bit of a high revision, would you prefer another?' ... The National Registry report states that the new statistics ... should show in the next few years. ... I was another ... statistic. ...*
>
> *This shouldn't have happened, he [the doctor] knew and that's why I am coming after him. ...*
>
> *[The Commission has] to bring this doctor to account ... [for] lying to me and not telling me that he knew. (Patient 02)*

The statement illustrates that the fact that the practitioner did not inform the patient that there was a problem, in other words, that the practitioner was not accountable to them, was the trigger for the complaint. The practitioner knew about an error with the equipment. The error was not his responsibility, as it was not caused by him or his action; nevertheless, to the patient he was the person accountable to tell them about the error.

Accountability in the patient's understanding was commonly linked with honesty and transparency, but also with the expectation that the practitioner should acknowledge the problem and manage it.

---

[21] I understand responsibility as feeling responsible for one's own actions, while accountability means that the practitioner is accountable to the patient. Often, responsibility for an action and being accountable to the patient overlap. However, there are occasions where one practitioner is responsible for the action that contributed or caused the incident, while the management or supervisor would be the person that is accountable to the patient and their family. In short, responsibility is an internal, subjective phenomenon, while accountability is an external, more objective phenomenon.

The main thing was that I wanted acknowledgement from him. ...
[F]or me he was a bad doctor. He put his tail between his legs and
has hidden from the whole thing. He is quite cowardly and he is
totally unprofessional. And that's what was really annoying me:
how unprofessional was this man. (Patient 14)

The patient perceived the practitioner's lack of accountability as unprofessional and subsequently generalised that the practitioner was a 'bad doctor', implying not only lack of accountability, but also lack of skill and competence.

In addition to the above themes, patients raised some less common reasons for making a complaint. These are summarised below.

3.5.8.5   Having to pay for substandard service

A side topic that emerged in a small number of patient interviews, but was also reflected in the interviews with practitioners as being considered a possible reason for a complaint, was paying for services that patients were disappointed with or perceived as being substandard.

And my own doctor charged, I don't know, it might have been
$63, compared to the other one's $80. So I thought, here I am get-
ting assistance from my doctor and it is cheaper than the other
one that was just money down the drain. I was very, very angry.
(Patient 14)

This may indicate an understanding of some patients that they are a health consumer. This means that where a payment for a service is made and the service is not up to their satisfaction, they complain. The practitioner becomes a health service provider in the sense that they provide a service of the quality that is paid for. Some interviews revealed that patients were willing to accept a lower level of competence and service from practitioners who bulk-bill, but on the other hand patients had higher expectations of practitioners who charged more than the scheduled fee, leaving them with a significant gap[22].

3.5.8.6 Ban practitioner from practising

Notably, only one patient said during the interview that they wanted to see the practitioner banned from practising in future.

> *Well, I think, he should have been ruled out of his profession, never ever [to] practise again. And I wrote that in one of the letters. ... I think he should be barred from acting as a doctor. Acting – I used the word acting. (Patient 21)*

The patient's use of the term 'acting' implies that she believed the practitioner was not skilled enough or fit to practise as a doctor.

3.5.8.7 Complaint easier compared to litigation

One patient said that making a complaint was faster and less costly than suing the practitioner.

> *Well, some wanted me to sue him. And I said, 'no, I'd never get anywhere. [It] probably takes up to ten years to go to court and then if I lost, I'd be out of pocket thousands of dollars.' So I said 'no, I won't sue'. But I made the complaint. (Patient 11)*

This was echoed by other patients who had considered and in some cases sought legal advice to sue the practitioner. Most of these patients decided against lodging a civil claim against the practitioner due to considerations of associated costs, length of proceedings and the adversarial nature of the proceedings. For those patients who had considered a civil claim, the cost of civil

---

[22] In the Australian health care system, medical practitioners are free to charge any fee for their service. For service recognised under the public health insurance scheme – Medicare – practitioners receive a benefit. Where practitioners charge the patient more than the patient can get refunded from Medicare, the patient is left with a gap payment, or out-of-pocket expense.

litigation was the most relevant factor when deciding against suing the practitioner.

> *I don't have enough money to hire a lawyer, because this would cost me $5000 maybe. [I] can't afford it. I just would like them [the HCCC] to treat it in a way so that somebody who has no money still has the right. (Patient 03)*

Making a complaint to the Health Care Complaints Commission meant that an authority knew about the practitioner and that it was assumed that it would take appropriate action to ensure it did not happen to anyone else in the future.

3.5.8.8   Getting reassurance

Some patients spoke about the possibility that there may be an explanation for the incident or the practitioner's action when making the complaint. One patient, who herself was a trained nurse, said that she did not intend to make a complaint but was seeking reassurance about the quality of care and treatment she had received.

> *I said to this person from the health care complaints commission, 'I am not writing as a complaint; I just want it to be checked.' ... At the end, I've got the letter stating that my file was checked by an independent doctor and the operation was performed correctly; how it should have been done. (Patient 19)*

Some of the patients felt uncomfortable making a complaint. The connotation of the word 'complaint' was often felt to be more serious and formal then simply having a concern. Using the term 'complaint' also implied that the patient had evidence to substantiate their concern, in other words, that their concerns were relevant and could be substantiated, rather than concerns being raised to get an explanation and trying to see whether or not they were justified.

3.5.8.9   Summary: Making a complaint

In summary, the motivation for people making a formal complaint was mainly a mixture of the wish to be heard, seeking acknowledgement of their concerns and getting an explanation of what had happened to them and why. Often associated with it was the stated aim of preventing others from having a similar experience. One patient said that the intention of making the complaint was to ban the practitioner from practising.

As mentioned, the interviewed patients did not easily make a complaint. In almost all cases, there had been interactions with the practitioner or their management in an attempt to get clarification, an explanation addressing the concerns the patient had. Where it was unsuccessful or insufficient, people made a complaint. Even then, some patients felt uncomfortable, feared retribution or were wary of creating problems for themselves in accessing care in the future.

> *I have got a lot of health problems, so I can't really rock the boat, because I am in and out of hospital with my condition all the time. So, because we are limited up here and people can't travel to another hospital, given the circumstances, I am stuck. So I can't. It was a big thing for me to actually put in the complaint about [Dr A] and the way I was treated. … I was labelled at the hospital as a hypochondriac. But I knew. (Patient 12)*

The most common reservation patients reported in relation to making a complaint was that they feared that it may mean that they could not access medical treatment in future when they needed it, not only from the practitioner complained about, but also other practitioners. Their assumption was that if they complained about one doctor, the practitioner would talk to colleagues and as a result, the patient could be banned from other health services, or be restricted in accessing other health service providers.

>   *And a lot of people [here] had the same thing and actually one fol-*
>   *lowed through with complaints and now can't even get in to any*
>   *doctors up here, because they don't want to touch her. That's the*
>   *other thing; I have to be really careful of, because I need my*
>   *health; I need the doctors. (Patient 12)*

In contrast, interviewed practitioners rarely mentioned that they spoke to a colleague about a complaint. When practitioners received a complaint they mainly spoke about it to their indemnity insurer and their family.

3.5.9   Outcome of the complaint

When asked about the outcome of their complaint, a number of patients were dissatisfied with the final outcome. Their ongoing dissatisfaction may have been the reason they participated in the research study, as some commented that they saw it as an opportunity to tell their 'side' of the story. Often, although the complaint had been closed by the Health Care Complaints Commission, it was not resolved for the patient. The incident and/or its consequences still had an impact on the patient's life.

The patient's reactions to the Commission's action varied. Where the Commission took no further action after assessing the complaint, those patients who made their complaint so that it was noted by an authority were satisfied. Also where the complaint related to a consultation for which the patient had incurred out of pocket expenses, the reimbursement of these fees was satisfactory to the patient. However, some patients did not feel that their complaint was taken as seriously as it should have been.

Where the Commission decided to refer the complaint to its Resolution Service to attempt a voluntary resolution process between the patient and the practitioner, the interviewed patients either had not consented to proceed with the resolution process as they believed that their complaint had not been taken seriously enough and warranted some type of action being taken against the practitioner, or others went through the resolution process, but were dissatis-fied with the outcome, as the practitioner became defensive or there were remaining open questions they had.

Where the complaint resulted in disciplinary action taken against the prac-titioner, either through referring the complaint to the former Medical Board, or the Commission prosecuting a practitioner, patients were satisfied with the outcome of their complaint. However, it should be noted that even in these cases, some patients reported not fully understanding the proceedings and the result.

> *I got a phone call from the physio and she has seen it in the local paper, and I went, 'what happened?' ... And she told me that [Dr A] had been struck off, since August this year, he is not allowed to practise and he had to go back and be completely retrained. That was on the front page of the paper. ... But the other day, I found out that he is actually still practising, but he has to have a supervisor standing right next to him all the time. (Patient 12)*

This patient described her physiotherapist informing her about the out-come of her complaint rather than the Commission. Another patient, whose complaint prompted proceedings before a disciplinary body, said that she would have been willing to give evidence, but was never asked to and felt that the practitioner's version was believed and as a result, no action was taken against him.

> *They believed everything that he said, so there was no opposition to him. (Patient 21)*

Overall, and independent of the actual outcome, a number of patients felt that it was difficult to initiate some type of disciplinary action against a practi-tioner.

> *The medical profession, they cover each other's backsides. It's*
> *very, very hard to get a complaint [through], unless you get a lot,*
> *a lot of people with the same or similar complaint. (Patient 01)*

A number of patients also commented that in their opinion, the practitioner had been dishonest or misleading, which had led to the complaint not going any further.

> *He is a very clever person and as you can see, he wants to wriggle*
> *out of whatever he can. (Patient 10)*

Overall, the majority of interviewed patients were dissatisfied with the outcome of their complaint to the Health Care Complaints Commission, mainly because their expectation of the outcome did not match the actual action taken.

3.5.10 Role of apologies

I was interested in how patients spoke about apologies by the practitioner or the lack thereof and how it affected their relationship with the practitioner. Mainly, patients said that they did not receive an apology from the practitioner at all, or where they did, it was some time after the incident, came from another person not the practitioner, or it was perceived as not being genuine.

The greatest number of patients spoke of not having received an apology and perceived this as a lack of acknowledgement of their experience. Some, however, did not expect an apology, but were seeking that their experience be acknowledged.

3.5.10.1 Lack of acknowledgment

Some patients said that they would not have expected an apology, if there had been a genuine acknowledgement by the practitioner that there had been an issue and an explanation.

> *[Y]ou don't need to say sorry. You just have to say something like 'I heard about you. I am glad that you are ok'. (Patient 03)*

Along similar lines, another patient said:

> *I was expecting not even an apology; [but] an explanation. 'ok, I had a bad day', or 'I didn't see it.' – an explanation. I wasn't expecting an apology, or anything. But he didn't even call [saying], 'I had a [bad] day, sorry about that.' [He] just lied to me. Just respond to me! I was expecting that; nothing else; not money; not an apology letter. (Patient 15)*

Both examples show that, where there has been an incident, patients expected acknowledgment and an explanation, and not necessarily an apology.

3.5.10.2 Lack of apology

Disappointment

While it seems from the above statements that for some patients it was most important to understand and be understood, for other patients, it was the practitioner offering an apology. Where this did not happen, patients were disappointed and upset.

> *I am quite prepared [to accept] that he is a human being; that he could have had a bad day; things went wrong; something terrible could have happened …. What upsets me is that the guy wasn't prepared to just apologise to me and say 'look, I am so sorry; it shouldn't have happened'. (Patient 06)*

The above statement illustrates that the patient was accommodating about the circumstances that could have explained the incident; however, the lack of an apology from the practitioner triggered an emotional response, and made the patient upset.

One patient reported that she was contacted by the hospital manager who offered support, but she states that the manager did not offer an apology.

> *The manager from the [local hospital] did ring me ... he didn't re-*
> *ally apologise. ... he just said, 'if there is anything we can do ...';*
> *but he didn't apologise, no. (Patient 16)*

The patient's almost neutral description may have been made because there was some level of acknowledgement through the offer of assistance, as well as because the manager was not the practitioner who was involved in the incident, but a third party.

Disbelief

Other patients responded with disbelief when their grievance was not acknowledged through an apology, as the following statement shows.

> *I was really quite stunned! I was going there with a genuine griev-*
> *ance and obviously was going through quite some grief and I just*
> *wanted an apology. I just wanted an acknowledgment. I suppose,*
> *I wished that there was a way that a doctor can say sorry without*
> *feeling like I am going to sue her, or whatever. I mean, I wasn't in-*
> *terested in that. I just wanted her to say, 'I am sorry.' (Patient 13)*

The patient acknowledged that the practitioner may have feared being sued if he apologised, but did not accept this as a valid excuse that would exempt the practitioner from having a duty to apologise to the patient. In another case where the patient did not get the apology they expected, it became the main issue of their complaint rather than the actual incident.

The main thing is: I didn't get an apology. I didn't get a word; not a word; not 'I apologise'; not 'I'm sorry that I put you through undue stress; not 'I'm sorry I couldn't help you any further'. (Patient 14)

Perception of denial, cover up and self-protection

In some cases, patients said that for them the lack of an apology was a sign that the practitioner tried to cover up their mistake.

I would not mind him to just see me and say, 'I am sorry, I gave you the wrong diagnosis'. But that's the way they work: they cover each other, 'well, we didn't do anything wrong'. (Patient 08)

The patient's statement implies that they believe there was a culture among medical practitioners to deny and cover up mistakes, and avoid apologising if there was an incident. The patient also implied that the practitioner's motivation for not apologising was to protect themselves and look after their own interests rather than the patient's best interest. This sentiment was repeated in a few of the patient interviews.

Lying in the bed as the patient, you are very vulnerable to the nurses and the doctors and you don't want to upset them. I didn't ring my buzzer, in case someone else had a more important problem. And I was concerned for others, not just demanding attention for myself, but I just was very disappointed with this man who was looking after his own self. He didn't even apologise to me in any way. (Patient 04)

This patient emphasised that she had been considerate of the nurses' and practitioner's needs, implying that she expected her needs to be respected in return.

3.5.10.3 Apology

Delay

In the few cases where patients had received an apology from the practitioner, most remained dissatisfied. One aspect that was mentioned by a number of patients was that although they received an apology from the practitioner, it came some time after the event. In one case, the practitioners were only aware of the incident when they were notified of the patient's complaint and apologised.

> *Then they ... contacted the doctors who both said that they were surprised and that they were sorry that it happened .... I just said to the complaints commission, I don't want it to go any further; all I want is [for] them to be aware of how badly I felt treated. I would hope they wouldn't treat another patient the same way ....*
> *(Patient 18)*

The patient accepted the apology, because although it was some time after the actual incident, it was promptly after the practitioners were made aware that the patient had had a bad experience. In other cases, patients viewed a delayed apology by the practitioner less favourably.

> *He [Dr One] didn't see me when I was in hospital. He rang me from his mobile phone. He kept away from me. ... It was 8 weeks after the operation. And he [Dr One] was 'I'm sorry'. ... I wanted to see him to ask, 'why couldn't you be honest with us'? Why couldn't he just have said: 'Look, I made a mistake, I am sorry', instead he lied all the time. (Patient 02)*

In the above example, the patient would have expected an apology sooner after the incident when it had been clear to the practitioner that an error had happened. Receiving no apology or explanation for the incident for two months was perceived by the patient as the practitioner being deliberately dishonest.

In one case, although the relevant practitioner had apologised to the patient within a couple of days for inadvertently forgetting to attend to them in the emergency department, the patient did not accept the doctor's apology.

> *It was eight hours ... Then we found out that our doctor went home. He forgot us. ... He rang me after a couple of days and said, 'look, I am really sorry about this.' ... He didn't care; he had to go home; he knocked off. (Patient 12)*

In this case, the patient's sense of urgency to be treated, exemplified by them attending the emergency department, was in stark contrast to the practitioner just forgetting them and going home. Here even a couple of days were perceived as too great a delay between incident and apology to be accepted by the patient.

In contrast, one patient reported that their practitioner had proactively and without delay apologised for misdiagnosing shingles. The patient [Patient 21] accepted the apology, commenting, 'See. I suppose, they are not perfect'. No complaint was made in this instance.

Apology appears forced or not genuine

Another reason why patients remained dissatisfied after a practitioner's apology was that they perceived the apology to be forced and not genuine, as the following example illustrates.

> *[O]nce, near the end of the [conciliation conference], he said in a roundabout way that he was sorry that it has come this, or something. He spoke so sharply and the chap from the complaints board even said that he was so surprised by the lack of empathy for me, in the way I am now. The word 'sorry' was mentioned once, but it was only on the side more or less. (Patient 11)*

The apology was delivered in a manner the patient perceived as being insincere. As a result, the patient was so stunned and disappointed that they decided not to continue with the resolution process. Reflecting upon this decision during the interview, the patient said that they did not feel they had achieved closure for themselves and now regretted not having pursued their complaint.

In another case, a patient reported that although the practitioner promptly apologised for having crossed personal boundaries, the same behaviour continued.

Apology without an explanation

In three instances, patients reported that the practitioner apologised, but did not provide an explanation of what exactly had happened. All of those patients were dissatisfied and found the apology incomplete due to the lack of fully understanding what had led to the incident. In the following example, a patient and his wife reflected on how they perceived the practitioner's apologies after the incident in which the husband suffered a brain injury due to the anaesthetics used during a routine operation to remove a skin cancer spot. Just after the incident, when it was still unclear whether the patient had suffered a stroke or another form of brain injury during the operation, the anaesthetist apologised to the wife for the first time.

> *I think the anaesthetist, he apologised. He did. He said, 'I'm really sorry.' About what I'm not sure. I think he was quite concerned. (Patient 22)*

At that stage, no further explanation was given regarding what could have been the reason for the incident. The wife commented that there was no explanation about what the practitioner was sorry for, but that she perceived that the practitioner was concerned. Shortly after, while the patient was still in hospital, the anaesthetist apologised a second time, attempting to explain what had happened.

Yes, he came another time and he apologised and he said, 'I'm re-
ally sorry. He was difficult to put under. He is a young man, he was
well. He was well. He was difficult to put under. His breathing …
he wasn't breathing …', but he never really went into it. …. I was in
shock, really. (Patient 22)

It was still not fully clear what exactly had happened to the patient during the surgery, and the wife was still in a state of shock. There was no further interaction between the anaesthetist and the patient and his wife during the patient's lengthy recovery. The private hospital where the incident happened did meet with the wife, but only after another practitioner had called the manager of the hospital on the family's behalf and expressed the view that this should never have happened and the treatment of the patient and his family was disgusting. As a result the wife was invited to meet with the management. She recalls:

So my son and I went in and it was very emotional. And they lis-
tened to all of it and I am sure that they thought that they were
going to be sued. And they sent a letter of apology and they do
admit; they investigated it. I must say that the man who is in
charge of the nursing section, I honestly believe that he was physi-
cally and emotionally [affected], he felt for us, because he actually
had started to cry. I think he probably could put himself into our
position. So I think he had a real understanding of what had hap-
pened and he promised that he would investigate the whole thing.
So he did and he sent me a letter and he rang me quite a few
times and he said that he had investigated it and it was true. The
sister in charge [did] apologise, she didn't get back to me and they
didn't have a proper hand-over, because they were busy and he
wasn't looked after properly and that they have put now into ef-
fect certain procedures that happen for someone who has had a
brain injury, or stroke. (Patient 22)

After the patient had made some progress in his recovery, the patient's wife made a complaint to the Health Care Complaints Commission. In response to it, the anaesthetist denied any wrongdoing and did not offer an apology. Instead, the patient was blamed for being over-anxious before the surgery. Some time after the complaint was closed without further action being taken, the anaesthetist called the patient's home:

> *[The anaesthetist] he did ring home one day and I answered the phone. It was totally unexpected. I actually thought he was a bit drunk. And it was in the evening and he had asked me how [my husband] was. And I said' [my husband is not well]; he is not working and things are not good'. And he apologised and he said he knows he is a really young man … and 'I am really sorry'. And I felt sorry for him. I actually felt sorry for him. And I said, 'I am sure you must be sorry. You must feel what it would be like. You are a father and the head of a family, so you must know how it would feel.' And that was it. He was really sorry. (Patient 22)*

Despite the discrepancy between the anaesthetist's behaviour directly with the family and the differing response to the formal complaint, which had angered the patient and his wife, it provided some type of closure.

What patients would have expected

Where no apology was offered, I asked patients what they would have expected from the practitioner. The responses showed that patients wanted an apology, together with a clear and honest explanation of what happened, why it happened and what would be done in future to prevent it from happening again. Several patients expected to see all these elements together, with the practitioner displaying a level of insight and humility.

He would have had to apologise in a very special way; he couldn't just say 'I'm sorry'. He would have to explain the whole situation; what went on with him and if it happened to be personal, so be it. He should have been able to tell me that, if he wanted me back. If he cared enough for me as a patient and as a person, I know that if I [were] a doctor – I just don't want people to ever see me badly – but if I were a doctor, a professional, I would surely make sure that that person would know exactly why I behaved that way and how out of line it was and would even say to them 'look, I am not expecting you to come back to me, but if you are prepared to give me another chance, I will never let that happen again'. ..., I would say 'I make sure that this will never happen again. And it was pretty despicable behaviour. If you give me a chance again, I will be very grateful, but if you do not, I also accept that.' I'd just be above all honest about it. So if he is really honest like that, I'd probably give him another chance and see how things went. (Patient 06)

What the statement also recognises is that even if the patient was to accept the apology, it was the patient's decision and right to decide whether or not to continue seeing this practitioner after the incident.

3.5.11 Impact on patient's behaviour in response to complaint

Analysing how the experience of the incident and the complaint had influenced the patients' behaviour in medical encounters in general, responses ranged from no change in the individual patient's attitude or behaviour to distrust of all health service providers and people in general.

The former end of the spectrum is represented by a patient who herself was a health practitioner and who felt that her experience was solely relevant to this particular practitioner and should not be generalised. At the latter end of the spectrum was the patient whose facial nerve was severed during surgery and where the practitioner had been dismissive and aggressive towards her afterwards. As her complaint had been discontinued by the Health Care Complaints Commission with the reason given that what she experienced was a rare, but recognised complication that had been mentioned according to the practitioner, she felt completely misunderstood and left alone, not only by the practitioner, but also the health system and the regulatory system as a whole. She said that as a result of the experience, she had become distrustful of every person, except her close family.

Although these extremes of patient behaviour in response to the complaint occurred, most commonly patients distinguished between their experiences with a particular practitioner and did not readily generalise it to other practitioners.

> *[Dr A] was [Dr A], I had not any problems about any other doctor but him – just him. And I'll probably end up dealing with [Dr B] now for any joints. He knows how to treat me. And the situation hasn't changed my opinion of doctors or staff. (Patient 12)*

Most patients said that they have become more active in that they ask more questions, seek a second opinion if uncertain and assert their rights as patients more often. The following statement summarises this position shared by the majority of interviewed patients:

> *When I am seeing a doctor, I still trust the doctor, I still respect [the doctor]. But what I do now is [seek a] second opinion – go for a second opinion. 'What do you think, and what do you think?' And please don't get offended, because I just would like to clarify that what you told me is really what I need to do. ... Even my GP now says, I am a very complicated patient, not because of the seriousness of my condition, it is more like 'why is this happening?' (Patient 03)*

In many cases, the negative experience has made patients become more involved in their own health care and the decision-making, taking on greater responsibility for treatment choices themselves.

3.5.12 Summary: Trust, the patient's perspective

Table 3.3 summarises the trust levels patients reported in relation to the practitioner complained about before and immediately after the incident, as well as at the time when the relationship ended and at the time of the interview.

Table 3.3   Trust levels reported by patients

Pa-tient	Trust level				Would you see the practition-er again?
	Initially-first consul-tation	Immediately after incident	When complaint made /end relation-ship	At the time of the in-terview	
Patient 01	8.5 - 9	4	1	0	no
Patient 02	10	10	0	0	no
Patient 03	9	-	-	0	no
Patient 04	10	8	0	0	no
Patient 05	9	5	0	0	no
Patient 06	8	Deteriorat-ed, but no	-	-	no
Patient 07	10	Still high, as doctor as-	-	0	no
Patient 08	8	-	-	-	no
Patient 09	-	-	-	-	no
Patient 10	10	Deteriorat-ed. no exact	-	Trust remains	no
Patient 11	8-9	2	-	2	no
Patient 12	2	0	-	-	no

Pa-tient	Trust level					Would you see the practition-er again?
	Initially-first consul-tation	Immediately after incident	When complaint made /end relation-ship	At the time of the in-terview		
Patient 13	9	3	-	0		no
Patient 14	2	1	-	0		no
Patient 15	-	-	-	-		no
Patient 16	Low (2.5)	Very low	-	-		no
Patient 17	5	-	-	0		no
Patient 18	10	7	-	1		no
Patient 19	8		0	0		no
Patient 20	8	6	1	0		no
Patient 21	-	-	-	-		-
Patient 22*	Felt com-fortable	-	-	-		no

Two of the 22 patients interviewed reported low trust levels at the initial consultation, while the vast majority reported high levels of initial trust in the practitioner. Immediately after the incident, all reported a decline in trust levels, but most did not describe a complete loss of trust. However, at the time of the interview, almost all did no longer trust the practitioner and all patients said that they would not return to see the practitioner.

It is important to note that most patients distinguished between their experiences with a particular practitioner and other practitioners. Patients may have become more suspicious and careful, but only one patient described being distrustful of all doctors and providers as a result of her experience.

Towards the end of each interview I asked patients to describe what the top three things were they were looking for in a doctor – it was a reflection on what would be their ideal doctor after they had the experience with the incident and complaint.

3.5.12.1 The ideal doctor

Patients mentioned all three areas – communication, care and competence – but with different prioritisations. Had the patient complaint been mainly communication related, then patients wished for a doctor who is a good communicator. Had the complaint been competence related, the priorities were that the practitioner had skill and competence. Had the complaint been triggered by the practitioner's perceived lack of care, especially after an incident, patients wished for a caring doctor.

Overall, the patients' responses had in common that they looked for a mix of attributes in a doctor. Most important were that they could trust the practitioner; that the communication would be open and honest; that the practitioner was skilled and competent to help them; and that the practitioner would take an interest in them as a person.

The following statement summarises the commonalities across patient answers. When asked what is most important to them in a doctor, it was the following:

> *Trust. That I can walk in there and I feel that I can be asking an honest question and I get an honest answer. And treating me as a human being. Not treating me any better, because I am rich, or any worse, because I am poor, but just treating everybody the same. ... And really looking after the patient; taking their interest into account, what that person needs. Talking to them as a human being. Give them the benefit of the doubt and talk to them as human beings. Just because some people may not be able to say something, does not mean they don't understand. So explain it to them as clear as it can be. Treat them fairly. Treat them honestly. Treat them with respect and dignity. Give them dignity and re-*

*spect, because being sick is very difficult, it is extremely difficult.
So, respect that in that person that they have to go through [that
illness]. Anything from stiches in the head, or you might have fall-
en over in a football game, or you might get an older lady and her
hair is falling out. That's her hair, so be respectful of that. And
treat her with the respect that she deserves. She had hair all her
life and her hair is falling out. Just care. Do the job that they aim
[you] to do from the beginning. Put all the paperwork and all the
bullshit aside, get all the insurance aside and all that out of [your]
head and treat the patient as a human being. (Patient 07)*

The characteristics of an ideal doctor described by patients mirror the
themes that emerged from the interviews, which were associated with enhancing trust. Honesty, empathy and using their competence in the patient's best
interest are most essential to patients. This emphasises that where patients
have a choice, they prefer a practitioner who they can trust.

3.6   Medical practitioners about errors

This section summarises the results of an anonymous survey of medical practitioners, in particular surgeons and general practitioners, which was administered in German in Saxony, Germany, and in English in New South Wales, Australia. The research question and underlining assumptions, introduced in Section 3.3.1, were reflected in the survey inquiring about medical practitioners'
attitudes to and experiences with medical errors. As is had been assumed that
the following six areas would relate to the willingness of a medical practitioner
to openly communicate about medical errors, the survey was structured along
those areas and results are also presented in the following sections:

3.6.2 General attitude towards medical errors

3.6.3 Communication about medical errors with patients

3.6.4 Experience with medical errors

3.6.5 Dealing with medical errors

3.6.6 Communicating about medical errors with others

3.6.7 Receiving information about medical errors

In addition, the respondents' demographic data was obtained.

The level of response for the German survey with 354 responses was significantly higher than for the Australian survey, where only 24 responses were received. I have decided to present the results separately, and use visualisation only in relation to the German responses. The Australian responses are included despite the small number of responses, as they indicate interesting trends particularly where they differ from the trends in the German survey responses.

3.6.1   Response rate and demographics

In Germany, a total of 3,211 survey packages were sent by mail to practitioners. In total, 354 responses were received, of which eight (2.3%) were submitted online. The overall response rate was 11%. The response rate was lowest among male general practitioners (10.6%) and highest among female surgeons (14.3%) [n=343]. There was no general reminder sent, as another research survey had been distributed by the Association of Statutory Health Insurance Physicians shortly after and the association wished not to overload and/or confuse practitioners.

By comparison, in Australia the professional colleges did not agree to distribute the surveys directly to their members, but promoted the survey through their newsletters and member updates. The College of General Practitioners advised that the information was sent to 5,500 members, while the College of Surgeons did not provide the specific number of recipients. According to the Royal Australasian College of Surgeons' activities report (2013, p. 36), at the time of the survey, there were 1,592 active fellows of the College in NSW. Hence, it is assumed that the invitation to participate in the survey was sent to over 7,000 practitioners in NSW. In total, 24 responses to the online survey were received from Australian practitioners.

3.6.1.1 Gender

In the German survey, 1,789 (55.7%) survey packages were sent to female practitioners and 1,422 (44.3%) to male practitioners. Of the 354 responses received, 191 (54.0%) were from female practitioners, and 153 (43.2%) from male
practitioners; 10 practitioners (2.8%) did not record their gender. According to
data provided by the Kassenärztliche Vereinigung Sachsen, the gender distribution among the respondents was representative of the gender distribution in
the sample.

In the Australian survey, according to the Royal Australasian College of
Surgeons' activities report (2013, p. 36), 8.8% of surgeons in NSW were female
at the time of the survey. According to the Australian Medical Workforce Advisory Committee (2005, p. 5), 37.0% of general practitioners in Australia were
female. Of the responses received, 11 (45.8%) responses were from female
practitioners and 13 (54.2%) from male practitioners. This means that compared to the overall gender distribution in the two professional groups, female
practitioners more commonly responded to the survey.

3.6.1.2 Professional speciality

The German survey was sent to 2,910 practitioners working in general practice,
which represents 90.6% of the full sample. The survey was also sent to 301
surgeons, accounting for 9.4% of the 3,211 practitioners to whom the survey
was sent in Germany. Of the surgeons, 86.7% were general surgeons, while the
remaining 13.3% were surgeons who were specialised in other areas, for example, cardiothoracic surgery.

In Germany, practitioners working in general practice represented 90.6%
of the sample and 89.5% of all respondents (n=352). This group of respondents
consisted of 218 general practitioners, 60 physicians working in general practice, 31 practitioners specialised in paediatrics and adolescent medicine and six

non-specialised practitioners. This group will be merged for the following analysis and referred to as general practitioners*[23].

37 surgeons responded to the survey, which represents 10.5% of all responses received. Surgeons represented 9.4% of practitioners in the sample. Of the surgeons who responded to the survey, 21 were general surgeons (56.6%) and 15 were specialised surgeons (43.4%). Notably, among the respondents, the proportion of general surgeons compared to specialised surgeons is 30.1% lower than in the overall sample.

Referring to the available data for the Australian workforce, 77.6% of Australian recipients were general practitioners and 22.4% surgeons. Of the Australian respondents, 25.0% were general practitioners, 33.3% surgeons and 41.8% did not specify their speciality. Due to the high proportion of respondents who did not specify their speciality, Australian results will not be further broken down by profession in the following sections.

3.6.1.3 Age

On average, German participating practitioners were 51.9 years old (n=343), which is almost one year younger than the average age of the practitioners the survey was sent to in Germany (52.8 years). The youngest respondents were female surgeons (50.3 years on average); the oldest male surgeons with an average of 55.4 years.

Table 3.4   Average age of German respondents by gender and profession

Profession	Gender	Sent	Received	Difference
General practi-	female	52.5 years	51.7 years	-0.8
General practi-	male	53.4 years	50.6 years	-2.8
Surgeon	female	52.8 years	50.3 years	-2.5
Surgeon	male	52.2 years	55.4 years	+3.4

---

[23] *For the purpose of summarising the results, 'general practitioner' is used as a collective term to include general practitioners as well as paediatricians and physicians who work in general practice.

The median age of German practitioners who responded was 51 years. The age of respondents ranged from 31 to 78 years of age.

Overall, Australian respondents were slightly younger than German respondents. The average age of Australian respondents was 50 years of age; the median age was 48 years, with the youngest respondent being 28 years old and the oldest 85 years.

3.6.1.4 Years in practice

On average, German respondents (n=343) had practised medicine for 21 years. Female respondents had worked for an average of 19.9 years, while male respondents had worked on average for 22.2 years. While being younger on average, Australian respondents (n=24) had practised for an average of 24.6 years, with female respondents having worked for 16 years and male respondents for 32 years, on average.

Among German respondents, the median time in practice was 20 years, with experience ranging from 0.3 years to 47 years. For Australian respondents, the median time in practice was 21 years, ranging from 5 to 62 years. On average, Australian practitioners had been practising for 25 years.

3.6.1.5 Primary place of work

German respondents (n=348) were primarily working in sole practices (71.8%), followed by shared practices (23.3%). Only 3.5% of the respondents primarily worked in hospitals and two respondents (1.4%) worked in multi-purpose facilities (Medizinische Versorgungszentren).

By contrast, Australian respondents (n=24) most commonly worked (41.7%) in a joint practice with other practitioners (41.7%) or in a public hospital

(41.7%). 8.3% of practitioners worked as sole practitioners or in a private hospital.

3.6.1.6 Proportion of clinical work

For almost two thirds of the German respondents (n=346), clinical work, as opposed to administrative or academic work, made up between 51% to 75% of their work. An additional 23.7% of respondents stated that the proportion of clinical work was above 76%.

Of the Australian respondents (n=24), 79.2% spent more than 76% of their time in clinical practice and a further 20.8% spent between 51% to 75%.

3.6.1.7 Summary: Response rate and demographics

The difference in response rates may indicate the relevance the topic has for the current practice of medical practitioners in Germany and Australia. Considering that in Germany, there was no incentive for practitioners to complete the survey and no reminder, the response rate is considered high given existing time pressures for practitioners. This may indicate that medical errors are a topic that practitioners are both interested in and wish to bring into an academic and/or professional discourse. In Australia on the other hand, it was both difficult to find partners interested in distributing the survey, but also the response rate was extremely poor. Even the added incentive of donating money to a charity for the completion of the survey did not make a significant difference. I believe that a combination of not having the opportunity to invite practitioners to participate by sending a personalised mail or email has had an impact on response rates. In addition, the poor response rate may indicate that Australian practitioners may feel that the topic of dealing with medical errors is no longer new in the academic and professional discourse, reflecting the amount of professional and policy debate about medical errors, quality and safety improvements and open disclosure that has already taken place here.

In relation to the demographic results, the German survey respondents' gender distribution was representative of the gender distribution in the sample, while among Australian respondents, female practitioners were slightly overrepresented. Respondents from Germany were slightly older than Australian respondents, despite Australian respondents reporting a longer time in practice. This may be a reflection of differences in education periods before entering the profession, for example, Australian students entering tertiary education earlier than their German counterparts and the length of university studies.

A significant difference between German and Australian respondents was in relation to their primary place of work, with German practitioners much more commonly working as sole practitioners, while Australian respondents most commonly working in shared practices or public hospitals. This may partially be due to the different structure of the health care systems in both countries.

A slight difference also was the amount of time practitioners spent on clinical patient care, which was higher among Australian practitioners than German practitioners. Again, the different way in health provision may play a role, whereby in Australia nurses, junior staff and allied health staff take on more complementary patient treatment and care tasks compared to these more often remaining with German practitioners themselves, rather than being delegated. This includes for example information about referrals, directing patients to other health service providers, in some instances for immunisations or chronic health care.

3.6.2   General attitude about medical errors

Chart 3.1   *German practitioners' agreement with the statement that medical errors are one of the most serious problems in health care*

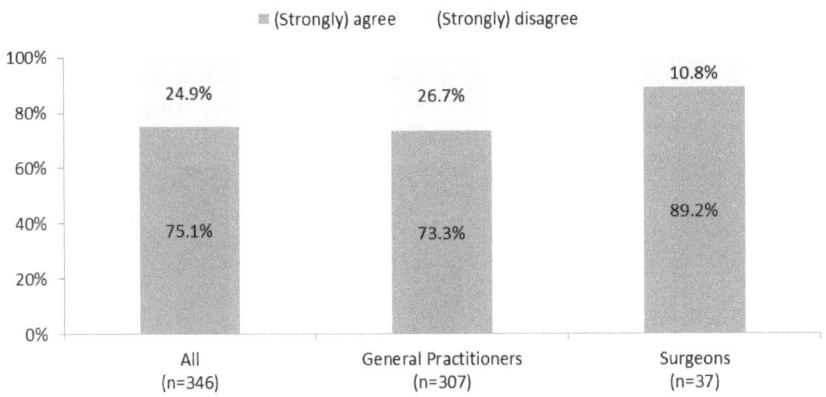

Three quarters (75.1%) of the German respondents (n=346) agreed or strongly agreed that medical errors are one of the most serious problems in health care. The proportion was significantly higher among surgeons, of whom 89.2% agreed with this statement.

In comparison, 50% of Australian respondents (n=24) agreed that medical errors are one of the most serious problems in health care.

Chart 3.2   *German practitioners' belief about proportion of patients in*
their area of practice that will experience an error

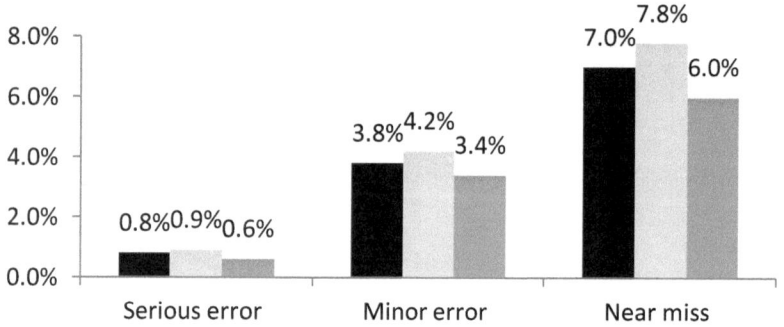

■ All (n=354)

Overall, German practitioners (n=354) estimated that 0.8 out of 100 patients in their area of practice will experience a serious error. Practitioners with up to 20 years of experience estimated the risk higher at 0.9 per 100 patients, while practitioners with more than 20 years of experience estimated that only 0.6 out of 100 patients will experience a serious error.

German practitioners estimated that 3.8 out of 100 patients will experience a minor error. Again, practitioners with up to 20 years of clinical experience estimated a higher risk (+0.8) for the patient than practitioners with more than 20 years of experience.

German practitioners estimated that 7 out of every 100 of patients in their area of practice would experience a near miss. In this category there is the biggest discrepancy between practitioners with up to 20 years of experience compared to those with more than 20 years (-1.8).

In general, German practitioners with more than 20 years of experience believed that the risk of patients experiencing any type of error is lower than their colleagues with less experience estimated it to be.

There were no such differences found when analysing the responses by profession. In relation to serious errors, surgeons estimated a higher risk for patients by 0.1 per 100 (0.9 v 0.8). The risk of a minor error was estimated to be the same by both professional groups (3.8). The estimated risk of experiencing a near miss differed by 0.3 percentage points between surgeons (6.8) and general practitioners (7.1).

Australian practitioners (n=24) estimated that for every 100 patients in their respective area of practice 2.4 will experience a serious error, 7 will experience a minor error and 6.8 will experience a near miss. Those estimates are significantly higher in relation to serious and minor errors than the estimates by German respondents.

German practitioners (n=354) believed that 8.3% of their peers will receive a complaint within the next year and 2.1% will be sued for malpractice or negligence. The numbers varied greatly between the professions. While general practitioners (n=315) believed that 6.4% of their peers would receive a complaint, surgeons (n=37) believed that almost a quarter (23.2%) of their peers would receive a complaint.

Similarly, general practitioners believed that the chance of a colleague being sued within the next year was 1.4%, while surgeons believed it would be as high as 7.8%. The risk of receiving a complaint was perceived to be four times higher for surgeons than for general practitioners. In relation to being sued, German surgeons believed it almost six times more likely than general practitioners that a peer would by sued.

Chart 3.3   *German practitioners' belief about proportion of their peers that*
                will receive a complaint or be sued in the next year

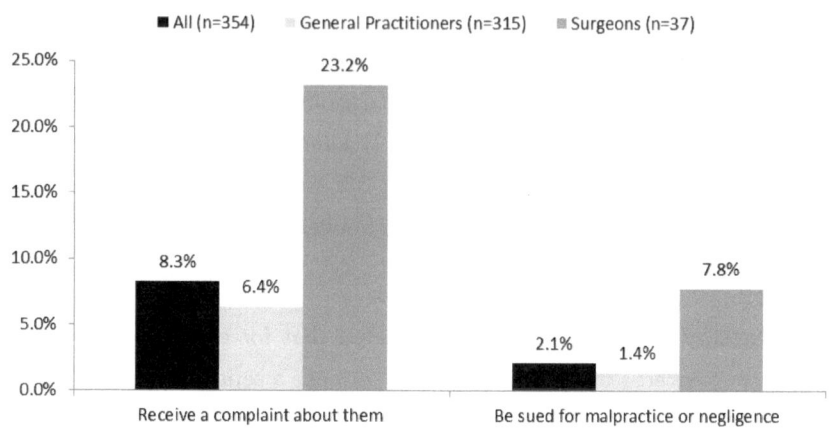

Australian respondents (n=24) believed that 19.5% of their colleagues would receive a complaint in the next year and that 8.2% would be sued. These are significantly higher estimates of the risk of receiving complaints or being sued compared to German respondents.

Notably, on average, German practitioners estimated their own risk to be higher than that of their peers. They believed that their own risk of receiving a complaint was 2.1 percentage points higher than for their peers, and the risk of being sued 0.7% higher than for their peers. Surgeons were the exception: They believed their own risk of being sued was 1.7% lower than that of their peers.

Chart 3.4   *German practitioners' belief about their own risk of receiving a*
complaint or being sued in the next year

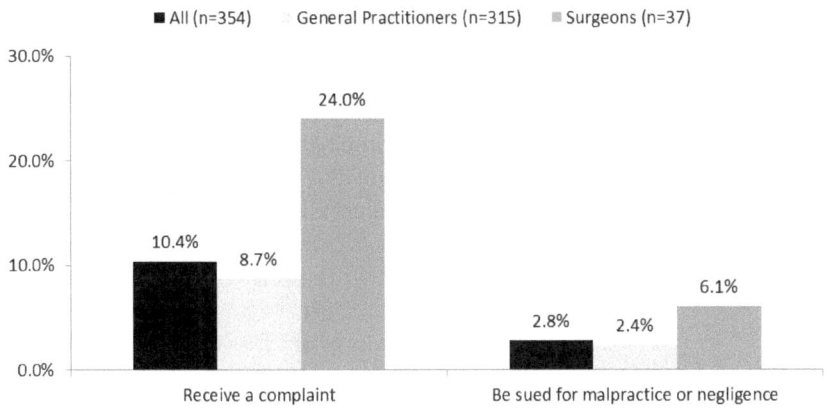

By comparison, Australian respondents estimated their own risk of receiving a complaint in the next year at 1.6%, and the risk of being sued at 5.9%. In contrast to German respondents, Australian respondents estimated their own risk to be lower than that of their peers. Significant is the difference in relation to complaints: Australian respondents believed that almost 20% of their peers would receive a complaint, but less than 2% of themselves.

Almost three quarters (71.1%) of the surveyed German practitioners (n=346) were of the opinion that the most likely cause of medical errors is a combination of system and individual failures. Almost one quarter (23.4%) nominated individual failure as the most likely cause. This compares with 98.8% of Australian respondents (n=24) nominating a combination of systemic and individual errors as the most likely cause of medical errors.

Chart 3.5   *German practitioners' belief about the most likely cause of medical errors (n=346)*

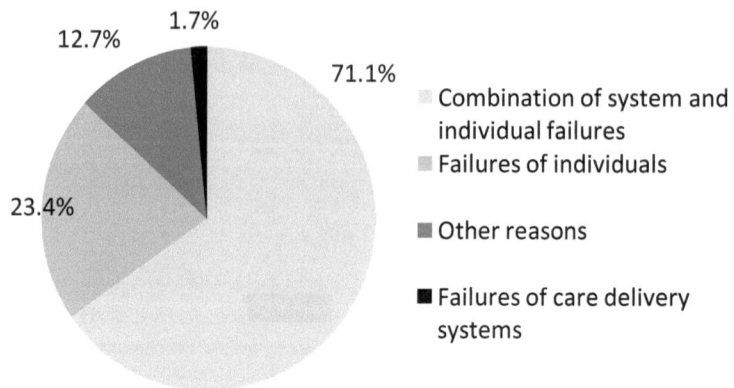

Some of the German respondents stated other reasons for medical errors, including stress, time and resource constraints, lack of communication and coordination between health services, as well as lack of patient compliance.

Practitioners also had the opportunity to make general comments about their attitude to medical errors. German practitioners noted a lack of transparency in dealing with medical errors, which would make it difficult to learn from errors. It was also mentioned that the perceived biased coverage of medical errors in the media and the perceived increase in patient claims were both reasons for the lack of transparency about medical errors. Comments from Australian respondents ranged from observing that medical errors are common, but mostly not serious, to the need to learn from mistakes and the opinion that the increasing fragmentation of medical service delivery increases the risk for errors. Another comment was that medical errors cause a minority of complaints and law suits.

3.6.2.1 Summary: General attitude about medical errors

German practitioners attributed a much higher significance to medical errors being a significant problem in health care provision than Australian respondents did, despite estimating the actual risk for serious errors and minor errors occurring to be much lower than their Australian counterparts did. German practitioners with more than 20 years of experience estimated the risk of errors occurring to be lower than less experienced practitioners did. This may indicate either a generational change in attitudes in that younger practitioners are more aware of the problem of medical errors, or it could indicate that practitioners believe that experience reduces the risk of medical errors, or it may indicate that with experience, medical practitioners may view the level of seriousness of certain errors differently.

Australian practitioners estimated their own or a colleague's risk of receiving a complaint or being sued as significantly higher than German practitioners. This may be a result of greater transparency of results, as medical court cases and disciplinary proceedings are regularly reported in the Australian media, but less commonly in Germany. German practitioners estimated the risk of surgeons being sued or complained about to be significantly higher than for general practitioners. This result accords with the analysis of patient claims made to German expert commissions instituted by the medical boards, which confirms that complaints about surgical procedures are the most common type of claim made by patients (Bundesärztekammer, 2013b).

In relation to the cause of medical errors, in both countries the vast majority of practitioners believed that a combination of individual and systemic failures cause medical errors. However, the proportion of German respondents who believed that errors are solely due to individual failures is significant while this belief is not shared among Australian respondents. The Australian result may be a reflection of the focus on creating a 'no blame' culture in the safety and quality discussions by concentrating on system failures as causes for patient incidents.

3.6.3   Communicating about medical errors with patients

The proportion of practitioners who supported the disclosure of an error grew with the increase in seriousness or severity of the error. Over 90% of German respondents supported disclosing serious errors (n=347) to patients, while only about one third (36.6%) agreed that near misses (n=353) should be disclosed to patients.

Chart 3.6   *German practitioners' opinion that errors should be disclosed to patients*

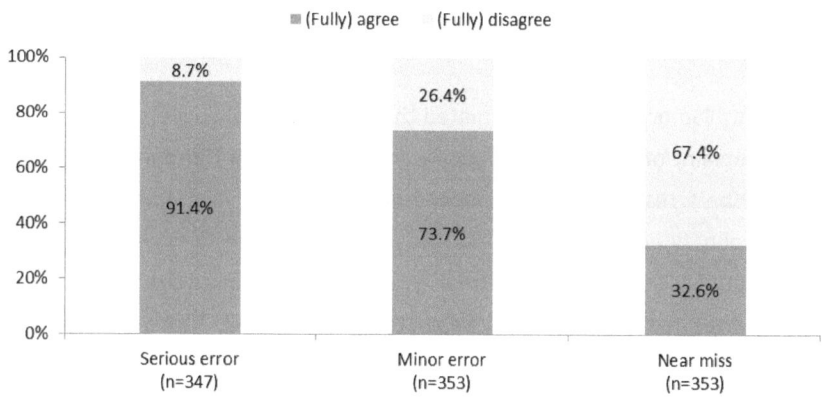

Australian respondents (n=24) showed higher rates of support for the disclosure of each type of error than the German respondents, with 95.8% supporting the disclosure of serious errors, 87.5% of minor errors and half (50%) of near misses.

Analysing the German responses by profession, length of clinical practice and gender highlight some differences. Surgeons tended to be less supportive of disclosure compared to general practitioners in relation to near misses (-3.1 percentage points) and minor errors (-4.7% percentage points). However, in relation to serious errors, it is the opposite, with 94.6% of surgeons (+3.7%

percentage points) agreeing that this type of error should be disclosed to the patient.

German practitioners with more than 30 years of experience were more willing to disclose near misses to patients than their colleagues with less experience. This difference is not noticeable in relation to minor errors. In comparison, in relation to serious errors, practitioners with less than 30 years of experience were more supportive of disclosure to the patient than their colleagues with more than 30 years of experience.

Analysing the preferences for disclosure by the gender of the practitioner, there is a trend among German female practitioners in general to being more supportive of disclosing medical errors. The difference in support compared to male practitioners increased with the seriousness of the error – from +0.5 percentage points for near misses, to +6.3 percentage points for minor errors and +7.1 percentage points for serious errors. Among Australian respondents, female practitioners were more supportive of the disclosure of near misses (+8.4 percentage points) and minor errors (+6.3 percentage points), but less supportive of the disclosure of serious errors (-9.1 percentage points) in comparison to male practitioners.

More than half of the German practitioners (55.0%, n=351) believe that disclosing a serious error to the patient would damage the patient's trust in their competence. Female practitioners (59.0%, n=188) were more likely to have this view than were their male colleagues (48.4%, n=153). Notably, a significantly higher proportion of general practitioners (56.6%, n=313) agreed with this statement in comparison to surgeons (41.7%, n=36). Analysing the responses by the length of clinical practice (n=340) shows that after an initial peak in the first three years of practice, practitioners with up to 15 years of clinical experience were less likely to agree than their peers that disclosing a serious error will damage the patient's trust in their competence.

Despite the view of the majority of the German practitioners that disclosing a serious error would damage the patient's trust in their skills, almost 60% (59.0%, n=351) thought that disclosing a serious error would make it less likely that the patient will make a complaint about them. The majority of practitioners (53.9%, n=349) also believed that it would be unlikely that the patient would sue them after they had disclosed a serious error.

Chart 3.7   *German practitioners' belief that disclosing a serious error would make it less likely that the patient would complain or sue (by length of clinical practice)*

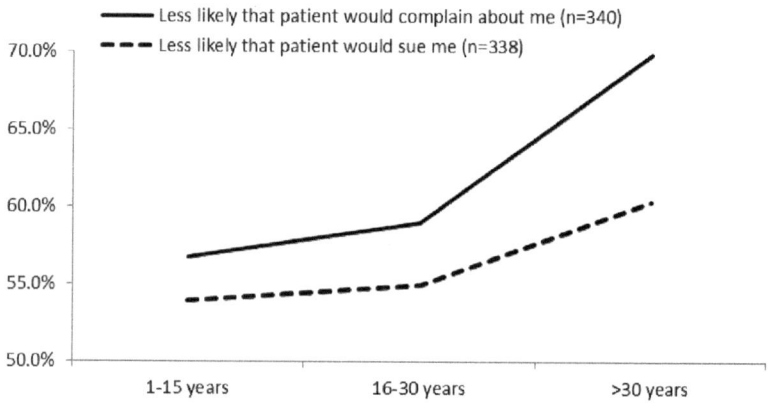

Of Australian respondents (n=24), one third believed that disclosing a serious error would damage the patient's trust in their competence, while two thirds (66.7%) did not think so. More than half (54.2%) believed that disclosing a serious error would make it less likely that the patient would complain and almost two thirds (62.5%) thought that disclosing such an error would make it less likely that the patient would sue.

Three quarters of the German practitioners (75.3%, n=336) stated that they would not disclose a serious error if they thought that the patient would not understand it. 43.5% would not disclose if they believed that the patient would not want to know about the error. Over one third (35.7%) would remain silent if the patient was unaware that an error had happened. Slightly less than one third (31.5%) would not disclose out of fear that they would be sued if they talked to the patient.

Chart 3.8   Factors nominated by German practitioners that would make it less likely that they would disclose a serious error to a patient (n=336)

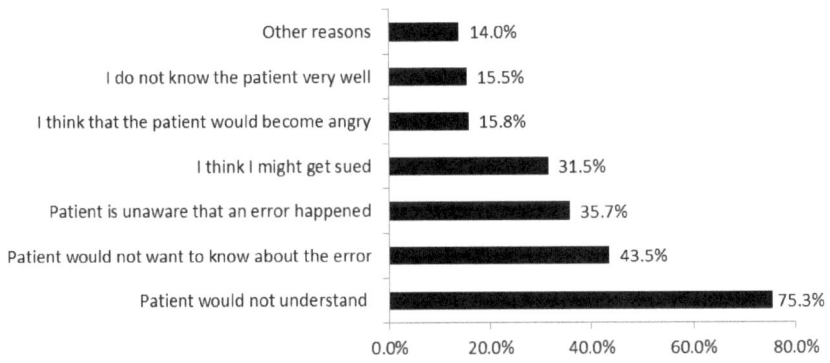

Other reasons — 14.0%
I do not know the patient very well — 15.5%
I think that the patient would become angry — 15.8%
I think I might get sued — 31.5%
Patient is unaware that an error happened — 35.7%
Patient would not want to know about the error — 43.5%
Patient would not understand — 75.3%

Other reasons stated by German respondents for not disclosing a serious error included that practitioners feared to lose their liability insurance cover; that the error did not have serious consequences for the patient; or that the patient has a terminal condition. Practitioners commented that the current legal environment and the position of the indemnity insurers would make it difficult to disclose serious errors. In particular, as at the time of the (potential) disclosure the final chain of causation is often not fully known, practitioners do not want to risk their insurance cover. The surveyed practitioners described a dilemma where on the one hand they are prohibited from disclosing an error by their indemnity insurer, and on the other hand, they feel that not disclosing the error would increase the risk of being sued. One practitioner commented that dealing with errors is always difficult, but self-respect and respecting the patient would mandate disclosing errors.

Similar to the German responses (75.3%), the most common reason Australian practitioners selected for not disclosing a serious error to patients was that they thought the patient would not understand (72.2%). This was followed by the thinking that the patient would not want to know (22.2%). Compared to German respondents, the same proportion of Australian respondents (16.7%) would not disclose a serious error because the patient was unaware of the error. Significantly fewer Australian (11.1%) than German (31.5%) practitioners would not disclose out of fear of being sued. Notably, a number of Australian practitioners specified they would always disclose, implying that none of the possible reasons would justify withholding disclosure from the patient. This was mirrored in the free comments practitioners made in relation to communication about medical errors with patients that overall showed support for open communication, but also linked the importance of communication after incidents to good communication with the patient before the incident.

3.6.3.1 Summary: Communicating about medical errors with patients

Overall, both German and Australian practitioners support disclosure, and their willingness to disclose increases with the seriousness of the error. There was a difference between respondents in both countries in relation to whether or not they believed that disclosing a serious error would damage the patient's trust in the practitioner. While the majority of German respondents thought it would affect the patient's trust, a minority of Australian practitioner shared this view. The majority of respondents in both countries believed that disclosing a serious error would make it less likely that the patient would make a complaint or sue them. Practitioners in both countries most commonly agreed that they may not disclose a serious error if they believed the patient would not understand. A significant proportion of German practitioners also thought that they would not disclose if they believed the patient would not want to know. This view was not shared by Australian practitioners.

3.6.4   Experience with medical errors

Almost three quarters of German practitioners (n=353) had experienced a near miss (74.5%) or minor error (69.7%). More than one quarter (27.8%) had experienced a serious error in their professional life, while 7.4% of practitioners stated that they had never been involved in any type of error; notably, those practitioners' experience in clinical practice ranged from two to 40 years.

Australian respondents also reported having been involved in near misses (66.7%) or minor errors (79.2%) in the past. Over half of these practitioners (54.2%) said that they had been involved in a serious error, which is double the proportion of the German practitioners.

3.6.4.1 Serious errors

Overall (n=336), one in five German practitioners (19.9%) had disclosed a serious error to a patient. This needs to be read in the context that about one quarter of German practitioners had experienced a serious error. Of the ones that had experienced a serious error, 61.9% had disclosed this to the patient. In addition, there were seven practitioners who had disclosed a serious error, although they had not been personally involved in a serious error, which suggests that they disclosed the error of another practitioner.

Of the Australian practitioners (n=23), 60.9% had disclosed a serious error in the past, of whom 21.4% had not been involved in the error themselves. Of the ones that had been involved in a serious error, 61.9% had disclosed the error to the patient.

Analysing the German responses by profession (n=334) shows that half of the surgeons among the respondents had already disclosed a serious error, while only 16.3% of general practitioners had. This is not unexpected given the nature of work in these professions and that it is more likely that serious errors are related to surgery. Looking solely at practitioners who had already been involved in a serious error, surgeons were much more likely to have disclosed the error to the patient (80.0%) than general practitioners (57.1%).

Chart 3.9   *Proportion of German practitioners who had been involved in a serious error and disclosed a serious error to the patient (by profession)*

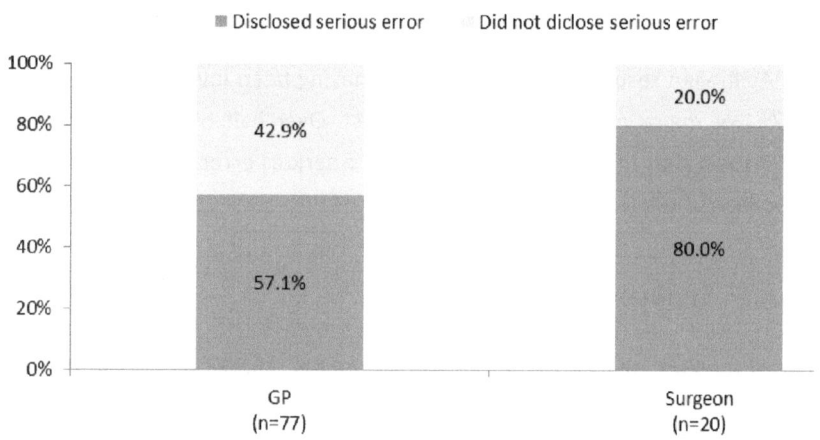

Of the German practitioners who had disclosed a serious error, over three quarters (76.6%) were satisfied with the disclosure conversation (n=64). For 42.2% (n=64) of these practitioners, the disclosure had a positive effect on their relationship with the patient. Another quarter (25.0%) stated that the disclosure had had no effect on their relationship with the patient. One third reported negative consequences from the disclosure (n=64). More than three quarters of German practitioners (76.9%, n=65) who had disclosed a serious error felt relieved after disclosing it to the patient.

All of the Australian respondents who had disclosed an error (n=13) were satisfied with their conversation with the patient. Over half of the Australian practitioners (53.9%) reported that the disclosure had a negative impact on their relationship with the patient, 38.5% reported no change and 7.7% said it had a positive effect. Almost two thirds (64.3%, n=14) were relieved after the disclosure.

3.6.4.2 Minor errors

Overall, three quarters of the German practitioners (n=345) had disclosed a minor error to a patient. There were six practitioners who had disclosed a minor error to the patient although not being involved in this type of error. Of the German practitioners who had been involved in a minor error (n=245), 88.6% had disclosed it. There was no such difference in disclosure rates across professions as had been the case for serious errors. 89.3% of general practitioners and 86.2% of surgeons who had been involved in minor errors did disclose them to the patient.

The vast majority of German practitioners who disclosed a minor error (88.5%, n=251) were satisfied with the disclosure conversation. A similarly high proportion (85.3%, n=251) felt relieved after they had spoken to the patient. Almost half of the practitioners (49.0%, n=251) stated that disclosing the error had had a positive impact on their relationship with the patient. An additional 41.8% of practitioners reported that the disclosure made no difference to the relationship. For less than one in ten practitioners (9.2%) the disclosure had a negative impact on their relationship with the patient.

In general, male practitioners tended more often to disclose serious (+14.5 percentage points) or minor (+9.7 percentage points) errors than their female colleagues did.

Among Australian respondents, 87.5% had disclosed a minor error to a patient in the past, with 14.3% of these disclosures related to errors the relevant practitioner had not been involved in. Where a practitioner had been involved in a minor error (n=19), 94.7% had disclosed the error to the patient. A high proportion of Australian practitioners (84.2%) who had disclosed a minor error were satisfied with how the disclosure conversation went. No respondent (n=20) reported any negative impact the disclosure had on their relationship with the patient, while the majority (65.0%) reported no change. However, some (35.0%) said that it had a positive effect on their relationship with the patient. In relation to minor errors, 85.0% of the practitioners (n=20) experienced relief after disclosing the error to the patient.

German practitioners commented in relation to their experience with medical errors that disclosure was desirable, but at the same time named several barriers that they perceived prevented them or other practitioners in general from disclosing errors to patients. These barriers included: the position of the indemnity insurers; the fear that the patient would sue after the apology for financial reasons; the awkwardness if the patient remains under their care; the difficulty in deciding which information is relevant to be disclosed to the patient; and the reaction of peers and supervisors, even if the patient appreciated the disclosure.

Australian practitioners commented that although they felt a responsibility to disclose, they experienced mixed emotions when disclosing errors and that the sense of relief was in comparison to non-disclosing, rather than actual relief.

3.6.4.3 Summary: Experience with medical errors

Involvement in minor errors and near misses were common among all practitioners. Australian practitioners reported much higher involvement in serious errors than German respondents. This may be due to their work environment, as a greater number of Australian respondents worked in public hospitals where the potential for serious errors due to the fragmentation of care and the seriousness of conditions treated is higher. In comparison, the vast majority of German respondents were sole general practitioners. This may also explain the smaller proportion of German practitioners who had ever disclosed a serious error compared to Australian respondents. Notably, the proportion of practitioners who both had been involved in a serious error and had subsequently disclosed the error was comparable in both countries, although significantly lower than the proportion who had supported disclosure of serious errors in general. There was a difference in the effect the disclosure had on the relationship with the patient, which was described more positively by German respondents, compared to Australian respondents. Despite this difference there was similarity in the high proportion of practitioners who felt relief after the disclosure, suggesting that even where the patient's reaction may have been negative, the practitioner felt relieved.

In relation to minor errors, actual disclosure rates by practitioners who had been involved in a minor error and who disclosed it to the patient were high among respondents from both countries. High levels of satisfaction with the disclosure conversation, the level of neutral or positive effects it had on the relationship with the patients, and a high proportion of practitioners who felt relief after the disclosure, were reported by respondents from both countries.

Among both groups there was a small number of practitioners who had disclosed an error they were not involved in, suggesting that they took the responsibility for disclosure although another provider had actually caused the error.

There was a difference in comments made by practitioners, with German practitioners raising what they perceived were barriers to disclosure, while Australian comments focussed on the emotional impact of disclosure.

3.6.5   Dealing with medical errors

Almost 90% (89.6%, n=354) of the German practitioners stated that they had never been trained in how to communicate about medical errors with patients. A similar high proportion of these practitioners would be interested in disclosure training (88.4%, n=353) or being supported by an expert in disclosure communication immediately after an incident (90.6%, n=351). Practitioners who had attended training in disclosure communication in the past stated that, on average, the last training was 7.5 years ago (n=34).

In comparison, 62.5% of the Australian practitioners (n=24) had received education on disclosing errors in the past, on average 6.5 years ago. Also, 79.2% of the Australian practitioners (n=24) would be interested in general education and training on disclosure and 91.7% indicated that they would welcome support by a disclosure expert after an incident.

When disclosing a serious error, German practitioners overall (n=351) reported that they would seek support most commonly from their indemnity insurer (50.7%), the medical board (50.4%) and/or a lawyer (48.4%), while 44.7% would seek the support of colleagues and peers or from professional bodies such as their College or association (31.3%). About a quarter of practitioners (27.4%) would talk to their family or friends when disclosing an error. Only 4.0% would not seek any support when disclosing a serious error. There are some notable differences in the responses from German practitioners when analysed by profession, as Chart 3.10 illustrates.

Chart 3.10   German practitioners' sources of support when disclosing a seri-ous error (n=349)

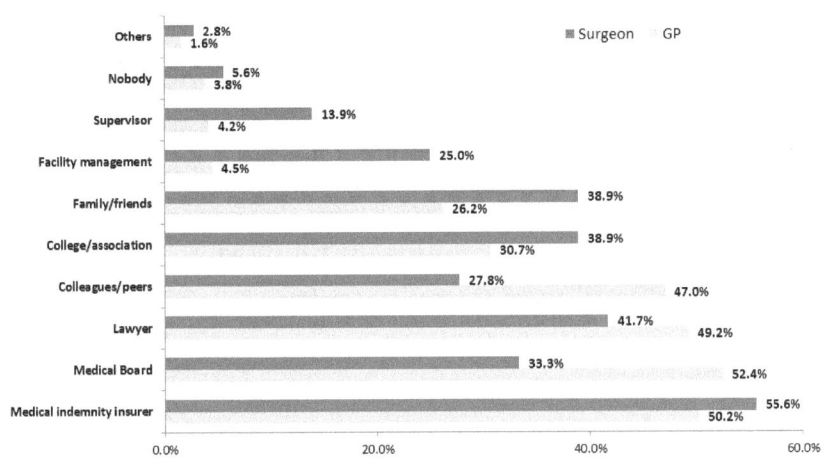

It appears that German surgeons (n=36) would be more likely to seek sup-port from different channels compared to the general practitioners (n=313). About one quarter of surgeons (27.8%) would seek the support of colleagues when disclosing an error, compared to almost half (47.0%) of general practi-tioners. Similarly, surgeons (33.3%) were less likely to approach the medical board for support than general practitioners (52.4%). More than half of German practitioners, both surgeons (55.6%) and general practitioners (50.2%), would seek support from their medical indemnity insurer when disclosing an error.

In comparison, the majority of Australian respondents (n=24) would seek support from their medical indemnity insurer (50.7%) or medical board (50.4%), followed by approaching a lawyer (48.4%), or colleagues and peers (44.7%). About one third would seek support from their professional college or associa-tion, and just over one quarter from family and friends. Least commonly, Aus-tralian respondents would seek help in dealing with disclosure from the man-agement of the health care facility they worked at.

3.6.5.1 Impact of serious errors

In response to the question of how a serious error had impacted on the practitioner, most commonly, German respondents (n=316) were anxious about future errors (42.1%). A similarly high proportion of practitioners had experienced
sleep problems (39.6%) and almost one in three practitioners (32.0%) stated
that the error had impacted on their confidence in their own skills. For almost a
quarter of the surveyed practitioners (23.4%), the error had negatively impacted on their job satisfaction. Only 4.1% said that the error impacted on their
professional reputation. Notably, almost one in five practitioners (18.4%) stated
that the error had no impact on any area of their life.

*Chart 3.11   Areas of life that German practitioners perceived were negative-
ly impacted after having been involved in an error (n=316)*

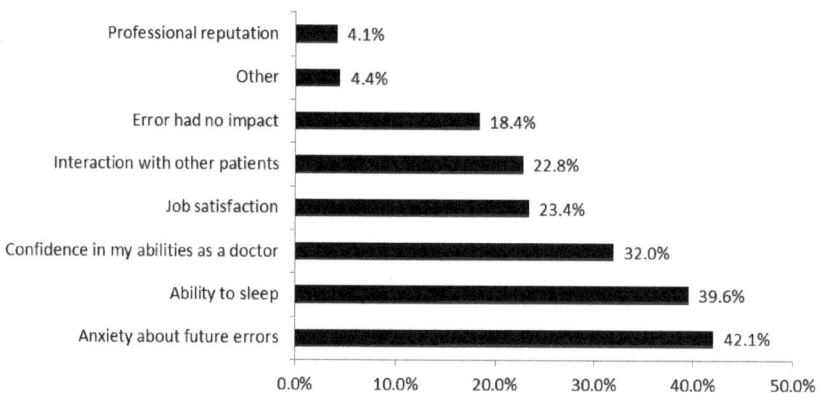

Among Australian respondents (n=24), the order of the different types of
impact an error had on them was overall the same as among German respondents, but the proportion who reported being anxious about future errors
(70.8%) was much higher than among German respondents. Similarly, the proportion of Australian practitioners reporting an impact on their ability to sleep
(54.2%), and their confidence in their abilities as a practitioner (58.3%) was
higher than among German respondents. Respondents also commonly reported

an impact on their job satisfaction (37.5%) and their interaction with other patients (29.2%). For 8.3% of respondents the error had no impact, while for 4.2%,
the error had impacted on their professional reputation.

Of the German practitioners (n=349) 80.5% would be interested in having
access to counselling if they were involved in a serious error, and female practitioners (88.7%) appear to be more interested in having access to counselling
after serious errors than their male colleagues (69.3%) (n=339). Only 1.7% of
the German practitioners had already had access to counselling.

Of the Australian practitioners (n=24) 78.3% were interested in counselling
after serious medical errors and 4.4% already had access to such counselling.

*Chart 3.12   Reasons nominated by German practitioners that would prevent
them from seeking counselling (n=342)*

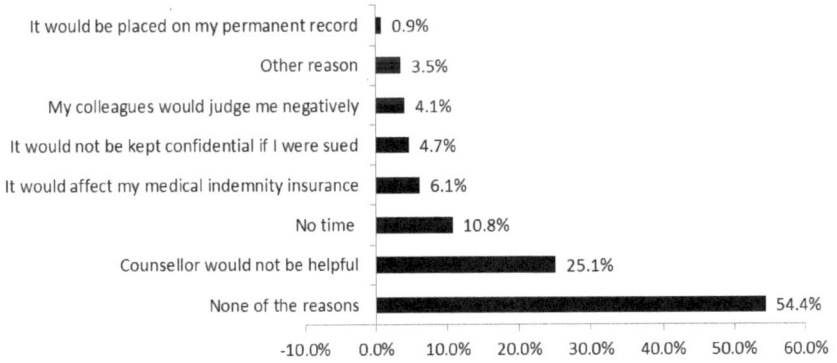

More than half of the German practitioners (54.4%) stated that there
would be no reasons that would prevent them from seeking counselling
(n=342). However, a quarter (25.1%) would not seek counselling, because they
believe that it would not be helpful. Other reasons that would prevent German
practitioners from seeking counselling included: they do not want to take time
away from their work (10.1%); they fear that it could affect their indemnity
insurance cover (6.1%); they fear that it would not remain confidential in case

they were sued (4.7%); or they believe that their colleagues would judge them negatively (4.1%).

Of Australian respondents (n=24), 29.2% would not seek counselling, believing that it would not be helpful. One quarter (25.0%) would not want to take time off work and 16.7% feared that seeking counselling could affect their medical indemnity insurance cover. Another 12.5% had concerns that it would be placed on their permanent record, or that it would not be kept confidential in the case of the patient suing them.

The surveyed practitioners had the opportunity to comment on dealing with medical errors. Analysing the comments of German respondents, two opposite views emerged: One view suggested that a more transparent approach to medical errors would be positive and that they would like to see the topic discussed as part of university training or continuing professional development. The other view that crystallised in the comments suggested that dealing with medical errors is a normal part of a practitioner's professional life and thus practitioners should be able to deal with errors without the need to seek help or support. Notably, the comments belonging to the first group that supports a more open approach and more communication about errors were all from female practitioners. Australian practitioners' comments included the observation that counselling was not available when the error occurred but would certainly have been helpful, while one made a reference to the coaching system at Harvard hospitals in Boston. Another comment suggested that medical errors are a part of professional life, and practitioners are being paid well to be able to deal with them.

3.6.5.2 Summary: Dealing with medical errors

While there is a significant difference in the proportion of practitioners in both countries who received training in how to deal with incidents and how to disclose them to patients, the majority of practitioners from both countries were interested in receiving future training and almost all wished to have access to a disclosure communication specialist directly after a serious incident happened.

Practitioners in both countries would seek support primarily from indemnity insurers, their registration authority and/or lawyers. This may be an indication of a shared legalistic and defensive approach to disclosing errors.

In relation to the impact a serious error had on the practitioner, practitioners in both countries most commonly reported being anxious about future errors; experiencing sleep problems; and experiencing a decreased confidence in their own skills. However, the proportion of Australian practitioners who had experienced such impacts was much higher than of German practitioners.

Most practitioners in both countries were interested in having access to counselling after serious errors and only a very small number in both countries reported that they already had access to such support. Barriers to seeking counselling most commonly related to personal reasons such as the belief it would not be helpful rather than being anxious that it may impact on their insurance cover or career.

Some practitioners in both countries commented that dealing with errors is part of professional life, while others were supportive of a more transparent and open approach to dealing with serious errors.

3.6.6 Communicating about medical errors with others

3.6.6.1 Disclosing errors to hospitals and health care organisations

Serious errors

Overall, 93.7% of German practitioners (n=348) agreed (66.4%) or strongly agreed (27.3%) that to improve patient safety, practitioners should report serious errors to their hospital or health care organisation. Of the Australian respondents (n=24), overall 87.5% agreed that practitioners should report serious errors to their hospital or facility.

Analysing the German responses by profession (n=346), a difference in the proportion of those who agree compared to those who strongly agree appears. While the distribution among general practitioners is close to the overall distribution, among surgeons 48.6% agree and 43.2% strongly agree that serious errors should be disclosed to the hospital or health care facility.

Analysing the German responses by the length of clinical practice (n=338), it appears that the longer clinicians were practising, the less likely they were to agree that disclosure of serious errors to their hospital or health care facility would enhance patient safety. No such distribution occurred in the Australian responses.

Chart 3.13   *Proportion of German practitioners who (strongly) agree that serious errors should be disclosed to their hospital or health care organisation to enhance patient safety (by length of clinical practice) (n=338)*

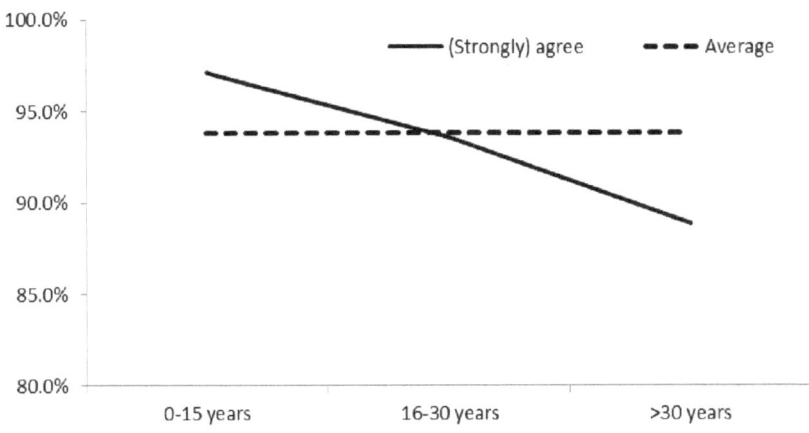

Minor errors

In relation to disclosing minor errors to the hospital or health care organisation to enhance patient safety, 64.5% of the German practitioners (n=347) and 66.7% of the Australian practitioners (n=24) agreed that this should be done.

Analysing the responses by the length of clinical practice, among German respondents (n=336) the lowest rate of support for disclosing minor errors was found in the group of practitioners with 16-30 years of practice (58.8%), while 72.1% of practitioners with less time in medical practice support it, as did 66.1% of practitioners with more than 30 years of practice.

Chart 3.14   *Proportion of German practitioners who (strongly) agree that minor errors should be disclosed to their hospital or health care organisation to enhance patient safety (by length of clinical practice) (n=336)*

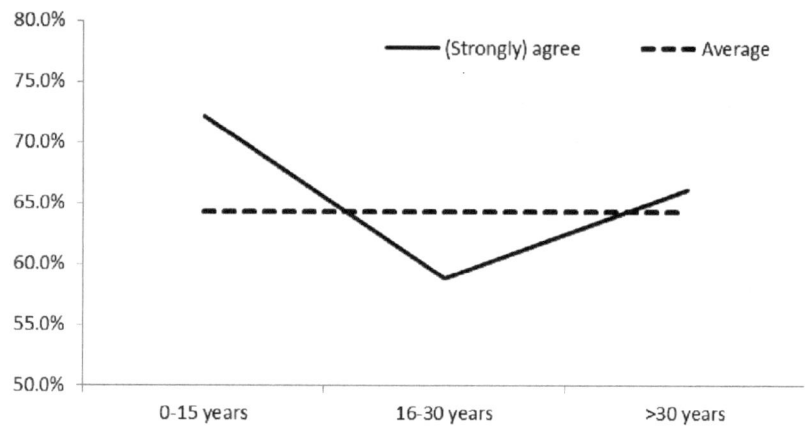

Female German practitioners (67.2%) were slightly more supportive of disclosing minor errors to the hospital or health care facility than their male colleagues (60.9%) (n=337).

3.6.6.2 Disclosing errors to colleagues

Serious errors

Overall, 90.6% of the German practitioners agree (62.2%) or strongly agree (28.4%) that serious errors should be discussed with colleagues to improve patient safety (n=352). As described above, a similar proportion of practitioners (91.4%) had agreed (58.8%) or strongly agreed (32.6%) that serious errors should be disclosed to patients (n=347). Of the Australian respondents (n=24), overall 95.8% agreed (45.8%) or strongly agreed (50.0%) to disclosing errors to colleagues.

Analysing the German responses by gender, female practitioners are slightly more supportive of discussing serious errors with colleagues, with 92.6% agreeing with this statement compared to 89.5% of male practitioners (n=342). A difference appeared between the professions, with 97.3% of surgeons supporting discussing serious errors with colleagues to enhance patient safety, compared to 90.1% of general practitioners (n=350).

There were inconclusive results when analysing the German responses by the length of clinical practice of the surveyed practitioners. The most supportive group among German respondents were practitioners with up to 15 years of experience (94.2%); the least supportive group were practitioners with 16-30 years experience, while 92.1% of practitioners with more than 30 years experience supported discussions with colleagues (n=341).

German practitioners working in sole practices were the least supportive of discussing serious errors with colleagues to improve patient safety, with 88.8% supporting it, compared to 100% of practitioners working in private or public hospitals, and 95.4% of practitioners working in shared practices (n=346).

Minor errors

Overall, 80.4% of the German practitioners (n=352) agreed (62.2%) or strongly agreed (18.2%) that minor errors should be discussed with their colleagues to improve patient safety. This result can be placed in the context that 73.7% of these practitioners had supported disclosing minor errors to patients, and 64.8% would disclose a minor error to the hospital or facility. When discussing minor errors with colleagues, there was no significant difference in support among female (81.2%) and male (80.1%) practitioners (n=342).

By comparison, 95.8% of the Australian respondents (n=24) agreed (70.8%) or strongly agreed (25.0%) that minor errors should be discussed with their colleagues to improve patient safety.

Chart 3.15   *Proportion of German practitioners who (strongly) agree to disclose errors to colleagues to enhance patient safety (by profession) (n=350)*

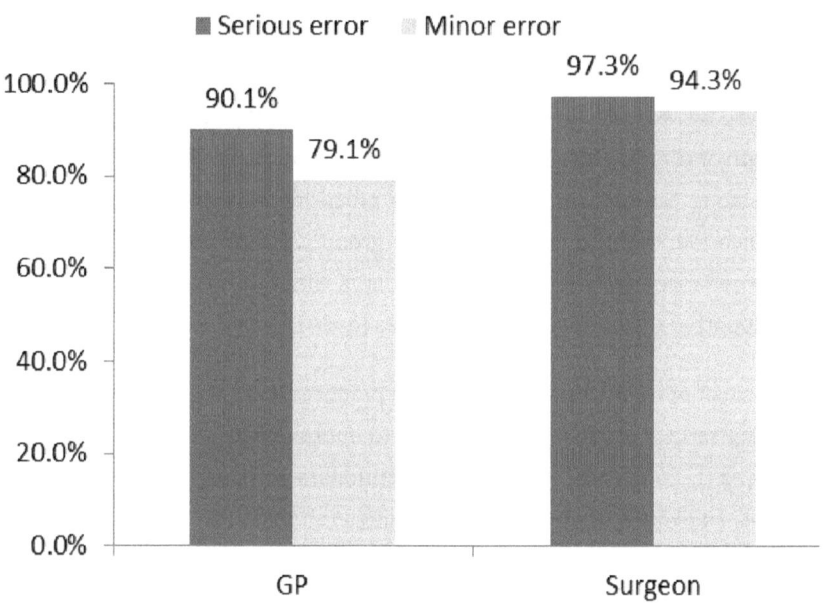

Analysing the German responses by profession (n=350), a difference between the professions emerged, with 94.3% of surgeons stating that minor errors should be discussed with colleagues to enhance patient safety, while only 79.1% of general practitioners agreed. Overall, surgeons were more likely to discuss both serious and minor errors with colleagues than general practitioners. There was no clear trend in relation to the willingness to discuss minor errors with colleagues when taking into account the time the practitioner had practised (n=341).

Similar to the results for disclosing serious errors, in relation to discussing minor errors with colleagues (n=346), German general practitioners working in sole practices were less likely to discuss minor errors with colleagues (79.5%)

than practitioners working in shared practices (82.8%) or public hospitals (87.5%).

3.6.6.3 Action taken when disclosing errors in the past

Disclosing their own error

When German practitioners were asked what action, if any, they had taken in the past when disclosing their own error (n=286), half of the practitioners had told their colleague (52.1%) and over one fifth (22.7%) had disclosed it to the patient and/or their family. 10.1% of practitioners had informed their medical indemnity insurance, and 7.3% had disclosed the error to their supervisors. 6.3% of respondents wrote a report and 2.1% told the management of the hospital or facility. 3.5% of respondents took other steps, including documenting the error in the patient's medical records, talking to the practitioner's own family, or reflecting on their own mistake. German practitioners reported taking action mostly in relation to near misses.

Focusing on those German practitioners who had been involved in a serious error (n=98), half of these practitioners (50%) had told a colleague about the error; 17.3% disclosed the error to the patient and/or the patient's family; 12.2% informed their medical indemnity insurer; and 10.2% told their supervisor. 6.1% of these practitioners wrote an incident report, 3.1 % told their management and 2.0% took other action. There is a discrepancy here with the results to an earlier question to which 61.9% of German practitioners who had experienced a serious error stated that they had disclosed the error to the patient or the patient's family.

In contrast, of the Australian practitioners who had been involved in serious errors, 61.9% had stated earlier in the survey that they had disclosed the error to the patient. When asked what action they took when disclosing serious errors (n=13), most had notified their medical indemnity insurer (69.2%), told their colleague (61.5%), or made an incident report (61.5%). Just under half

(46.2%) of these practitioners had told the patient or the patient's family about the serious error and about one third (30.8%) told an executive of the hospital or health organisation. The discrepancy in the proportion who said that they had disclosed the error to patients was less among Australian practitioners than among German practitioners.

As a result of the action taken in relation to their own error, German practitioners described a broad and mixed range of positive and negative outcomes. Notably, the majority of comments about the outcomes of their action related to practitioners who had discussed the error with their colleagues. Among these, they commented that the discussion with their colleagues helped analysing the causes of the error, provided feedback on the practitioner's perception of the severity of the error and ways it could or could not have been prevented. Overall, talking to colleagues appeared to be the most common action taken. It was used to validate the practitioner's own analysis and interpretation of the error, helped them in finding solutions or prepared them for disclosing the error to the patient or facing a legal claim. In comments, discussions with colleagues were described as a learning tool.

Of the practitioners who had told the patient or their family about their error, most commented that they experienced understanding and positive feedback from the patient or family. Overall, only a few comments described a negative outcome, for example, that the patient did not wish to see the practitioner again and moved to another doctor. Three of the Australian respondents stated that the error led to litigation.

Of the practitioners who had reported the error either to management or their supervisors, most reported a positive outcome, mainly that causes were analysed. In this group, two comments from German practitioners stood out: One practitioner reported that when they informed their supervisor, the supervisor advised the practitioner to remain silent about the error. Despite this advice, the practitioner informed the management, who together with the practitioner then proceeded to inform the patient. Another comment described the experience of the practitioner who when admitting an error was accused of incompetence by their supervisor in front of other staff.

Disclosing a colleague's error

In relation to an error caused by another practitioner, over two thirds of German practitioners (n=152) discussed the error either with the responsible practitioner (29.5%) and/or another practitioner (40.2%).

Chart 3.16   Action taken by German practitioners after own and other practitioners' errors

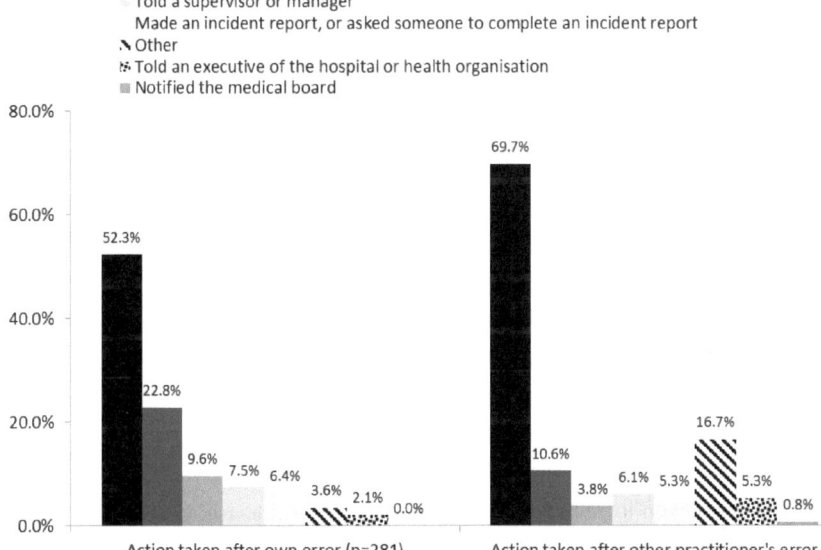

The above chart illustrates the difference in action taken by German practitioners depending on whether it was the practitioner's own fault, or whether they became aware of an error that was caused by another practitioner.

In both situations, talking to a (or the responsible) colleague was the most common action taken in response to becoming aware of the error. Most notable is the difference in the number of practitioners who disclosed the error to the patient and their families: while almost one quarter of practitioners discussed their own error with the patient, only one in ten did so in relation to an error caused by another practitioner. A considerable proportion of practitioners who became aware of an error caused by another practitioner responded that they did not take any action. Practitioners who either had talked to the responsible colleague or another of their colleagues overwhelmingly commented that it had helped them to analyse the error and learn from it. Interestingly, the error being a learning opportunity was commented on independently whether the error was caused by the surveyed practitioner or someone else.

Australian practitioners were more specifically asked about the action taken in relation to a *serious* error by another practitioner with 80% (n=15) telling a/or the responsible colleague. Just under half of those practitioners (46.7%) made an incident report and one third (33.3%) told their supervisor. Just over a quarter (26.7%) of practitioners told the patient or the patient's family, the same proportion of practitioners notified the medical indemnity insurance. 20.0% informed the hospital management. In contrast to action taken after serious errors they themselves were involved in, Australian practitioners less commonly told the patient and their family, but more commonly told a supervisor or manager.

A few of the German practitioners commented on negative outcomes of their action taken in relation to a colleague's error, including that the responsible practitioner stopped referring patients to the surveyed practitioner after being made aware of their error. In the overall comments made regarding communicating about medical errors with others, practitioners showed a wish for and willingness to be part of a more transparent and constructive handling of errors. One comment specifically stated that talking about the error with others is essential to regain professional confidence. Another practitioner noted that the currently existing structures in the primary and secondary health care sector were not supportive of a transparent and constructive discussion and handling of errors.

Some Australian practitioners commented that as a result of their disclosure of errors, the relevant practitioner was trained, and changes made to processes. However, some commented that there was no change or that management did not take any action against the practitioner.

3.6.6.4 Summary: Communicating about medical errors with others

Overall, there is a high level of support among practitioners in both countries for the disclosure of serious errors to hospital management to enhance patient safety and the majority of practitioners support the disclosure of minor errors. There is a slight tendency of surgeons overall being more supportive of disclosure, but the support for disclosing errors decreases slightly with the length of practice, which may suggest a certain level of disillusionment with the action taken or lack of action by hospital management in the past in response to disclosure.

There is also a high level of support for disclosing errors to peers to enhance patient safety, and practitioners in public hospitals appear to be most supportive. Australian respondents supported the disclosure of minor errors to colleagues more strongly than their German counterparts.

Amid these high levels of support for disclosure of errors to enhance patient safety, and in principle, support for disclosure of errors to patients, when listing actual action taken in the past in response to their own or another practitioner's error, disclosure to patient and their families was much less common. This may partly be explained by the fact that although practitioners were able to select multiple responses regarding what actions were taken after a medical error, some might only have selected the most important action they took in response to an error. Overall, the action taken after errors concentrated on internal and inter-professional avenues of disclosure and much less commonly included external disclosure to patients or external bodies. There appeared to be a discrepancy between the practitioners' wish for more transparent handling of errors and the actual action taken in reality.

3.6.7   Receiving information about medical errors

The survey also inquired about practitioners' current and preferred avenues to access information about medical errors.

Following the assumption that reliable information about errors can only be provided if errors are routinely reported, practitioners were asked which features a reporting system should possess to increase their willingness to report errors to improve patient safety.

German respondents (n=340) most commonly sought a reporting system to be inaccessible to lawyers (65.3%); allowing anonymous reporting (61.8%); and that there are no negative consequences (61.5%) for both the reporting and involved practitioners. Around half of the German practitioners also found it important that the reporting system would be accessible and easy to use (52.9%) and that there would be evidence that the reports are actually used for quality improvements (49.4%). Some practitioners commented that they wanted a system to be directly accessible by practitioners, but not accessible by authorities.

Chart 3.17   Features of a reporting system that would increase German practitioners' willingness to report errors to improve patient safety (n=340)

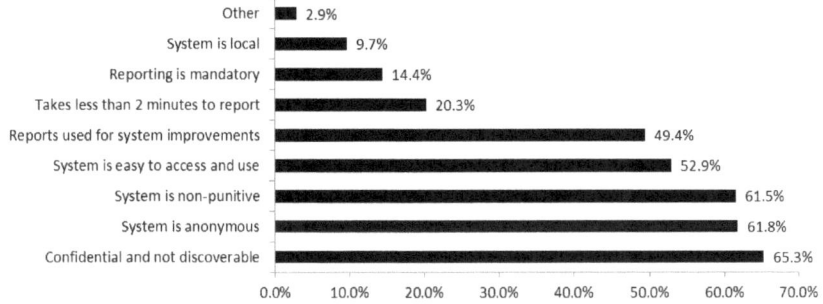

For Australian respondents (n=22), it was equally most important (81.8%) that the reporting system would be easy to access and use, non-punitive and that there would be evidence that the information was actually being used for quality and safety improvements. Almost two thirds of Australian respondents (63.6%) preferred the reported information to be confidential and inaccessible to lawyers. Half of practitioners stated that they would appreciate the reporting to take less than two minutes. The proportion of Australian practitioners preferring an anonymous system (40.9%) was lower than for German respondents (61.8%). Notably, almost one in four of the Australian respondents (22.7%) stated that mandatory reporting requirement would increase their willingness to report, which is a higher proportion than for German respondents (14.4%).

Overwhelmingly, both German (n=351, 90.6%) and Australian practitioners (n=24, 95.8%) agreed that to improve patient safety, they needed to know about medical errors that occur in their hospital or health organisation.

There appeared to be a difference between the current sources of information about medical errors and the source that practitioners would prefer, as illustrated in Chart 3.18.

Chart 3.18   *Current and preferred source of information about medical errors*

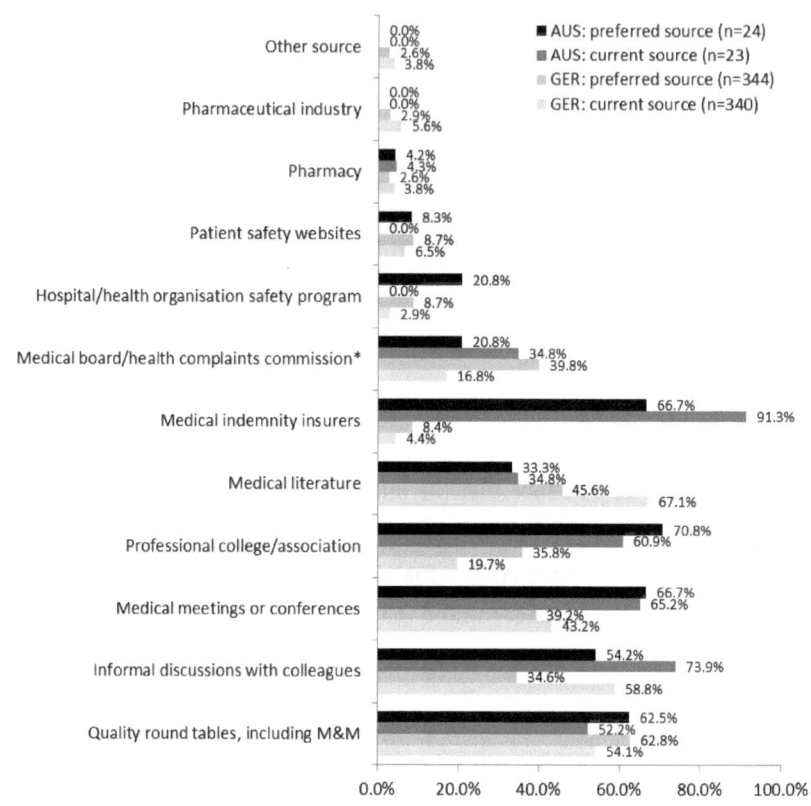

*applies to Australian surveys only

Looking at preferred sources of information about medical errors overall, Australian practitioners nominated more sources from which to receive information than their German counterparts. There appears to be a preference to receive such information from professional peers or bodies. In particular, quality roundtables and morbidity reviews (GER: 62.8% / AUS: 62.5%) were named, as well as the medical board (GER: 39.8% / AUS: 20.8%), medical meetings and conferences (GER: 39.2% / AUS: 66.7%) and professional colleges and associations (GER: 35.8% / AUS: 70.8%). A notable difference existed between German and Australian practitioners' preferences to receive such information from indemnity insurers, with 8.4% of German respondents preferring it as a source of information compared to 66.7% of Australian practitioners. However, the proportion of German practitioners currently receiving such information from indemnity insurers was at a low level (4.4%) compared to a high level of 91.3% among Australian respondents.

The biggest potential for German sources of information, calculated as the difference between current and preferred sources of information about medical errors, was accorded to the medical board (+23.0 percentage points), professional colleges and associations (+16.1 percentage points) and quality rounds and tables (+8.7 percentage points). The greatest discrepancy among the German responses was recorded in relation to discussions with colleagues, which were currently named as the second most common source of information about medical errors (58.8%), but were nominated as the preferred source by only a third of German practitioners (34.6%; -24.2 percentage points). The second greatest discrepancy between current and preferred source of information about medical errors was recorded in relation to medical literature, which currently was named the most common way for German practitioners to inform themselves about medical errors (67.1%), but was the preferred source for only 45.6% (-21.5 percentage points) of surveyed German practitioners.

The biggest potential for Australian sources was recorded in regard to information provided by hospital safety programs, from which none of the respondents currently received information, but one in five (20.8%) would prefer in the future. In comparison, Australian practitioners preferred less information from medico-legal (-24.6 percentage points) and regulatory bodies (-14.0 percentage points) about medical errors in the future.

Peer-based sources, including medical meetings and conferences, quality round tables and professional associations, appear to be the overall preferred sources of information about medical errors for practitioners from both countries.

When asked whether the current ways of informing practitioners about medical errors were adequate, over two thirds (67.1%) of German practitioners (n=346) and 52.2% of Australian practitioners (n=23) (strongly) disagreed.

When asked what type of information practitioners would like to receive about errors, 86.9% of German practitioners (n=350) and 79.2% of Australian practitioners (n=24) wanted information about how to prevent common serious errors. The demand for information about preventative measures was higher than information on past errors.

A similar picture emerged in relation to practitioners' preference regarding information about minor errors, with 60.4% of the German respondents (n=351) and 70.8% of Australian respondents (n=24) preferring information about how to prevent these types of error. Practitioners also appeared to be interested in information about serious (GER: 56.6% / AUS: 66.7%) and minor (GER: 47.9% / AUS: 62.5%) errors that affect their own patients.

There was overall slightly less interest in receiving information about serious or minor errors affecting patients such as theirs or in regard to all patients. Notably, 2.9% of German practitioners did not want any information about serious errors and 10.5% (AUS: 4.2%) did not want any information about minor errors.

When given the opportunity to add further comments in relation to receiving information about medical errors, some of the German practitioners stated that they supported an open and transparent handling of medical errors. In the comments, practitioners noted that for a transparent discussion about medical errors, meetings or organisations at a professional level would be more appropriate and thus more acceptable to practitioners, than discussions in the media, general public or through the legal system and bodies.

3.6.7.1 Summary: Receiving information about medical errors

Practitioners' willingness to report errors was supported by reporting systems that were convenient, confidential and non-punitive. Specifically for Australian practitioners it was very important that there was evidence that the reported information was actually being used for quality and safety improvements. Almost all practitioners agreed that to improve patient safety, they must be aware of errors in their work environment.

In relation to sources of information about medical errors, overall peer-based bodies or mechanisms appeared to have the greatest relevance for practitioners in both countries. There was a notable difference in medico-legal and regulatory bodies being a current or preferred source of information, suggesting that Australian practitioners much more commonly receive information about medical errors from these bodies than their German counterparts.

Questioned about what type of information about medical errors would be most relevant to practitioners, responses from both countries showed similar results with a clear preference for information about error prevention.

3.6.8 Summary: Medical practitioners' attitudes to and experiences of medical errors

The survey revealed that medical errors are considered significant in the professional life of medical practitioners, although more significant to German practitioners. Amid medical errors being less often and less openly discussed in Germany, German practitioners estimated errors to occur less often than Australian practitioners.

In both countries, practitioners see a combination of individual and systemic failures as the main cause of medical errors, although the proportion of German practitioners attributing errors primarily to personal failures is significantly higher than of Australian respondents, which may indicate a difference in the safety culture that has largely concentrated on a no-blame environment and focus on system improvements in Australia in past years.

Overall, practitioners appear to be willing to disclose errors to patients, their willingness increasing with the severity of the error. However, there appears to be a difference between a generally transparent attitude and actual experiences with practitioners reporting not to have disclosed a significant proportion of errors to patients. The most common reason why they would not disclose was that they thought the patient would not understand, which, in the context of patient health literacy and the practitioner's role in providing information appropriately and adequately, reveals a shortcoming. While German practitioners highlighted legal and organisational barriers to disclosing errors, Australian practitioners focused on the emotional impact of disclosure. All practitioners who had disclosed an error in the past reported some type of impact on their lives, most commonly anxiety, sleep problems and decreasing confidence in their professional skills.

Although the levels of previous training in disclosure varied, overwhelmingly practitioners supported timely support by a disclosure expert immediately after an error had occurred. In relation to information about medical errors, peer-based sources were most relevant and information about error prevention the most sought after, highlighting the wish to know what solutions and changes have worked to address errors.

Chapter 4   Discussion

4.1   Introduction

In this chapter, I will summarise my main findings and relate those to the existing literature. The chapter consist of four sections. In the first section I will reiterate the main conclusions drawn from my review of the literature that provided a framework for my understanding of interpersonal trust in this book and the design of the empirical studies.

In the second section, I will discuss the key findings of the explorative interviews with patients and practitioners, contrasting their perceptions and narratives and relate them to the model of trust dynamics that I introduced in Chapter 2.

In the third section I will discuss the results of the anonymous survey of medical practitioners that inquired into their experiences with and attitudes to medical errors. Placing findings from this study into the context of existing research will help to identify areas that remain obstacles for practitioners to safely disclose errors in their professional practice, and to inform possible strategies to overcome these.

In the last section of the chapter, I will return to my overall research question and offer a response to what the relationship between interpersonal trust in the doctor-patient relationship and communication in the context of health care incidents appears to be. I will conclude this book in the following chapter by offering my perspective on key issues derived from my findings and their relevance for medical practitioners, patients, policy makers, educators and regulators of the medical profession.

4.2 Building a framework from the review of relevant literature

In Chapter 2, I introduced existing approaches to trust in general (Giddens, 1990; Hardin, 1992; Luhmann, 1973, 1979), and interpersonal trust in particular (Coleman, 1990; Jones, 1996; Thom et al., 2004; Trachtenberg et al., 2005), to form my own understanding of interpersonal trust as *a dynamic and voluntary process, involving both cognitive and affective elements that shape a positive expectation of a future outcome and enables cooperation by accepting vulnerability posed by associated risks.*

Applying this understanding of trust to the patient-practitioner relationship in health care, I distinguish different types of typical patient-practitioner interactions, with their inherently different roles and unique expectations (Arora et al., 2005; Ende et al., 1989; Lee & Lin, 2009) when attempting to understand how trust between the patient and practitioner is formed or destroyed. To illustrate my understanding, I introduced a dynamic model, consisting of two circles. The inner circle represents the patient-practitioner relationship while the outer circle represents the continuous cycle of information and knowledge, which shapes expectations and ultimately, these expectations are used to evaluate actual outcomes. I argue that where expectations are matched by outcomes, trust will be enhanced, while where the outcome or behaviour does not concur with the expectations, trust starts to deteriorate. Communication plays an essential part in the model, in that it is interdependent with trust. Where trust deteriorates, communication suffers, meaning it becomes less open and information is selected in a manner to fit negative perceptions. In contrast, where trust grows, the quality of communication improves by being more open (Macintosh, 2007) which in turn makes it more likely to achieve a mutual understanding of information and to find common ground as to what can be expected in the relationship.

In the literature, it was suggested that trust is self-enforcing (Hardin, 1992) meaning that existing trust makes it more likely that information and behaviour is interpreted in a manner that enhances trust. Referencing Festinger's (1962) theory of cognitive dissonance, I argue that communication, similar to trust, is self-enforcing, and good communication facilitates better communication.

Applying my understanding of the interpersonal trust dynamics to situations where an incident in the care or treatment of the patients occurred, it appears that trust levels before the incident are particularly relevant to the quality of communication after the incident. According to my argument, high levels of trust before the incident enable the communication immediately after the incident to be based on goodwill of both sides, which makes it more likely that full information is provided to and accepted by the patient. In contrast, where trust deteriorates, because expectations are continuously not met, the quality of communication deteriorates in that information becomes limited or is being withheld and the patient perceives the information provided as inadequate or misleading. Given this dynamic, I suggest that prompt and effective open disclosure after incidents is crucial to restore trust and to enable effective communication about the incident with a high level of understanding and acceptance of the information that arises. On the other hand, without adequate disclosure, the dynamic would swing to the negative side starting a cycle of negative perceptions, leading to negative expectations, and if confirmed, to the deterioration of trust that may ultimately lead to distrust.

The literature review revealed multiple barriers exist in practice that either stop practitioners from disclosing incidents, or that cause them to be guarded or incomplete in their communication with the patient (Gallagher et al., 2003; Gallagher, Garbutt et al., 2006; Gallagher, Waterman et al., 2006; Iedema et al., 2008b; Iedema, Allen, Britton, & Gallagher, 2011; Iedema, Allen, Britton, Grbich et al., 2011). According to my model, both types of reaction to an incident ultimately contribute to deterioration in the trust relationship. I further argue that making a formal complaint to a third party can be considered a sign that the relationship has become untenable and the opportunity to restore trust directly between the patient and practitioner is minimal or lost. Daniel et al. (1999) found that most patients who had made a complaint would not consider return- ing to the practitioner for further treatment. This finding was replicated in the empirical data derived from the interviews with patients, which I refer to in more detail later in this discussion.

After conceptualising the relevance of interpersonal trust for the success- ful management of incidents – 'successful' implying that no formal complaint is made and a level of interpersonal trust is maintained or restored – I then re- viewed relevant empirical studies that had researched interpersonal trust in the patient-practitioner relationship. What I found was that most empirical studies related to trust in routine situations (Anderson & Dedrick, 1990; Kao, Green, et al., 1998; Thom, 2001; Thom et al., 2002) and mainly used a snapshot approach to ascertain trust levels at a given point of time in the relationship. I found exist- ing studies unsuitable to support or discredit the trust dynamic that I had con- ceptualised. So I aimed to explore this uncharted area in my fieldwork.

The way I designed the empirical study allowed me to discover factors that patients and practitioners thought to be relevant to the trust dynamic after incidents. I inquired about both sides' experiences and perceptions using mini- mal pre-defined categories. Nevertheless, as I stated above, I assumed the emerging themes to broadly relate to the areas of competence, communication and care, which was indeed the case as I will discuss further in this chapter. Secondly, I had assumed that a mismatch between expectations and actual outcomes would have a negative impact on trust levels, while where expecta- tions were met or exceeded, it would have a positive impact on reported trust levels. As I will discuss in more detail in this chapter, I was able to confirm the first part of the assumption relating to the trust deterioration, but given the unique characteristic of the sample, the assumed link between met expecta- tions and a positive impact on trust could not be confirmed; nevertheless, the data also did not include evidence that would have discounted this part of my assumption.

I complemented the findings from the explorative interviews with a quantitative survey of practitioners that focussed on one particular, but nevertheless fundamental, aspect in my understanding of how trust could be maintained or restored after incidents – the practitioner's willingness to disclose incidents to patients.

As outlined above, there was a multitude of possible barriers to disclosure and I wanted to establish which were most relevant to surgeons and general practitioners in Germany and Australia. As Gallagher, Waterman, et al. (2006) found when they compared the attitudes of US and Canadian practitioners, there were few differences in their willingness to disclose and reported reasons for not disclosing, despite differences in the medico-legal environment. Gallagher, Waterman, et al. (2006) suggested that 'these beliefs may relate to norms, values and practices that constitute the culture of medicine' and that 'the finding that physician attitudes generally varied more by speciality than by country further supports the role of medical culture in shaping these views' (p. 1609). Given the results of the survey I conducted with German and Australian practitioners broadly mirrored the results of Gallagher's earlier study in this regard, it supports their view that a responsive and supportive medical culture is required to underpin open disclosure in practice.

4.3 Discussion of findings from the explorative interviews

In the following section, I will discuss the key findings from the explorative interviews to establish what factors patients and practitioners perceived to be relevant in the building or the deterioration of interpersonal trust and what from their perspectives triggered a formal complaint. I will pay particular attention to the perception of apologies after incidents, related emotions and their influence on the relationship and trust levels.

4.3.1   Does trust matter?

From the review of relevant literature, I concluded in Chapter 2 that interpersonal trust is fundamental to an effective relationship between patients and practitioners (Benedetti, 2011) in that it enhances the quality of communication, facilitates cooperation (Gambetta, 1988; Macintosh, 2007) and enhances patient satisfaction, compliance and continuity of care (Krupat et al., 2001; Lee & Lin, 2009; Macintosh, 2007; Trachtenberg et al., 2005) leading to overall better health care outcomes for patients. What was unclear to me was the exact mechanism that would explain those correlations and I offered a possible explanation by outlining my understanding of the interdependence between communication and trust in Chapter 2.

In the interviews I conducted, practitioners opined that trust in general matters, because they felt that it was easier to treat and care for patients who they felt trusted them. Practitioners also reported feeling more comfortable to extend their care beyond the problem the patient presented with and proactively explore other health issues in the patient's best interest. These findings concur with the understanding by Jones (1996), who described that in a relationship trust enables a person displaying overall goodwill towards another person and vice versa. When practitioners perceive the patient to be trusting, they reported being more open in their communication with patients about uncertainties or risks associated with the proposed treatment. While it has been suggested that trust is a vehicle that allows people to make decisions amid risks and uncertainty (Luhmann, 1979), the above findings expand this view and suggest an indirect mechanism: trust enables transparent communication about risks, which then enables a mutual understanding of risks and facilitates cooperative (Gambetta, 1988) decision-making. I want to clarify this dynamic further and suggest that a shared feeling of trust facilitates openness in communication about all, including negative, aspects of care and as such is a mechanism to manage expectations and find a mutual understanding of what can realistically be achieved.

Notably, despite practitioners describing trust as beneficial in their relationship with a patient they did not believe it to be 'essential' to treat a patient, stating that they have an 'obligation' to treat people, independent of whether or not they feel they have established a trusting relationship. This attitude mirrors the professional duty medical practitioners have, which is 'caring for people who are unwell and seeking to keep people well' (Australian Medical Board, 2010, p. 2) and to make decisions 'about patients' access to medical care ... free from bias and discrimination' (Australian Medical Board, 2010, p. 3). Interestingly, it emerged during the interviews that some patients had voluntarily sought and accepted treatment from practitioners they did not trust (importantly, also did not mistrust) under certain circumstances. Patients rationalised their decision by either citing a lack of access to alternative practitioners or for reasons of convenience, including that the practitioner was located close by or did not charge additional fees. However, these patients reported being cautious in their interaction with the practitioner they did not trust and attempted to minimise their reliance upon their advice, for example by limiting the services they sought to routine prescriptions or the management of non-serious, common health conditions, and by confirming information provided by the practitioner through other sources, including the internet, pharmacists or other practitioners. This finding suggests that cooperation without or with low levels of trust is possible in the patient-practitioner relationship, if the associated risks are perceived to be minimal. This implies that there might be a threshold of risk, unique to every person or situation, up to which cooperation without trust is possible. However, I would argue that even in those situations, trust is instrumental in making such interactions easier, more effective and efficient. In contrast, once the individual threshold of risk management is reached, trust becomes essential to further cooperation. Practitioners, in line with Luhmann's (1979) understanding of trust as a complexity reducing mechanism, highlighted the importance of trust to ease patients' navigation of complex and fragmented modern health care delivery by overcoming the asymmetry in information and knowledge between patient and increasingly specialised practitioners and thus accepting vulnerability (Rousseau et al., 1998).

It seems this observation becomes even more relevant after incidents when patients reported feeling particularly uncertain and anxious and trust would enhance the openness of communication and the willingness to cooper-ate (Gambetta, 1988). Indeed, practitioners reported that when they perceive a patient trusts them, they are more willing to openly talk about the incident with the patient and expect the patient to be more accepting and understanding of what happened. This finding was mirrored in the patient interviews where pa-tients reported reserving judgement about what had happened, because they trusted the practitioner and believed that there must be an explanation for what had occurred. Those findings support the link between interpersonal trust and open disclosure, in that without trust, disclosure will either not take place or may be limited or ineffective. This conclusion changes the direction of the common conception that trust is one possible outcome of successful open dis-closure (Berlinger, 2005; Fallowfield & Fleissig, 2003; Wojcieszak, Banja, & Houk, 2006) and turns it around to suggest that trust is a facilitating factor for open disclosure. In line with this conclusion, patients reported that the per-ceived trustworthiness of a source of information influences what credibility is assigned to the information and how it is prioritised in the decision-making process. This finding confirms my earlier conceptualisation whereby trust levels influence both the selection and interpretation of information and offers an-other perspective in explaining how trust is linked to successful open disclosure.

A finding that stood out from the patient accounts was the influence gen-eral practitioners' judgement and advice have on the patient's decision-making, not only about what care to seek and by whom, but importantly after incidents, regarding what action to take or abstain from. The value patients placed on their general practitioner's opinion of another practitioner supports Coleman's

(1990) idea that trust can be influenced beyond face-to-face interaction by relying on the judgement of an intermediary.

The interviews confirmed that immediately after an incident, patients feel uncertain and wish to understand what had happened. At this point in time in the relationship there appears to be a window of opportunity for the practitioner to preserve the patient's trust, as patients reserve judgement until they have some information that helps them to make sense of their experience. If the practitioner can provide the information in a manner that is adequate and respectful of the patient's situation and needs, it is an opportunity to maintain and increase trust. However, where the information comes from other sources, is incomplete, or contradicts previous information provided by the practitioner, this can adversely affect patient trust.

4.3.2   Relation of trust, perception and behaviour

When I approached my fieldwork, I assumed that people's perception of another person or situation would shape their communication and behaviour towards that person. Both practitioners and patients confirmed this assumption by reporting that the first impression sets the tone for the unfolding relationship. In general, positive first impressions described in the interviews correlated with high levels of reported trust, while negative or inconsistent first impressions correlated with low levels of patient trust. These findings support the notion that trust is self-enforcing (Jones, 1996), in that it fosters behaviour associated with further enhancing trust.

Where the practitioner's first impression of the patient was negative or inconsistent, they reported treating the patient with caution and were expecting some type of (communication) issue to arise. Notably, practitioners formed their first impressions based on the perception of the person during the first encounter, including reference to body language, as well as contextual information, including the patient's medical history, or the opinion of other people.

Practitioners reported having a negative first impression where they perceived the patient as demanding, questioning the practitioner or being disrespectful.

In comparison, patients reported negative first impressions where practitioners appeared to dismiss their health complaints or were seen as unwilling to help, which was interpreted as being uncaring; where the consultation was rushed; or where the practitioner did not communicate adequately. In contrast, positive first impressions were associated with the practitioner being a good communicator, being responsive to the patient's needs, appearing confident and competent, and working in a professional and clean environment. Overall, the interviews confirmed that first impressions influence the perception of the other person and have an impact on the unfolding relationship and reported trust levels, including after incidents.

Over time, how both sides perceive their interaction after an incident becomes increasingly influential in the dynamics of trust. Patients who eventually made a complaint viewed the practitioner after the incident to be unhelpful, unresponsive, unsupportive, and did not feel understood and in some cases abandoned, despite the majority of patients reporting a positive experience and perception of the practitioner before the incident.

After incidents, practitioners described being careful and feeling worried in their interaction with the patient. Practitioners also reported feeling not understood by the patient, or perceiving the patient as unresponsive or unhelpful. These findings may suggest that after the incident, both sides had to deal with complex emotional impacts from the incident which had the effect of decreasing the transparency of communication, and in return decreased the opportunity to find a shared understanding of what had happened and its impact on both the patient and the practitioner. With reference to Luhmann's (1979) conception of trust as a mechanism to reduce complexity, Lewicki et al. (2006) note that trust allows the possibility of undesirable behaviour by the other to be removed from considerations, whereas distrust reduces complexity by allowing undesirable conduct to be seen as likely (if not certain). (p. 1002)

Instinctively, practitioners appear to often withdraw from the relationship and become cautious in their communication with the patient. Ironically, this behaviour exactly appears to accelerate the deterioration of trust, in that a lack of communication increases the risk of misunderstandings and misconceptions and decreases the opportunity to clarify these in order to develop a shared understanding of the situation.

4.3.3   Factors influencing interpersonal trust

In the explorative interviews with patients and practitioners, the themes that emerged and appeared to influence interpersonal trust related to communication, competence and care. This is consistent with the conceptualisation of Thom (2001) and key findings from an explorative study by Mechanic and Meyer (2000), which explored how patients who had been diagnosed with either breast cancer, Lyme disease or mental illness assessed trust in their practitioners.

In the following section, I compare and contrast patients' and practitioners' perceptions of communication, care and competence related factors and how they associate them with enhancing or deteriorating trust.

Overall, the comparison of perceptions reveals a widespread mismatch between expectations on both sides which may be a contributing factor for the deterioration of interpersonal trust in the patient-practitioner relationship. Given that all interviewed patients and practitioners had been involved in a complaint, which as I suggested above may be an indication that the relationship had deteriorated to a point were minimal or no trust remained, the analysis focussed on factors contributing to the deterioration of trust. Where pa-

tients spoke about factors that positively influenced their trust levels, they usually related to their interaction with the practitioner before the incident, or
interactions with other practitioners. For the clarity of the discussion, I will refer
to each of the three areas – competence, communication and care – separately,
but acknowledge that in practice, they are often intertwined and interdependent.

4.3.3.1 Competence

The patient's positive perception of the practitioner's competence was positively associated with reported trust in the practitioner. Patients opined that technical brilliance and good health outcomes can counteract perceived flaws in
communication or care. Practitioners also nominated competence related factors to be most essential for a trustful relationship between patients and practitioners. However, it is important to note that it is the perceived competence of
the practitioner that influences trust levels, which may or may not mirror their
objective competence. What makes a practitioner competent in the patient's
eye may differ completely from what makes a practitioner competent in their
own or their peers' eyes. To explain this notion: commonly, patients, although
knowing that mistakes can happen, do not expect them to happen to them, and
as a result view the absence of complications or negative side effects as normal
rather than a sign of the practitioner's competence. In contrast, practitioners,
being well aware of the inexact nature of medicine and having a higher level of
contextual knowledge as to the expected risks for certain treatment or procedures, more commonly view the absence or low level of complications or negative side effects as related to the level of competence.

Perceptions of competence were either established proactively, based on
reputation, or retrospectively, by evaluating the extent of overlap between
prior expectations and actual outcomes.

Reputation, understood as the opinion of others about a person, appears to play a significant role in whether or not initial trust is established, particularly in the absence of prior direct interaction (Teacy, Patel, Jennings, & Luke, 2006). Patients stated that they would not consult a practitioner with a negative reputation. This is in line with Coleman's (1990) conceptualisation of trust through intermediaries whereby the trustee relies on the judgement of the intermediary to place or not to place trust in another person. Patients most commonly relied on other practitioners' judgement to evaluate a practitioner's competence before the first encounter, while after their own (negative) experiences; they more commonly sought the advice and reassurance from family, friends and other patients. Referring to Coleman (1990), it could be argued that the negative experience with the practitioner has shattered their trust in the intermediaries – the general practitioner's – judgement, and they shift seeking advice to other intermediaries – friends, family or other patients. Overall, it appears that patients relied upon reputation more in the initial stages of their relationship with the practitioner, while after repeated encounters, their own experiences took precedence in evaluating the relationship.

To illustrate how subjective perceptions can be relevant, I reiterate that several of the interviewed patients expected the practitioner to at least 'take a look' and physically examine them if they presented with a physical ailment. Where information about a physical illness was obtained solely verbally, it negatively impacted on the patient's perception of the practitioner's competence. This finding is important as physical examinations are not considered essential by practitioners. One obvious example is the accepted practice of telecommunication-based health care provision, particularly in Australia (Medicare Australia, 2014), where a number of health conditions can be diagnosed and treated based on observations, medical information, including test results, and verbal information provided by the patient without the need for a physical examination. However, I note the findings of Reilly (2003) who in an observational study established that physical examination in a significant number of hospital patients led to a correction or change of treatment, suggesting the importance of physical examinations to confirm diagnosis and treatment advice that may have been determined by other means.

I assumed that in the trust dynamic, perceived trust levels are influenced both by proactively checking the alignment between reputation and expectations, and retrospectively, by evaluating actual outcomes against prior expectations. I suggest that the greater the overlap, the greater the trust. The latter assumption was underpinned by the finding that patients reported taking into account the final health outcome to rationalise their level of confidence in a practitioner. In contrast, patients associated poor treatment outcomes or side effects with declining trust. In some cases, it was the scope of the expectation that was broader than what the practitioner could provide. Where the practitioners successfully treated a specialised part of the patient's conditions, but the overall well-being of the patient did not improve significantly, the patient reported being dissatisfied with the practitioner and less confident in their abilities. This finding qualifies the general link between patient satisfaction and trust (Krupat et al., 2001; Trachtenberg et al., 2005) by suggesting that the scope of the patient's satisfaction is relevant. An interesting difference in patients and practitioners' perceptions of competence was that practitioners distinguished between ability and judgement. In other words, practitioners saw competence as twofold, consisting of both what practitioners could technically do, but also how and when they would use their skills. This distinction was not found in the patients' accounts, which indicates that patients assume that the practitioner will use their skills in the patient's best interest, hence differentiating between skill and judgement became irrelevant.

Patient complaints about incidents were often unexpected by practitioners (see also Jain & Ogden, 1999) and often prompted the practitioners to reflect on their interaction and with the patient. While for patients it was more commonly the incident that prompted them to rationalise their trust in the practitioner by evaluating their interaction, expectation and outcomes, for practitioners it was the time of the complaint. Again this may be the difference in expectations about health care, with patients not expecting something bad to happen to them, so the incident is an unexpected event that triggers the described trust dynamics. Practitioners on the other hand are much more familiar with the possible side effects and complications that arise out of or are associated with health care and thus do not view the incident the unexpected event, but the complaint. Complaints often 'forced' the practitioner to take notice, something that patients commonly aimed to achieve by making the complaint. The misalignment in perceptions may also partially explain the difficulty in successfully disclosing incidents, as practitioners may not pay sufficient attention to addressing the patient's surprise and associated emotions, while focusing on factual information about the suspected causes of the event. Although incidents prompted both patients and practitioners to rationalise prior, and often subconsciously held, beliefs and trust dispositions, they did so at different times.

In the interviews, practitioners described how, prompted by the complaint, they reflected on their interaction with the patient and in most cases could empathise with the patient's perceptions. This reflective process, which usually followed an initial feeling of anger and feeling treated unfairly in response to the complaint, enabled the practitioners to make sense of why the patient had made the complaint. Commonly, practitioners suggested that a mismatch between the level of care and the outcome that the patient expected and the level that, in their opinion, was realistically achievable, contributed to the decline in trust. In this context, practitioners commented that it is often difficult to have a real sense of the patient's expectations, given that some expectations or influencing factors, such as irrational fears or unrealistic expectations of 'perfection' in medicine, may not be clear to the practitioner. Again this finding highlights the importance of open communication between patient and practitioner beyond the exchange of medically relevant facts.

All complaints had been closed at the time of the interview and the above accounts often reflected a sense of resolution that the practitioner had achieved as a result of their own reflection and sense-making. Jain and Ogden

(1999) identified in their study how general practitioners usually react to patient complaints in three typical stages. Initially, practitioners feel shocked and
overwhelmed when they receive a patient complaint. This was followed by a
sense of anger and antagonism towards the patient, before eventually reaching
a sense of resolution in the last stage. Importantly, the strong emotional reactions experienced in the first two stages pose a significant challenge to practitioners being open and responsive to a patient's complaint. Finding from a
study among New Zealand practitioners (Cunningham, 2004) also suggest that
when a complaint is made, the practitioner's trust in the patient is negatively
affected and goodwill displayed towards the patients decreases. This in turn
makes the restoration of trust at that stage more unlikely.

Overall, perceptions of competence related to reported trust levels, but
varied as to which competence related factors contributed to the deterioration
of trust between patient and practitioner.

4.3.3.2 Communication

In the interviews, practitioners suggested that respecting the patient's expectations would in their view contribute positively to a trusting relationship and
reflected whether or not they had been able to match the patient's expectation. Despite both practitioners and patients valuing honesty and transparency
in their relationship, practitioners commonly assumed what they believed the
patient wanted, rather than proactively inquiring about it. Communication related themes in the interview with practitioners foremost focussed on medical
information and less commonly on the impact of the treatment on the life of
the patient. Practitioners often may not know the individual circumstances of a
patient, but it appears not to be a priority for them to obtain such information.
Considering that unique life circumstances may impact on patients' preferences, this finding is problematic and, as Weston and Belle Brown (1989) suggested, explanations and treatment must at least be consistent with the patient's point of view to make sense to them.

Inconsistency in information was described by both practitioners and patients as an issue that influences trust levels. The findings suggest that horizontal inconsistency, between information from different sources, is less relevant
for the trust dynamic than vertical inconsistency in information provided by the
same person over a period of time. Notably, patients perceived as more trustworthy practitioners who referred to other sources, such as internet pages or
brochures, to back up the information they provided verbally to the patient. In
an age of increasing use of the internet by patients to research medical information, practitioners have a greater opportunity to increase consistency in
advice (Sillence, Briggs, Harris, & Fishwick, 2007) and thus enhance patient trust
if they proactively direct them to suitable resources (McMullan, 2006) that
support their own advice.

'Explaining' was one of the most prevalent themes during the patient interviews. Where patients described their practitioner taking time to explain the
diagnosis and proposed treatment, patient trust was high and those practitioners were also perceived as caring. From a practitioner's point of view, where
they were open about the limitations of their knowledge, but spent time explaining the reasons to the patient, they reported no negative impact on the
patient's trust level. Patients on the other hand reported appreciating that
diagnosis and treatment is based on information available at the time and may
change. Those findings suggest that despite the risk of vertical inconsistencies in
information provided to the patient, when it is explained adequately it may not
negatively impact on patient trust.

After incidents, patients reported that the lack of explanation about what
had happened had been a significant factor associated with deterioration of
trust and for their decision to make a complaint. This finding is in line with the
complaint statistics of the NSW Health Care Complaints Commission according
to which communication issues are the second most common type of issue
patients complain about (HCCC, 2013, p. 103) and often communication issues
relate to treatment or conduct issues (Kable et al., 2014), suggesting a link be-

tween an actual outcome and the way it was communicated to the patient. In cases where the patient did receive information, but felt misled, the perceived dishonesty significantly contributed to declining trust levels. The perception of being provided with misleading or wrong information was considered a deliberate act and often coincided with the patient describing the practitioner denying any wrongdoing or becoming defensive. Findings by Mechanic & Meyer (2000) suggest that patients anticipate that practitioners are always honest; therefore a perceived breach of their most basic assumption has a significant impact on their trust level. Notably, where patients reported mistrusting the practitioner at the time of the interview, they re-interpreted the incident as a deliberate act, implying that the practitioner intended to hurt them. One possible explanation for why patients thought they were being deceived was that none of the interviewed patients received a full and genuine apology. As Wu et al. (2009) found in their study about how patients perceive apologies, patients respond more favourably to practitioners who apologised and took responsibility and that 'after an adverse event, the patient's perception of what was said appeared to be more important than what was actually said' (p. 1015).

Many of the interviewed patients stated that by making the complaint, they wanted the practitioner to take notice, to no longer be able to brush them aside or ignore what happened to them and at the same time, take back some power and control in the relationship. Complaints were commonly triggered by a sense of powerlessness experienced by the patient: not being able to get the explanation they need to understand what had happened; not being treated respectfully, which mainly related to the reported lack of an apology and the unwillingness of the practitioner to engage with the patient after the incident. At the time when patients decided to make a complaint, their attention had often shifted from the actual incident towards being dissatisfied with their interaction with the practitioner after the incident. Coinciding with this shift in attention was a shift in the outcomes sought from primarily wanting an explanation and apology immediately after the incident to forcing the practitioner to engage and in some cases penalise them for their behaviour.

Rather than the adequacy of explanation provided, practitioners perceived that a major contributing factor to the decline of the relationship with the patient were opinions of other practitioners that contradicted the original practitioners' advice or conduct. The contrasting 'expert' opinion, in their view, contributed significantly to the patient losing trust and as a result not being willing to accept their own explanations relating to the incident. Indeed, patients disclosed that in many cases they were encouraged by others, including other practitioners, to make a complaint about their experience.

Overall, the discussion revealed that where incidents led to complaints, a multitude of differences in perceptions about the quality and adequacy of the patient-practitioner communication exist in general and are linked by both sides to deteriorating trust levels.

4.3.3.3 Care

In relation to aspects of care, again there was an overall misalignment of patient and practitioner perceptions of what contributes to good care and how it influences the relationship.

Not surprisingly, general practitioners, more commonly than surgeons, prioritised care in their relationship with a patient. Practitioners' understanding of being caring was primarily skills and competence related: being comprehensive, accessible and proactive in their treatment advice. In comparison, patients' perceived practitioners to be caring when they felt listened to, their wishes and preferences respected, and felt being treated as a human being.

On the other hand, where practitioners associated a perceived lack of care with the deterioration of their relationship with the patient, they assumed it was because the patient had to wait, felt rushed during the consultation, did not get what they wanted from the practitioner, or were charged for a service they were not happy with. By contrast, patients associated the perceived lack of empathy by the practitioner, a dismissive attitude and treating the patient as a medical problem rather than a person with deterioration in the relationship.

Practitioners suggested that in their view a single episode of dissatisfaction can cause the patient to start interpreting their following experiences in a negative way similar to the effect of a snowball. This view gives support to Festinger's theory of cognitive dissonance (1962) which argues that where perceptions did not align with prior expectations, people tend to either interpret the new experience in a way that fits their existing preconceptions or change their existing consecptions in the light of the new experience. Overall, practitioners believed that rarely a single care related factor, but rather a combination of dissatisfaction with different aspects of the care, communication or competence, would trigger patient complaints.

Overall, there was an obvious discrepancy in the perception of patients and practitioners in relation to care factors they associated with trust building or deterioration. In general, practitioners tend to view the encounter in the context of their professional routines as 'normality', while patients perceived medical encounters more commonly as an exception in their lives.

So far, the discussion of the results of the explorative interviews supports the conclusion that, in practice, differences in perceptions can appear in relation to multiple aspects of communication, competence and care and are considered to influence the trust relationship between patient and practitioners. This supports the conclusion that working towards a shared meaning of health conditions and proposed treatments is only one aspects of a trusting patient-practitioner relationship. In addition, both sides must endeavour to align patient and practitioner preferences and understandings regarding care and communication. Being as open and responsive as possible in their interactions with each other seems fundamental to be able to achieve this.

4.3.4　Apologies

As mentioned above in the discussion of communication related factors, most patients who made a complaint did not receive an apology after the incident despite several authors suggesting that when something goes wrong patients want an apology (Berlinger, 2005; Hobgood et al., 2005; Wojcieszak et al., 2006; Woods, 2007).

Notably, from the interviews it emerged that it is not only important that the practitioner apologises, but also the timing of the apology. Where the apology was delivered immediately after the incident or immediately after the practitioner became aware that there was a problem, patients accepted the apology and interpreted the incident as an honest mistake or unfortunate event, rather than a deliberate error, a finding in line with Wu et al. (2009). Patients who had received a prompt apology also confirmed that they did not make a complaint in those cases, supporting Woods (2007) who states that apologies, disclosure and relationship all affect the patient's decision to take legal action. In contrast, where an apology was not offered, was delayed, or contradicted the practitioner's behaviour, such apologies were perceived as insincere and non-genuine by the patient and did not change their mainly negative perception of the practitioner. These findings contradict suggestions by Lazare (2004, 2010) who recommends withholding an apology until all the facts are clear. Notably, almost all patients expected both an apology and an explanation from the practitioner, which suggests that an apology alone would be insufficient to repair the relationship. While Lazare (2010) considers that the apology should include an expression of regret as well as an explanation of the facts that led to the incidents and steps taken to prevent future re-occurrence, the Australian open disclosure framework (ACSQH, 2013) defines an apology as an expression of regret once the harm to the patient is recognised, independent of whether the surrounding facts are established at that stage or not. According to the framework, causes of and actions taken in response to the incident are separate elements in the open disclosure process, complementing the apology. It appears that the Australian framework's approach to apologies is more in line with patient expectations expressed in the interviews than Lazare's (2004, 2010).

Practitioners reported not having apologised to the patient after the incident, because they did not have a chance, for example, if the patient had left their care; because they were advised by their indemnity insurer against apologising; or because they were too busy and forgot to do it. In the practitioners' view their lack of apology was the result of external advice or was inadvertent. There was no case where practitioners reported that they did not apologise because they felt they had done nothing wrong. The Australian open disclosure framework (ACSQH, 2013) mandates that an apology should be part of any open disclosure; however, it seems that practitioners may have to become more aware that apologising is an essential part of disclosure and it seems some indemnity insurers may also have to be reminded of this, despite most insurers publically advocating open disclosure (AVANT, 2014; MIGA, 2005).

Where practitioners apologised to the patient, their motivations varied. Some tried to calm down the patient in order to then be able to defend themselves, others apologised to acknowledge the patient's poor experience. In one case, the practitioner apologised with the intent of ending the relationship and bring closure to the incident by saying 'sorry there is nothing more I can do'. Overall, the apologies as described by practitioners in the interviews were instrumental rather than a reflection of genuine care and empathy for the patient, which suggests that more work is required beyond mandating that practitioners apologise (ACSQH, 2013a), to assist them in doing it appropriately.

4.3.5   Impact of the incident

Both patients and practitioners reported that their incident experience prompted them to be more aware and cautious in patient-practitioner interactions overall. Despite this generalised change in behaviour, where both sides reported having residual negative emotions, these related to the specific practitioner or patient involved in the particular incident and were not generalised. This finding lends some support to my view that interpersonal trust and related dynamics are foremost an interpersonal phenomenon to be understood in the context of a specific relationship in a specific situation, an understanding shared by Candlin and Crichton (2013).

It is important to remember that only a small number of health care incidents prompt formal complaints. Complaints usually are a sign that the patient's trust in the practitioner has deteriorated significantly (Daniel et al., 1999), and can trigger the practitioner no longer wanting to continue the relationship (Cunningham, 2004). Where no or low levels of trust remain, patients appear to prefer discontinuing the relationship (Daniel et al., 1999), while practitioners' responses in the interviews exposed a dilemma between feeling professionally obliged to continue treating a patient who complained, while acknowledging that they would expect to have a difficult relationship with the patient and ultimately would prefer if the patient decided, or accepted a recommendation to see another practitioner.

Most of the interviewed patients, who had complained to the Health Care Complaints Commission, were not satisfied with the outcome. The issues that triggered the complaint often remained unresolved from the patients' point of view, despite the Commission having closed the case. One possible explanation is that only patients who felt there were outstanding issues volunteered to participate in the research, and indeed, some disclosed this as their motivation to participate in the study. Another explanation could be that the role and the function of the Commission (HCCC, 2014a) and its focus on dealing with serious issues of public health and safety seems misaligned with individual patients' perceptions of the incident and related expectations of what should happen in response. This misalignment between patients' wishes and Commission actions may be that the patient wants an apology, but the Commission is unable to direct the practitioner to apologise; or that the patients want to meet with the practitioner to make them understand what impact the incident had on their life, but the practitioner declines to participate in the voluntary resolution process (HCCC, 2014b).

Overall, the findings suggest that at the time when patients lodge a complaint, their relationship with the practitioner has deteriorated to an extent where either no or only a low level of trust remains. Formal complaint processes (HCCC, 2014c) seem unsuitable to restore trust after incidents. Rather, adequate open disclosure immediately following incidents, at a time when patients appear to reserve their judgement and practitioners don't feel forced to engage in an adversarial formal complaint process, provide an opportunity to maintain and restore trust.

The discussion so far has shown that in general, patient and practitioner perceptions of communication, competence and care related aspects in medical encounters differ, specifically after incidents. In addition, the priorities assigned to particular factors differ, as does the perception of the impact on the trust relationship. On the other hand, both sides tend to put their experience of an incident and complaint into a broader context spanning the whole relationship from first encounter until the time of the complaint. As such, the incident or complaint constitutes a point in the relationship at which prior expectations and perceptions are rationalised, which can change the dynamics of the relationship. This conclusion supports my understanding of trust dynamics, introduced in Chapter 2, and supports its value in explaining the development of interpersonal trust both in routine situations, as well as after incidents.

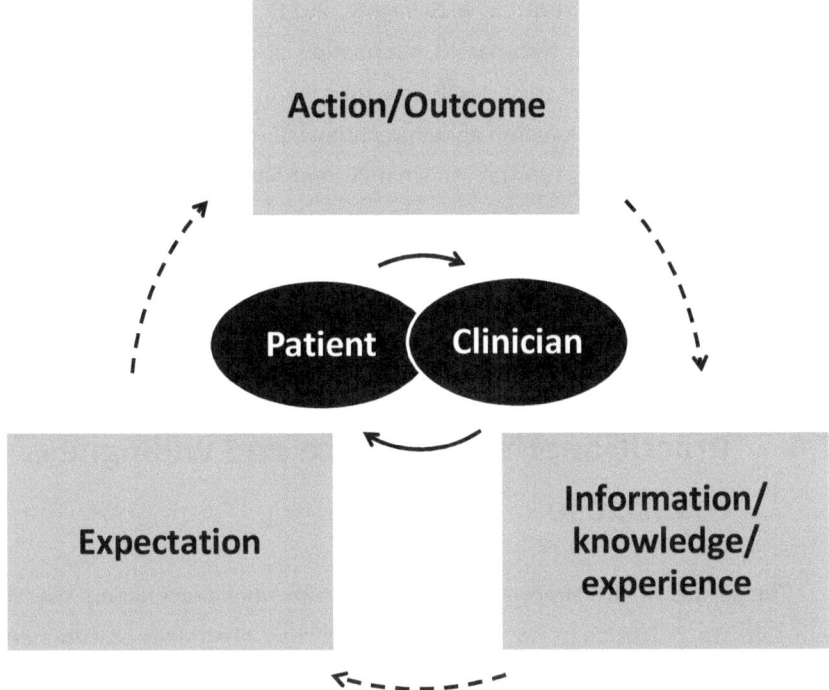

Figure 4.1   Dynamic process model of trust (adapted from Beitat et al., 2013, 81; reprinted with permission)

However, the findings from the explorative interviews support a refinement of the model to reflect that competence, communication and care related aspects influence all stages of the circular trust process. According to the model, to build or maintain trust, patients and practitioners have to share a mutual understanding of relevant information; they have to align their expectations about what can or cannot be achieved in the treatment and they need to establish a mutual interpretation of the outcomes and evaluate them against prior expectations. During all stages of the dynamic process, open and responsive communication appears essential to achieve alignment of knowledge, expectations and interpretation of outcomes. For communication to be successful it has to establish an ongoing shared understanding not only on the factual level, but also contribute to an understanding of each other's emotions, perceptions and priorities (Iedema, Allen, Britton, & Gallagher, 2011). Thus acknowledging the importance of open and transparent information after incidents to maintain and restore interpersonal trust, I will now turn my attention to the results of the second study, which inquired about practitioners' experiences and attitudes towards disclosing errors to establish what current barriers to open communication exist from a practitioner's point of view. By being aware of existing barriers, appropriate measures can be designed to facilitate open communication after incidents and support practitioners in feeling safe and equipped to have those conversations with patients.

4.4 Practitioner's experience and willingness to disclose

The results of the anonymous survey illustrate that practitioners overall, with German practitioners to a greater extent than Australian practitioners, tend to underestimate the risk of medical errors. While estimates of serious or minor errors occurring in their area of practice ranged from under 1% to 7% of health encounters, according to the World Health Organisation (2014), about one in ten – or 10% – of patients who are hospitalised are being harmed by a medical error. Although this number only applies to hospitalised patients, it is significantly higher than surgeons estimated in their responses to the survey. An early study from 1991 (Brennan, Leape, Laird, Hebert, Localio, & et al., 1991) that reviewed over 50,000 randomly selected medical records of emergency patients found that on average, 3.7% of patients would experience a medical error. Other reports (The National Academy of Science, 2006) have suggested that medication related errors alone, which are one of the most common type of errors, would occur on average at least once a day in hospitalised patients. Although there is no consensus on error rates, it appears that overall practitioners underestimate the risk of errors occurring.

On the other hand, the surveyed practitioners perceived themselves being at a high risk of receiving a patient complaint or being sued. Here, their estimates were much higher than complaint statistics of the NSW Health Care Complaints Commission would suggest. In 2012-13, the Commission (HCCC, 2013) put the risk of a medical practitioner receiving a formal complaint at 0.05%[24]. Similarly, according to statistics released by the German Bundesärztekammer (2013b, 2013c), the risk for German practitioners having a claim lodged against them with one of the expert assessor boards was 0.03% in 2012[25]. The discrepancy between practitioner perception and actual complaint numbers may partially be explained by assuming that the surveyed practitioners also referred to complaints that were made directly to them or the management of the health facility they work for, rather than to an independent third party. Surveyed practitioners believed that the overall risk of surgeons receiving either a complaint or claim from patients is significantly higher than it is for practitioners in general practice. This concurs with statistics from the Bundesärztekammer (2013b, p. 9) that lists surgery on top of all areas to which claims are related, despite a smaller number of practitioners working as surgeons compared to general practitioners (Bundesärztekammer, 2013c, p. 125).

It appears that surgeons are more vulnerable to complaints given the nature of the service they provide, which is associated with higher than average risks of complications or side effects, and when they eventuate they are usually more obvious to the patient than incidents that occur in general practice. Despite the higher risk of being complained about or sued, surgeons were more supportive of disclosing serious errors both to patients as well as to the facility management to enhance patient safety. The wide acceptance of morbidity and mortality reviews (Travaglia & Debono, 2009) that often involve surgical cases

---

[24] Calculation based on the Commission's Annual Report 2012-13 (HCCC, 2013) that states that 30,333 (p. 108) medical practitioners were registered with a principal place of practice in NSW and the Commission received 1,616 complaints about medical practitioners (p. 106).

[25] 12,232 complaints were made about medical practitioners in 2012 to one of the expert commissions or state based medical boards (Bundesärztekammer, 2013b, p. 3), and a total of 348,700 medical practitioners worked as at 31 December 2012 (Bundesärztekammer, 2013c, p. 123), calculating a risk for a medical practitioner to receive a complaint or claim at 0.03% in 2012.

may be a factor that contributes to a higher level of willingness and acceptance of disclosure and learning from errors, compared to general practitioners.

Interestingly, despite the majority of the surveyed practitioners believing that disclosing a serious error would damage the patient's trust in their skills, a majority also thought that disclosing a serious error would make it less likely that the patient would complain about them or sue them. Relating this to the earlier findings from patient interviews that found that immediately after the incident patients rationalised their trust which usually resulted in a small dip in reported trust levels, it implies that practitioners believe that a temporary dip in trust levels immediately after the incident can be counteracted by open disclosure. As discussed above though, the quality and appropriateness of the disclosure are major factors in whether or not the trust can be restored.

Given that most practitioners revealed not having received specific training in disclosing incidents and errors to patients, it was not surprising that overwhelmingly, practitioners were interested in having access to a disclosure communication specialist immediately after the incident. Most training on open disclosure to date, where it exists, is either by self-learning, or in the form of seminars or workshops (ACSQH, 2013b; Cognitive Institute, 2014). Some of these training programs use case studies or role play, but the training is delivered outside real-life situations. This is in contrast with the survey findings that suggest that practitioners overwhelmingly would welcome expert assistance in real-life situations at the time of the incident.

The majority of practitioners also acknowledged that errors have an impact on both their professional confidence and their personal life and would like to have access to counselling after a serious incident – a finding in line with Wu's (2000) assertion that practitioner are the 'second victim' of incidents. In Germany, general guidelines on open disclosure do not exist at this point in time. Open disclosure policy in NSW, Australia so far has focused on patients', rather than practitioners' needs. Although the current guidelines applicable to health staff in public facilities in NSW acknowledges that:

> When an incident occurs, the clinicians involved in the incident
> and in the open disclosure process may require emotional and
> psychological support and advice on how to deal with their re-
> sponse to the incident. (NSW Health 2007c, p. 12)

The advice further suggests that support could be provided by medical indemnity insurers and local employee assistance programs, 'particularly for staff
who are interviewed during an incident investigation' (NSW Health 2007c, p.
12). This suggests that the assistance is intended to manage practitioners' anxiety relating to possible disciplinary or legal findings rather than dealing overall
with the patient's and their own emotions relating to the incident. Particularly
female practitioners appear to be interested in having access to counselling
after incidents, which, given the increasing feminisation (Australian Institute of
Health and Welfare, 2009; Brooks, Lapsley, & Butt, 2003) or as Markwell (2011)
refers to it, the 'normalisation' of the medical workforce, such support systems
may be even more relevant in future.

Overall, practitioners appear to overestimate their risks of receiving complaints or being sued after incidents, which may inhibit their willingness to disclose incidents to patients, despite being generally supportive of disclosure.
Practitioners did not feel well equipped for open conversations with patients
after medical errors, had no or little training in open disclosure and reported
that errors had multiple negative effects on both their professional confidence
and personal lives. Those findings suggest that more needs to be done to help
practitioners in practice to feel safe to disclose, support them to do it well and
to assist them in dealing with the impact of the incident.

4.4.1   Overcoming barriers to disclose

My intention when conducting the survey was practical in that I wanted to identify existing barriers to disclosure in practice with the intention of formulating
strategies to overcome these. Being aware that a gap in disclosure existed (Gal-

lagher, Waterman et al., 2006; Levinson, 2009), I was interested in how it could be overcome.

In the discussion above, I concluded that practitioners in practice, primarily in Germany where the majority of respondents came from, do not feel safe, well equipped or well supported to confidently disclose errors or incidents to patients. I now shift my focus towards how these identified barriers can be overcome.

The survey results offer some direction, in that they reveal that after serious errors, practitioners primarily sought support from their indemnity insurer, the medical board and/or a lawyer, which reflects a legalistic and defensive approach. It seems that practitioners prioritise information and advice from these bodies after medical errors, which in turn make them suitable bodies to target as they appear to influence practitioners' decision-making regarding whether or not to disclose and apologise. Most practitioners described the current ways of informing practitioners about errors, and their prevention, as inadequate.

Despite a high proportion of practitioners reporting disclosing and discussing errors among peers, they also expressed that they would prefer more formal and transparent forums to discuss errors and incidents. They also expressed their belief that an open and constructive management of errors could decrease the risk of future repetition and could help them in regaining their professional confidence. A wider forum would also allow contextualising incidents by considering a broader range of systemic and personal factors that might have contributed to the incident. With the majority believing that errors are caused by a combination of individual and systemic errors, any action taken to reduce the risk of future errors would have to address both individual and systemic factors. Contrasting the overall support for disclosure that practitioners expressed, a minority did not want any information about medical errors. This group may require specific attention to overcome their current disinterest and to involve them in quality and safety improvements.

4.5   Summary

In response to my research question – What is the relationship between interpersonal trust in the doctor-patient relationship and communication in the
context of health care incidents? – I conclude that trust facilitates open communication after incidents, but also is restored as a result of successful open
disclosure.

The discussion of the empirical findings broadly supports and expands the
dynamic model of trust that I introduced at the beginning of this book. Emerging from the explorative interviews with patients and practitioners who had
been involved in a formal complaint relating to a health care incident was that
the cycle of information, expectation and evaluation of outcomes is influenced
by communication, competence and care related aspects.

The dynamic process of trust appears to be similar in routine situations and
after incidents in that factors that were associated with trust building and deterioration broadly fall into those three areas: communication, competence and
care. However, overall there appears to be a difference in the perception of
patients and practitioners of what constitutes good communication, what is
considered competence and what is perceived as caring. Comparing the narratives offered by practitioners and patients it became clear that not only perceptions differed, but also the priorities assigned to these in the individual decision-
making.

This book has offered an additional reason why practitioners should engage in open disclosure. So far, it has been argued that being open about incidents is an ethical obligation; is an extension of obtaining informed consent
from the patient; is what patients want; and may prevent costly and lengthy
complaints and legal proceedings. I now add to this that open, timely and responsive communication about incidents poses a unique opportunity to restore
the patient's trust which becomes more unlikely as time passes without an
adequate explanation and almost impossible by the time a formal complaint

has been made. Although open communication about an incident that is responsive to the patient's expectations and adequate for the patient's needs may restore, although not guarantee, patient trust, the interpersonal trust before the incident also influences the communication after incidents.

Thus trust becomes a facilitator or prerequisite for successful open disclosure, as it ensures the goodwill in striving to be aware and align the differences in perceptions, which need to be addressed to find a common understanding of what happened and how to move forward.

Given that the findings suggest that the trust relationship is formed at the first encounter and builds or deteriorates with every interaction, we have to extend our view on incident management by looking at the overall quality of the relationship and the overall quality of communication, and view the incident as part of the patient's journey rather than something separate from it.

Having established the general importance of patient expectations being met to sustain trust, open disclosure appears to be a suitable mechanism to be responsive to patient expectations after incidents and thus restore trust. However, in practice barriers exist that prevent practitioners from disclosing incidents, or where they do disclose, the communication and action taken may not meet the patient's expectation. No or inadequate disclosure can trigger the relationship between patient and practitioner to deteriorate and ultimately may prompt the patient to make a complaint, often to 'force' the practitioner to take notice and provide answers. Complaints often trigger the practitioner's goodwill towards the patient to deteriorate. In addition, the current structure of the complaint system concentrates on the factual level, evaluating the adequacy of the medical treatment and does not substantially address the wider emotional issues and the impact the incident had on both the patient's and practitioner's lives. Thus, complaint processes may bring closure, but rarely restore trust.

The discussion underpinned the importance of a local, open and timely response to incidents. Any delay in open communication increases the risk that the patient's trust in the practitioner deteriorates, which in turn will influence negatively the way the patient perceives information or explanation provided at a later stage. Similarly, where the open disclosure is inadequate in responding to associated emotions and in acknowledging the broader impact the incident had on the patient's life, the same dynamic will apply, decreasing the opportunity to prevent and resolve conflicts.

With this in mind, the results from the anonymous survey are particularly relevant to understanding the key areas that influence the willingness of practitioners to engage in local disclosure processes. Practitioners' remaining fears of negative consequences of disclosure for their professional life and the perceived lack of support after incidents stood out.

In the following chapter, I conclude this book by using the insights I have gained throughout the studies to offer some suggestions to practitioners, patients, researchers and policy makers.

Chapter 5   Reflections and Recommendations

5.1   Introduction

At the conclusion of my book, I reflect upon the insights that I have gained about interpersonal trust and ask myself, as the reader may do, how do they matter?

In this chapter, I will offer some suggestions why I believe the findings of this book matter: for patients, for practitioners, and for researchers who are interested in interpersonal trust, and for policy makers and regulators in the medical arena.

Before doing so, I would like to reiterate that my motivation starting this book was grounded in practice: I aimed to gain a better understanding of the functioning of real-life interactions between patients and practitioners. So, I now endeavour to reflect on my findings from a similar, practical view point, anticipating that some of the following suggestions will undergo a process of consensus finding, before and if adopted in practice. However, if one practitioner will take the time to reflect on their interactions with patients, acknowledges the influence their and patients' perceptions can have and as a result, attempts to be as transparent and responsive as possible in their communication to align perceptions in order to build trust, I have achieved my goal.

This book embraced the complexities of real life, and throughout the book, I have acknowledged that when attempting to explain what interpersonal trust is and how it influences relationships, one should not separate such analysis from the persons involved and the unique situation they are placed in. As Jackson (2013) concluded, 'trust is context- and situation-specific and never a case of 'one size fits all'' (p. 327).

Nevertheless, the unique narratives provided by people about their relationships include patterns that can be discovered and although not identical,
some are alike and repeated across different relationships, which can offer
some insight in what factors may influence trust dynamics in general. This book
sought to make a contribution to the existing research in interpersonal trust by
exploring a specific situation – patient-practitioner relationships after incidents
– and providing empirical evidence about how trust evolves, after incidents
have been experienced differently by patients and practitioners in real life.

Essentially, I now understand that both patients and practitioners influence the trust dynamics through their perceptions, communication and actions,
but at the same time, there are differences in the nature of and priority assigned to those. Ultimately, it seems that the challenge in building and maintaining trusting relations long-term is to firstly, being aware of those differences
and secondly, to try to come to a mutually shared understanding. Communication appears to be essential to facilitate this ongoing process of negotiating a
mutual understanding.

My original contribution to the research on interpersonal trust has been to
introduce and support a model to explain the dynamic of trust development
and deterioration. In the context of patient-practitioner relationships, I identified patterns in patient and practitioner accounts that I used to refine the model to consider three areas – communication, competence and care – that appear to influence the trust dynamic, which itself is a cycle consisting of perceptions, expectations and outcomes. The model appears to be transferrable to
different situations in health care and, I would argue, other fields or disciplines.

5.2   Limitations and recommendations for future research

Before suggesting how my research could benefit future research, I will acknowledge its limitations. Firstly, the empirical data from the explorative interviews is limited as it stems from a small subset of patients and practitioners – those who had been involved in a formal complaint. In addition, the participants may not be representative of patients and practitioners involved in a complaint in general, given that incidents and complaints are both topics that harbour negative associations, which people usually may not wish to be reminded of, unless they have not achieved a sense of closure yet. I have acknowledged this in the discussion of my findings.

Another limitation of my study is that the perceptions were self-reported at the time of the interviews. As discussed in the context of my methodological approach, I consider that perceptions of events change over time depending on the factors taken into account by the person. Nevertheless, as I outlined in Chapter 3, I consider that it is relevant to inquire about perceptions, as, in my conceptualisation, they shape expectations and ultimately behaviour. For future research, I suggest inquiring into the possibility of researching the trust dynamic in real-time, shadowing real-life interaction and using a multi-level approach to compare self-reported perceptions of an interaction with researcher observations of the same interaction. I acknowledge that such research has multiple ethical and risk implications, but these could potentially be addressed by using a video-ethnographic (Iedema, Mesman, & Carroll, 2013) approach. Such an approach would also be responsive and able to capture the complexity of real-life interactions and trust developments within these, as well as offer the opportunity to contrast self-reported perceptions and video-reflexive findings.

A further limitation of my study was that the patient and practitioner narratives that I compared did not relate to the same incident. As mentioned in Chapter 3, it was my initial intent to include both sides' perspectives to the same incidents, but in practice, either the patients or the practitioners did not agree to participate in the research. The suggested real-time approach may address these issues, as the trust dynamic could be studied before an incident results in a complaint, which appears to be the end of the relationship and thus at a time when it is highly unlikely to expect cooperation from both sides.

Given the sample consisted of patients and practitioners involved in formal complaints, I was not able to confirm the assumed positive trust dynamic, meaning the assumption that where after incidents patient and practitioner perceptions, expectations and outcome are aligned, trust can be restored. The assumed trust dynamic may inform and be validated by future research on the implementation of open disclosure.

Lastly, the results of the two studies – the explorative interviews and the anonymous survey – did not complement each other to the extent I had hoped and did not allow a full comparison of findings in different cultural and medico-legal environments, due to the poor response rate in Australia. Here prior assurance of key regulatory bodies to assist in the implementation of the research in Australia may have been beneficial before designing the comparative study.

On a positive note, I am satisfied that the dynamic model of trust that I developed in Chapter 2 to guide my fieldwork has been supported by the findings and, most importantly, not been contradicted by them. In that, this model offers a new way to conceptualise the dynamic nature of interpersonal trust relations and its elements appear to apply to different situations. In the case of patient-practitioner relations, the model was useful in understanding trust in normal, routine situations as well as after incidents and complaints.

The model appears sufficiently broad to allow it to be transferred to other interpersonal trust contexts and I would encourage other researchers to draw on the model for future studies.

5.3   Recommendations for policy makers and regulators

Several aspects of this research may be relevant to policy makers and regulators in the context of incident management, open disclosure and complaint handling. Firstly, I have established that trust and communication are closely related. In the context of incidents this means that continuing trust is not only a possible outcome of successful open disclosure (Wu et al., 2009), but is also a pre-requisite. This is a new perspective that leads to the suggestion that open disclosure policy must attempt to create an environment that is perceived as safe and supportive by both patients and practitioners alike, to enable them to engage in open communication about incidents. As I have briefly outlined in Chapter 2, in reality there exist multiple barriers that prevent practitioners from disclosing incidents at all, or may lead to the disclosure being incomplete, which in turn might be perceived as deceptive by the patient and can trigger a complaint. From a policy and regulator's perspective that means addressing the legal environment that hinders openness in the communication after incidents (AVANT, 2013; Doms, 2010), but also supports the practitioners feeling safe and equipped to have such difficult conversations, and lastly, to de-brief them, so that they are able to improve their disclosure skills in future.

Practical support, such as the contribution by Truong et al. (2011) or the Australian framework for open disclosure (ACSQH, 2013a), is a suitable starting point, but needs to be underpinned by training and support at the time of incidents in real life. The open disclosure policy that is currently being drafted in NSW (NSW Health, 2014b), seems a step in the right direction by offering broad support to 'do' open disclosure in the first place and to assist practitioners to 'do it well'.

The findings of the explorative study have also suggested that existing complaint mechanisms seem unsuited to facilitate the restoration of trust when often at a time when a complaint is made, the trust between patient and practitioner has deteriorated to such an extent that its restoration seems unlikely or would require repeated positive experiences to change negative perceptions into positive ones. Nevertheless, independent complaint bodies play a role in bringing closure to conflicts that stem from incidents after which trust could not be restored.

5.4   Recommendations for practitioners and education

As mentioned above, real-time training applicable to real situations appears to be sought by practitioners to support them in disclosing incidents and errors to patients in practice. The results of the survey reveal that advice is primarily being sought from legal and health professional bodies, suggesting that advisory and training services offered by these bodies would likely be accepted by practitioners. However, given the clarity with which the interviews showed the difference in perceptions between patients and practitioners and the importance of being responsive to the patient's perceptions in order to avoid the deterioration of trust, it seems of the utmost importance that patients and consumers are involved in the creation of training material and activities. In real-life disclosures, this may mean seeking and being responsive to patient input throughout all stages of the disclosure process, as well as providing them with an opportunity to give feedback.

Some practitioners are great communicators, but for others, it is a skill that can be acquired. Education programs directed at practitioners and other clinicians should include dedicated modules to improve clinician skills in communicating with patients beyond ascertaining medically relevant facts to inquiring about their perceptions and expectations as to the treatment and care. This is in line with a patient-centred approach to health care that is being promoted in Australia (ACSQH, 2008, 2011) and in Germany by the introduction of the *Patientenschutzrecht* (Bundesministerium für Gesundheit, 2013). After incidents, communication is often more difficult given the practitioner's and the patient's emotions related to the incident. The reluctance of some practitioners to offer an apology after incidents may be an indication of how difficult they find it to respond to the emotional impact of an incident. Practitioners should be given the opportunity to acquire specific skills on how to appropriately communicate in such difficult situations. In addition, such skills need to be refined in practice, which may for example mean involving junior staff in open disclosure so that they can learn from senior staff. An open debriefing after disclosure conversations can also help to improve practitioners' confidence in engaging in open disclosure in the future.

5.5   Recommendations for patients

Lastly, the research has not only highlighted patient perceptions and expectations, but it also suggests that different types of patient seek different levels of involvement and control in their health care relationships. Being open about their preferences will enable the practitioner to respond appropriately. Patients who have experienced incidents should also provide feedback about their experience to the provider, their management or an independent body. Only where practitioners, policy makers and regulators are aware of the patients' issues can appropriate action be taken. Where patients seek to continue their relationship with a practitioner, they should expect that it may take some time, goodwill and willingness on both sides to openly engage with each other to facilitate a mutual understanding that would allow the restoration of trust.

5.6   Final remarks

This book has looked at the nucleus of health care delivery – the patient-practitioner relationship. I have only considered external influences to the relationship in passing, for example, the reliance on the judgement of others and the implications that incident experiences can have on the broader life of both patients and practitioners. There are certainly more factors that influence the trust dynamic, for example, inter-professional relationships practitioners have with other clinicians, or the dynamics in interpersonal trust relations when care and treatment is fragmented and involves a number of clinicians caring for the same patient.

Nevertheless, I hope that this book will contribute to the academic debate, and also enrich discussions about how to improve patient-practitioner relationships and how to adequately and appropriately manage incidents in health care with the aim of preserving or restoring the patient's trust in the practitioner, which has wider implications for future health care encounters.

References

Allen, J., & Brock, S. A. (2000). Health care communication using personality types: Patients are different. London, Philadelphia: Routledge.

Anderson, L. A., & Dedrick, R. F. (1990). Development of the trust in physician scale: A measure to assess interpersonal trust in patient-physician relationships. *Psychological Reports, 67,* 1091-1100.

Arora, N. K., Ayanian, J. Z., & Guadagnoli, E. (2005). Examining the relationship of patients' attitudes and beliefs with their self reported level of participation in medical decision making. *Medical Care, 43* (9), 865-872.

Ärzte Zeitung (2008, 21 November). *Eine Entschuldigung bei Behandlungsfehlern ist möglich* [Apology about medical errors is possible]. Retrieved at http://www.aerztezeitung.de/praxis_wirtschaft/praxisfuehrung/article/5 22224/entschuldigung-behandlungsfehlern-moeglich.html

Atkinson, P., Coffey, A., Delamont, S., Lofland, J. , & Lofland, L. (Eds.). (2001). *Handbook of ethnography.* Thousand Oaks: Sage.

Atkinson, P., & Silverman, D. (1997). Kundera's immortality: The interview society and the invention of self. *Qualitative Inquiry, 3.* 304-325.

Australian Bureau of Statistics (2014, 7 February). *Population clock.* Retrieved from http://www.abs.gov.au/ausstats/abs%40.nsf/94713ad445ff1425ca25682 000192af2/1647509ef7e25faaca2568a900154b63?OpenDocument

Australian Commission on Safety and Quality in Health Care (ACSQH) (2008). *Australian Charter for Health Care Rights.* Sydney: Australian Commission on Safety and Quality in Health Care.

Australian Commission on Safety and Quality in Health Care (ACSQH) (2011).
   *Patient-centred care: Improving quality and safety through partnerships
   with patients and consumers.* Sydney: Australian Commission on Safety
   and Quality in Health Care.

Australian Commission on Safety and Quality in Health Care (ACSQH) (2012).
   National safety and quality health service standards. Sydney: Australian
   Commission on Safety and Quality in Health Care.

Australian Commission on Safety and Quality in Health Care (ACSQH) (2013a).
   Australian Open Disclosure Framework. Sydney: Australian Commission
   on Safety and Quality in Health Care.

Australian Commission on Safety and Quality in Health Care (ACSQH) (2013b).
   Open disclosure: Just-in-time information for clinicians. Sydney: Australian Commission on Safety and Quality in Health Care.

Australian Commission on Safety and Quality in Health Care (ACSQH) (2014, 7
   May). The Australian Open Disclosure Framework. Retrieved from
   http://www.safetyandquality.gov.au/our-work/open-disclosure/the-
   open-disclosure-framework/

Australian Department of Health (2014, 7 February). *Legislation administered by
   the Minister for Health and the Minister for Mental Health and Ageing.*
   Retrieved from
   http://www.health.gov.au/internet/main/publishing.nsf/Content/health
   -eta2.htm

Australian Institute of Health and Welfare (2009). *Australia's welfare 2009: The
   ninth biennial welfare report of the Australian Institute of Health and
   Welfare.* Canberra: Australian Institute of Health and Welfare.

Australian Medical Board (2010). *Good medical practice: A code of conduct for
   doctors in Australia.* Retrieved from http://www.medicalboard.gov.au/

Australian Medical Workforce Advisory Committee (2005). *The general practice workforce in Australia: Supply and requirements to 2013*. Sydney: Australian Medical Workforce Advisory Committee

AVANT Medical Indemnity Insurance (AVANT) (2013). *Practitioner indemnity insurance policy*. Retrieved from
www.avant.org.au/WorkArea/DownloadAsset.aspx?id=17179869362

AVANT Medical Indemnity Insurance (AVANT) (2014, 1 March). *How to say sorry safely*. Retrieved from
http://www.avant.org.au/uploadedFiles/Content/Resources/Member/How-To-201005-How-To-Say-Sorry-Safely-All-Specialties.pdf

Axelrod, R. (1984). *The evolution of cooperation*. New York: Basic Books.

Babrow, A. (2001). Uncertainty, value, communication, and problematic integration. *Journal of Communication, 51* (3), 553–573.

Bachmann, R., & Zaheer, A. (Eds.). (2006). *Handbook of trust research*. Cheltenham, Northampton: Edward Elgar.

Baker, G. R., Norton, P. G., Flintoft, V., Blais, R., Brown, A., & et al. (2004). The Canadian adverse events study: The incidence of adverse events among hospital patients in Canada. *Canadian Medical Association Journal, 170* (11), 1678-1686.

Banja, J. D. (2005). Does medical error disclosure violate the medical malpractice insurance cooperation clause? In K. Henriksen, J. B. Battles, E. S. Marks, & D. I. Lewin (Eds.), *Advances in patient safety: From research to implementation* (Volume 3: implementation issues*)*. Rockville (MD): Agency for Healthcare Research and Quality (US). Retrieved from
http://www.ncbi.nlm.nih.gov/books/NBK20549/

Barach, P., & Cantor, M. D. (2007). Adverse event disclosure: Benefits and drawbacks for patients and clinicians. In S. Clarke, & J. Oakley (Eds.), *Informed consent and clinician accountability: The ethics of report cards on surgeon performance* (pp. 76-90). Cambridge University Press.

Barnard, A., McCosker, H., & Gerber, R. (1999). Phenomenography: A qualitative research approach for exploring understanding in health care. *Qualitative Health Research, 9,* 212-226.

Beach, M., Sugarman, J., Johnson, R. L., Arbelaez, J. J., Duggan, P. S., & Cooper, L. A. (2005). Do patients treated with dignity report higher satisfaction, adherence, and receipt of preventive care? *Annals of Family Medicine, 3,* 331–338.

Becker, L. C. (1996). Trust as noncognitive security about motives. Symposium on trust, University of Chicago. *Ethics 107* (October 1996), 43-61.

Beitat, K. (2004). *Politische Skandale in den Medien. Der Fall Jürgen Möllemann [Political scandals in the media. The case of Jürgen Möllemann].* Leipzig: University of Leipzig.

Beitat, K., Bentele, G., & Iedema, R. (2013). Trust after medical incidents. In C. N. Candlin & J. Crichton (Eds.), *Discourses of trust* (pp. 70-85). Palgrave studies in professional and organizational discourse. Basingstoke: Palgrave Macmillan.

Benedetti, F. (2011). *The patient's brain.* Oxford: Oxford University Press.

Bentele, G. (1998). *Der Faktor Glaubwürdigkeit [The factor credibility].* In O. Jarren, U. Sarchinelli, & U. Saxer(Eds.), *Politische Kommunikation in der demokratischen Gesellschaft: Ein Handbuch mit Lexikonteil [Political communication in the democratic society: A handbook with lexicon]* (pp. 305-311). Opladen: Westdeutscher Verlag.

Bentele, G. (2008). *Objektivität und Glaubwürdigkeit: Medienrealität rekonstruiert [Objectivity and credibility: Media reality reconstructed].* Wiesbaden: Verlag für Sozialwissenschaften.

Bentele, G., & Seidenglanz, R. (2005). Vertrauen und Glaubwürdigkeit [Trust and trustworthiness]. In: G. Bentele, R. Fröhlich, & Szyszka, P. (Eds.), *Handbuch der Public Relations: Wissenschaftliche Grundlagen und berufliches Handeln [Handbook of public relations: Scientific fundamentals and professional behaviour]* (pp. 346-360). Wiesbaden: Verlag für Sozialwissenschaften.

Berg, B. L. (2009). *Qualitative research methods for the social sciences* (7th ed.). Boston, MA: Allyn & Bacon.

Berlin, L. (2006). Will saying 'I'm sorry' prevent a malpractice lawsuit? *The American Journal of Roentgenology, 187* (1), 10-15.

Berlinger, N. (2005). *After harm: Medical error and the ethics of forgivenness.* Baltimore: Johns Hopkins University Press.

Bhattacharya, R., Devinney, T. M., & Pillutla, M. M. (1998). A formal model of trust based on outcomes. *Academy of Management Review 1998, 23* (3), 459-472.

Bismark, M. M., & Micalizzi, D. A. (2011). Informed choice: The meeting point of law, medicine, and person-centred care. *Health Issues, 107,* 24-27.

Blendon, R. J., DesRoches, C. M., Brodie, M., Benson, J. M., Rosen, A. B., & et al. (2002). Views of practicing physicians and the public on medical errors. *New England Journal of Medicine, 347,* 1933-1940.

Boll-Palievskaya, D. (2005). Zusammenprall der Kulturen [Clash of cultures]. *Deutsches Ärzteblatt, 102* (10), 654-656.

Boulware, L. E., Cooper, L. A., Lloyd, E. R., LaVeist, T. A., & Powe, N. R. (2003). Race and trust in the health care system. *Public Health Reports, 118,* 358-365.

Braithwaite, J., Iedema, R., & Jorm, C. (2007). Trust, communication, theory of mind and the social brain hypothesis: Deep explanations for what goes wrong in health care. *Journal of Health Organization and Management, 21* (4/5), 353 – 367.

Braun, V., & Clarke, V. (2006). Using thematic analysis in psychology. *Qualitative Research in Psychology, 3,* 77-103.

Brennan, T. A., Leape, L. L., Laird, N. M., Hebert, L., Localio, A. R., & et al. (1991). Incidence of adverse events and negligence in hospitalized patients: Results of the Harvard medical practice study I. *New England Journal of Medicine, 324,* 370-376.

Britten, N. (1995). Patients' demands for prescriptions in primary care. *British Medical Journal, 310,* 1084–1085.

Brooks, P. M., Lapsley, H. M., & Butt, D. B. (2003). Medical workforce issues in Australia: 'tomorrow's doctors — too few, too far'. *Medical Journal of Australia, 179* (4), 206-208.

Bryant, A., & Charmaz, K. (2007). Grounded theory in historical perspective: An epistemological account. In A. Bryant, & K. Charmaz (Eds.), *The SAGE Handbook of grounded theory* (pp. 31-57). Los Angeles: Sage.

Bryant, A., & Charmaz, K. (Eds.) (2007). *The Sage handbook of grounded theory.* London, Thousand Oaks, Singapore, New Delhi: Sage.

Buetow, S. (2010). Thematic analysis and its reconceptualization as 'saliency analysis'. *Journal of Health Services Research & Policy, 15* (2), 123–125.

Bundesärztekammer (2006). *Grundsätze ärztlicher Ethik (Europäische Berufsordnung). [Principles of medical professional practice (European code of conduct)].* Retrieved from http://www.bundesaerztekammer.de/page.asp?his=1.100.1142.1145&al l=true

Bundesärztekammer (2010). *Statistische Erhebung der Gutachterkommissionen und Schlichtungsstellen für das Statistikjahr 2009 [Statistics of the expert assessor commissions and medication bodies for the year 2009]*. Retrieved from http://www.bundesaerztekammer.de/downloads/gutachterkommission_statistik_2009.pdf Bundesärztekammer (2014, 6 February). *Adressen bei den Landesärztekammern [Addresses at the state medical boards]*. Retrieved from http://www.bundesaerztekammer.de/page.asp?his=2.59.5301.5361

Bundesärztekammer (2011). *(Muster-)Berufsordnung für die in Deutschland tätigen Ärztinnen und Ärzte (Stand 2011) [(Model) code of conduct for medical practitioners practising in Germany (2011)]*. Retrieved from http://www.bundesaerztekammer.de/page.asp?his=1.100.1143

Bundesärztekammer (2013a). *Gutachterkommissionen und Schlichtungsstellen bei den Ärztekammern: Ein Wegweiser [Expert assessor commissions and mediation bodies at the medical boards: A guide]*. Retrieved from http://www.bundesaerztekammer.de/downloads/Brosch_Gutachterkommissionen_14062013.pdf

Bundesärztekammer (2013b). *Statistische Erhebung der Gutachterkommissionen und Schlichtungsstellen für das Statistikjahr 2012 [Statistics of the expert assessor commissions and medication bodies for the year 2012]*. Retrieved from http://www.bundesaerztekammer.de/downloads/Erhebung_StaeKo_mit_Zahlen_2012_komplett.pdf

Bundesärztekammer (2013c). *Tätigkeitsbericht 2012 [Performance report 2012]*. Retrieved at http://www.bundesaerztekammer.de/page.asp?his=0.1.1610.11207

Bundesministerium für Gesundheit (2013). *Patientenrechtegesetz passiert den Bundesrat [Patient protection law passes upper house]*. Retrieved from http://www.bundesgesundheitsministerium.de/ministerium/presse/pres semitteilungen/2013-01/patientenrechtegesetz-im-bundesrat.html

Bundesministerium für Gesundheit (2014a, 7 February). *Staatliche Ordnung: Staat [Governmental structure: Government]*. Retrieved from http://www.bmg.bund.de/gesundheitssystem/staatliche-ordnung/staat.html

Bundesministerium für Gesundheit (2014b, 7 February). *Staatliche Ordnung: Bundesländer [Governmental structure: Federal states]*. Retrieved from http://www.bmg.bund.de/gesundheitssystem/staatliche-ordnung/bundeslaender.html

Bundesministerium für Gesundheit (2014c, 7 February). *Grundprinzipien: Freie Arztwahl [Basic principles: Freedom to choose medical practitioner]*. Retrieved from http://www.bmg.bund.de/krankenversicherung/grundprinzipien/freie-arztwahl.html

Calnan, M., & Rowe, R. (2004). *Trust in health care: An agenda for future research*. London: The Nuffield Trust.

Calnan, M., & Rowe, R. (2006). Researching trust relations in health care: Conceptual and methodological challenges – an introduction. *Journal of Health Organization and Management, 20* (5), 349-358.

Candlin, C. N., & Crichton, J. (Eds.). (2013). *Discourses of trust*. Palgrave studies in professional and organizational discourse. Basingstoke: Palgrave Macmillan.

Cave, J, & Dacre, J. (2008). The competent novice: Dealing with complaints. *British Medical Journal, 336*, 326-328.

Chan, D. K., Gallagher, T. H., Reznick, R., & Levinson, W. (2005). How surgeons disclose medical errors to patients: A study using standardized patients. *Surgery, 138*, 851-858.

Clinton, H. R., & Obama, B. (2006). Making patient safety the centerpiece of medical liability reform. *New England Journal of Medicine, 354*, 2205-2208.

Cognitive Institute (2014, 1 March). *Open disclosure series.* Retrieved from http://www.cognitiveinstitute.org/Courses/OpenDisclosureSeries.aspx

Coleman, J. S. (1990). *Foundations of social theory.* Cambridge: Boston: Harvard University Press.

Coulter, A., Entwistle, V. A., & Gilbert, D. (1999). Sharing decision with patients: Is the information good enough? *British Medical Journal, 318*, 318-322.

Crotty, M. (1998). *The foundations of social research: Meaning and perspectives in the research process.* Crows Nest: Allen & Unwin.

Crusius, A. (2009). *Statement zur Pressekonferenz der Bundesärztekammer: Fehlerhäufigkeiten und Fehlerursachen in der Medizin* [Statement at the press conference of the federal medical board: Occurrence and causes of medical errors]. Retrieved from http://www.bundesaerztekammer.de/downloads/Statement_Dr._Crusiu s_edg.pdf

Cunningham, W. (2004). The immediate and long-term impact on New Zealand doctors who receive patient complaints. *The New Zealand Medical Journal, 117* (1198). Retrieved from http://journal.nzma.org.nz/journal/117-1198/972/.

Cutcliffe, J. R. (2005). Adapt or adopt: Developing and transgressing the methodological boundaries of grounded theory. *Journal of Advanced Nursing, 51* (4), 421-428.

Damasio, A. (2005). *Descartes' error: emotion, reason, and the human brain*. London: Penguin books.

Daniel, A. E., Burn, R. J., & Horarik, S. (1999). Patients' complaints about medical practice. *The Medical Journal of Australia, 170* (12), 598-602.

Das, T. K., & Teng, B.-S. (1998). Between trust and control: Developing confidence in partner cooperation in alliances. *Academy of Management Review, 23* (3), 491-512.

Denzin, N. K., & Lincoln, Y. S. (2000). *Handbook of qualitative research (2nd ed.)*. Thousand Oaks, London, New Delhi: Sage.

Deppermann, A. (1997). *Glaubwürdigkeit im Konflikt: Rhetorische Techniken in Streitgesprächen: Prozessanalysen von Schlichtungsgesprächen [Credibility in conflicts: Rhetorical techniques in conflict discussions: Analyses of processes in mediations]*. Frankfurt a. M., Berlin, Bern, New York, Paris, Wien: Lang.

Dervin, B. (1998). Sense-making theory and practice: An overview of user interests in knowledge seeking and use. *Journal of Knowledge Management, 2* (2), 36-46.

Deutsch, M. (1958). Trust and suspicion. *Journal of Conflict Resolution, 2,* 265-279.

Deutscher Bundestag (2007, 23 November). Gesetz zur Reform des Versicherungsvertragsrechts [Act reforming the insurance contract legislation]. Bundesgesetzblatt, I S. 2631 (59).

Dirks, K. T. (2006). Three fundamental questions regarding trust in leaders. In R. Bachmann & A. Zaheer (Eds.), *Handbook of trust research* (pp. 15-28). Cheltenham, Northampton: Edward Elgar.

Dirks, K. T. & Ferrin, D. L. (2001). The role of trust in organizational settings. *Organization Science, 12,* 450-467.

Doms, T. (2010). Behandlungsfehler: Was der Arzt sagen darf [Medical error: What the doctor is allowed to say]. *Deutsches Ärzteblatt, 107* (50), 2529-2530.

Duclos, C. W., Eichler, M., Taylor, L., Quintela, J., Main, D. S., & et al. (2005). Patient perspectives of patient-provider communication after adverse events. *International Journal for Quality in Health Care, 17* (6), 479-486.

Duden (2014, 1 February). *Vertrauen [Trust].* Retrieved at www.duden.de

Earle, T. C., & Siegrist, M. (2006). Morality Information, performance information, and the distinction between trust and confidence. *Journal of Applied Social Psychology, 36* (2), 383-416.

Encinosa, W. E., & Hellinger, F. J. (2008). The impact of medical errors on ninety-day costs and outcomes: An examination of surgical patients. *Health Services Research, 43,* 2067–2085.

Ende, J., Kazis, L., Ash, A., & Moskowitz, M. A. (1989). Measuring patients' desire for autonomy: Decision making and information seeking preferences among medical patients. *Journal of General Internal Medicine, 4,* 23-30.

Engel, K. G., Rosenthal, M., & Sutcliffe, K. M. (2006). Residents' responses to medical error: Coping, learning, and change. *Academic Medicine, 81,* 86-93.

Entwistle, N. (1997). Introduction: Phenomenography in higher education. *Higher Education Research & Development, 16* (2), 127-134.

Entwistle, V. A., & Quick, O. (2006). Trust in the context of patient safety problems. *Trust in health care organizations, 20* (5), 397-416.

Erdem, S. A., & Harrison-Walker, J. (2006). The role of the internet in physician-patient relationships: The issue of trust. *Business Horizons, 49,* 387-393.

Fallowfield, L., & Fleissig, A. (2003). *Communication with patients in the context of medical error: Final report*. London: Psychosocial Oncology Group Brighton & Sussex Medical School, University of Sussex; National Patient Safety Agency.

Festinger, L. (Reprinted). (1962). *A theory of cognitive dissonance*. Stanford: Stanford University Press.

Fontana, A., & Frey, J. H. (2000). The interview: From structured questions to negotiated text. In N. K. Denzin & Y. S. Lincoln (Eds.), Sage *handbook of qualitative research* (2nd ed.) (pp. 645-672). Thousand Oaks, London, New Delhi, Singapore: Sage.

Friedman, H. S. (1979). Nonverbal communication between patients and medical practitioners. *Journal of Social Issues, 35*, 82-99.

Gallagher, T. H., Garbutt, J. M., Waterman, A. D., Flum, D. R., Larson, E. B., & et al. (2006). Choosing your words carefully: How physicians would disclose harmful medical errors to patients. *Archives of Internal Medicine, 166* (15), 1585-1593.

Gallagher, T. H., Studdert, D., & Levison, W. (2007). Disclosing harmful medical errors to patients. *New Englang Journal of Medicine. 356*, 2713-2719.

Gallagher, T. H., Waterman, A. D., Ebers, A. G., Fraser, V. J., & Levinson, W. (2003). Patients' and physicians' attitudes regarding the disclosure of medical errors. *Journal of the American Medical Association 2003, 289* (8), 1001-1007.

Gallagher, T. H., Waterman, A. D., Garbutt, J. M., Kapp, J. M., Chan, D. K., & et al. (2006). US and Canadian physicians' attitudes and experiences regarding disclosing errors to patients. *Archives of Internal Medicine, 166* (15), 1605-1611.

Gambetta, D. (Ed.). (1988). *Trust: Making and breaking cooperative relations*. New York: Basil Blackwell.

Gambetta, D. (2000). Can we trust trust? In D. Gambetta (Ed.), *Trust: Making and breaking cooperative relations* (pp. 213-237). Electronic edition, Department of Sociology, University of Oxford. Retrieved at http://www.sociology.ox.ac.uk/papers/gambetta213-237.pdf

Ganther, J. M., Wiederholt, J. B., & Kreling, D. H. (2001). Measuring patients' medical care preferences: Care seeking versus self-treating. *Medical Decision Making, 21* (2), 133-140.

GfK Verein (2014). *Trust in professions 2014*. Retrieved from http://www.gfk-verein.org/

Giddens, A. (1990). *The consequences of modernity*. Stanford: Standford University Press.

Giddens, A. (1991). *Modernity and self identity: Self and society in the late modern age*. Cambridge: Polity Press.

Gigerenzer, G., & Edwards, A. (2003). Simple tools for understanding risks: From innumeracy to insight. *British Medical Journal, 327*, 741-744.

Gilbert, D. T., Fiske, S. T., & Gardner, L. (Eds.). (1998). *The Handbook of Social Psychology (4ᵗʰ ed.)*. New York: Oxford University Press.

Glaser, B. (1998). *Doing grounded theory: Issues and discussions*. Mill Valley: Sociology Press.

Glaser, B., & Strauss, A. (1967). *The discovery of grounded theory*. Chicago: Aldine.

Goleman, D. (2006). *Social intelligence: The new science of human relationships*. London: Hutchinson.

Grbich, C. (2007). *Qualitative data analysis: An introduction*. London, Thousand Oaks, New Delhi: Sage.

Grey, C. ,& Garsten, C. (2001). Trust, control and post-bureaucracy. *Organisational studies 2001, 22* (2), 229-250.

Guijarro, P. M., Andrés, J. M. A., Mira, J. J., Perdiguero, E., & Aibar, C. (2010). Adverse events in hospitals: The patient's point of view. *Quality and Safety in Health Care, 19*, 144-147.

Günterberg, K., & Beer, C. (2010). Das Einkommen niedergelassener Ärzte. PaPfleReQ, 4, 87-93.

Hall, M. A., Dugan, E., Zheng, B., & Mishra, A. K. (2001). Trust in physicians and medical institutions: What is it, can it be measured, and does it matter? *The Milbank Quarterly, 79* (4), 613-639.

Hammersley, M. (1992). *What's wrong with ethnography: Methodological explorations*. Routledge: London.

Hardin, R. (1992). The street-level epistemology of trust. *Analyse & Kritik, 1992, 14*, 152-176.

Hardin, R. (2001). Conceptions and explanations of trust. In K. S. Cook (Ed.), *Trust in society* (pp. 3-39) Russell Sage Foundation series on trust (v. 2). New York: Russell Sage Foundation.

Hargie, O., Saunders, C., & Dickson, D. (1994). *Social skills in interpersonal communication* (3rd ed.) London, New York, Routledge.

Harms, L. (2007). *Working with people*. South Melbourne: Oxford University Press.

Health Insurance Act 1973 (Commonwealth). Retrieved on 13 January 2014 at http://www.austlii.edu.au/au/legis/cth/consol_act/hia1973164/

Health Insurance Regulation 1975 (Commonwealth). Retrieved on 13 January 2014 at http://www.austlii.edu.au/au/legis/cth/consol_reg/hir1975273/

Health Practitioner Regulation National Law (NSW). Retrieved on 13 January 2014 at http://www.legislation.nsw.gov.au/maintop/view/inforce/act+86a+2009+cd+0+N

Healthcare Commission (2005). *Primary care trust survey of patients 2005*. London: Healthcare Commission.

Hesse, B. W., Nelson, D. E., Kreps, G. L., Croyle, R. T., Arora, N. K., & et al. (2005). Trust and sources of health information: The impact of the internet and its implications for health care providers: Findings from the first health information national trends survey. (reprinted). *Archives Internal Medicine, 165*, 2618-2624.

Heyl, B. S. (2001). Ethnographic interviewing. In P. Atkinson, A. Coffey, S. Delamont, J. Lofland, & L. Lofland (Eds.), *Handbook of ethnography* (pp. 369-383). Thousand Oaks: Sage.

Hickson, G. B., Clayton, E. W., Githens, P. B., & Sloan, F. A. (1992). Factors that prompted families to file medical malpractice claims following perinatal injuries. *Journal of the American Medical Association, 267* (10), 1359-1363.

Hobgood, C., Tamayo-Sarver, J. H., Elms, A., & Weiner, B. (2005). Parental preferences for error disclosure, reporting, and legal action after medical error in the care of their children. *Pediatrics, 110* (6), 1276-1286.

Holstein, J. A., & Gubrium, J. F. (1995). *The active interview*. Thousand Oaks: Sage.

Hurley, C., Baum, F., Johns, J., & Labonte, R. (2010). Comprehensive primary health care in Australia: Findings from a narrative review of the literature. *Australasian Medical Journal, 2*, 147-152.

Iedema, R. (2014). Open disclosure. In T. Levett-Jones (Ed.), *Critical conversations for patient safety: An essential guide for health professionals* (pp. 74-82). French Forest: Pearson.

Iedema, R., Allen, S., Britton, K., & Gallagher, T. (2011). What patients know about problems and failures in care. *BMJ Quality and Safety, 12*, 198-205.

Iedema, R., Allen, S., Britton, K., Grbich, C., Piper, D., & et al. (2011). Patients'
and family members' views on how clinicians enact and how they should
enact open disclosure: The '100 patient stories' qualitative study. *British
Medical Journal, 343*, doi: 10.1136/bmj.d4423.

Iedema, R., Mallock, N. A., Sorensen, R. J., Manias, E., Tuckett, A. G., & et al.
(2008a). The national open disclosure pilot: Evaluation of a policy implementation initiative. *Medical Journal of Australia, 188* (7), 397-400.

Iedema, R., Mallock, N., Sorensen, R., Manias, E., Tuckett, A. G., et al. (2008b).
Final report: Evaluation of the national open disclosure pilot program.
Sydney: The Australian Commission on Safety and Quality in Health Care.

Iedema, R., Mesman, J, & Carroll, K. (2013). *Visualising health care practice
improvement: Innovation from within.* London: Radcliffe Publishing.

Iedema, R., Sorensen, R., Manias, E., Tuckett, A., Piper, D., & et al. (2008). Patients' and family members' experiences of open disclosure following adverse events. *International Journal for Quality in Health Care, 20* (6), 421-
32.

Immel-Sehr, A. (2011). Reden ist Gold. [Talking is golden]. *AOK-Magazin Gesundheit und Gesellschaft, 7–8*, 32-35.

Institute of Medicine, Committee on Quality of Health Care in America (2000).
To err is human: Building a safer health system. Washington D.C.: National Academy Press.

Jackson, H. (2013). Talking and doing trust in community relations. In: C. N.
Candlin, & J. Crichton (Eds.*), Discourses of trust* (pp. 315-329). Basing-
stokes: Palgrave Macmillan.

Jain, A., & Ogden, J. (1999). General practitioners' experiences of patients' complaints: Qualitative study. British Medical Journal, 318, 1596.

Jones, K. (1996). Trust as an affective attitude. Symposium on trust, University
of Chicago. *Ethics 107*, 4-25.

Kable, A., Farmer, W., & Beitat, K. (2014). Why do patients complain about how health professionals communicate? In T. Levett-Jones (Ed.), *Critical conversations for patient safety* (pp. 26-36). French Forest: Pearson.

Kao, A. C., Green, D. C., Davis, N. A., Koplan, J. P., & Cleary, P. D. (1998a). Patients' trust in their physicians: Effects of choice, continuity, and payment method. *Journal of General Internal Medicine, 13*, 681-686.

Kao, A. C., Green, D. C., Zaslavsky, A. M., Koplan, J. P., & Cleary, P. D. (1998b). The relationship between method of physician payment and patient trust. *Journal of the American Medical Association, 280*, 1708-1714.

Kassenärztliche Vereinigung Sachsen (2010). Über medizinische Fehler sprechen – wie stehen Sie dazu? [Talking about medical errors: What is your perspective?] *KVS Mitteilungen, 12*, 6. Retrieved from http://www.kvs-sachsen.de/mitglieder/kvs-mitteilungen/2010/12-2010/meinung/

King, R., & Green, P. (2012). Governance of primary healthcare practices: Australian insights. *Business Horizons, 55* (6), 593-608.

Kirschning, S., Michel, S., & von Kardorff (2004). Der online informierte Patient: Offener Dialog gesucht [The online informed patient: Looking for open dialogue]. *Deutsches Ärzteblatt, 101*, 3090-3092.

Kraman, S. S. (2010). *Proactive reporting, investigation, disclosure, and remedying of medical errors leads to similar or lower than average malpractice claims costs.* Rockville (MD): US Department of Health and Human Services. Agency for Healthcare research and quality. Retrieved at http://www.innovations.ahrq.gov/content.aspx?id=2731#a3

Kraman, S. S., & Hamm, G. (1999). Risk management: Extreme honesty may be the best policy. *Annals of Internal Medicine, 131*, 963-967.

Kramer, R. M. (1996). Divergent realities and convergent disappointments in the hierarchic relation: Trust and the intuitive auditor at work. In R. M. Kramer & T. Tyler (Eds.), T*rust in organisations* (pp. 216-245). Thousand Oaks: Sage.

Kramer, R. M. (2006). Trust as situated condition: An ecological perspective on trust decisions. In R. Bachmann & A. Zaheer (Eds.), *Handbook of trust research* (pp. 68-84). Cheltenham, Northampton: Edward Elgar.

Krupat, E., Bell, R. A., Krawitz, R. L., Thom, D., & Azari R. (2001). When physicians and patients think alike: Patient-centered beliefs and their impact on satisfaction and trust. *The Journal of Family Practice, 50* (12), 1057-1062.

Lamb, R. (2004). Open disclosure: The only approach to medical error. *Quality and Safety in Health Care*, 13 (1), 3-5.

Lange, A. (2007). Arzt-Patient-Beziehung: Gelungene Kommunikation fängt mit gutem Zuhören an [Doctor-patient-relationship: Successful communication starts with good listening]. *Deutsches Ärzteblatt, 104* (40), 107.

Langfred, C. W. (2004). Too much of a good thing? Negative effects of high trust and individual autonomy in self-managing teams. *Academy of Management Journal, 47*, 385-399.

Lazare, A. (2004). *On apology.* New York: Oxford University Press.

Lazare, A. (2010). The apology dynamic. AAOS Now (May 2010). Retrieved from http://www.aaos.org/news/aaosnow/may10/managing5.asp

Leape, L. (2011). Foreword. In R. D. Truog, D. M. Browning, J. A. Johnson, & T. H. Gallagher (2011). *Talking with patients and families about medical error: A guide for education and practice* (p. vii-ix). Baltimore: The Johns Hopkins University Press.

Leape, L., Berwick, D., Clancy, C., Conway, J., Gluck, P., & et al. (2009). Transforming healthcare: A safety imperative. *Quality and Safety in Health Care, 18*, 424-428.

Leavitt, J., & Leavitt, F. (2011). *Improving medical outcomes: The psychology of doctor-patient visits.* Lanham, Boulder, New York, Toronto, Plymouth: Rowman & Littlefield.

LeDoux, J. E. (1996). *The emotional brain: The mysterious underpinnings of emotional life*. New York: Simon & Schuster.

Lee Y-Y., & Lin, J. L. (2009). Trust but verify: The interactive effect of trust and autonomy preferences on health outcomes. *Health Care Annals, 17*, 244-260.

Levett-Jones, T., Macdonald-Wicks, L., & Oates, K. (2014). The relationship between communication and patient safety. In T. Levett-Jones (Ed.), *Critical conversations for patient safety* (pp. xviii – 11). French Forest: Pearson.

Levinson, W. (2009). Disclosing medical errors to patients: A challenge for health professionals and institutions. *Patient Education and Counseling, 76*, 296-299.

Levinson, W., & Gallagher, T. (2007). Disclosing medical errors to patients: A status report in 2007. *Canadian Medical Association Journal (CMAJ), 177* (3), 265-267.

Levinson, W., Lesser, C. S., & Epstein, R. M. (2010). Developing physician communication skills for patient-centred care. *Health Affairs, 29* (7), 1310-1318.

Lewicki, R. J., Tomlinson, E. C., & Gillespie, N. (2006). Models of interpersonal trust development: Theoretical approaches, empirical evidence, and future directions. *Journal of Management 2006, 32*, 991-1022.

Lewin, K. (1943). Defining the 'field at a given time.' *Psychological Review, 50* (3), 292-310.

Lewis, J.D., & Weigert, A. (1985). Trust as a social reality. *Social Forces, 63*, 967-985.

Löfstedt, R. E. (2005). *Risk management in post-trust societies*. London: Palgrave Macmillan.

Loh, A., Simon, D., Kriston, L., & Härter, M. (2007). Patientenbeteiligung bei medizinischen Entscheidungen [Patient involvement in medical decision making]. *Deutsches Ärzteblatt, 104* (21), 1483-1488.

Longhurst, M. F. (1989). Physician self-awareness: The neglected insight. In M. Stewart, & D. Roter (Eds.), *Communication with medical patients* (pp. 64-72). Sage series in interpersonal communication 9. Newbury Park, London, New Delhi: Sage.

Luhmann, N. (1973). *Vertrauen. Ein Mechanismus der Reduktion sozialer Komplexität*, Stuttgart: Enke.

Luhmann, N. (1979). *Trust and power: Two works by Niklas Luhmann* (reprinted 2005), Chichester, New York, Brisbane, Toronto: John Wiley & Sons.

Luhmann, N. (1984). *Soziale Systeme: Grundriß einer allgemeinen Theorie [Social systems: Outline of a general theory]*. Frankfurt a. M.: Suhrkamp.

Luhmann, N. (2000). Familiarity, confidence, trust: Problems and alternatives. In: D. Gambetta (Ed.), *Trust: making and breaking cooperative relations* (pp. 94-107). Electronic edition, Department of Sociology, University of Oxford, Retrieved from http://citeseerx.ist.psu.edu/viewdoc/download?doi=10.1.1.23.8075&rep =rep1&type=pdf&a=bi&pagenumber=1&w=100

Macintosh, D. (2007). Trust and the limits of knowledge. In S. Clarke & J. Oakley (Eds.), *Informed consent and clinician accountability: The ethics of report cards on surgeon performance* (pp. 157-166). Cambridge: Cambridge University Press.

Madden, B., & McIlwraith, J. (2008). *Australian medical liability*. Chatswood: LexisNexis.

Maguire, S., Phillips, N, & Hardy, C. (2001). When silence=death, keep talking: Trust, control and the discursive construction of identity in the Canadian HIV/AIDS treatment domain. *Organization Studies, 22* (2), 285-310.

Markwell, A. (2011, *26 September*). More than a woman. *Australian Doctor*. Retrieved from http://www.australiandoctor.com.au/opinions/guest-view/more-than-a-woman

Marton, F., Dall'alba, G., & Beaty, E. (1993). Conceptions of learning. *International Journal of Educational Research, 19* (3), 277-300.

Mazor, K. M., Reed, G. W., Yood, R. A., Fischer, M. A., Baril, J. , & Gurwitz, J. H. (2006). Disclosure of medical errors: What factors influence how patients respond? *Journal of General Internal Medicine, 21* (7), 704-710.

Mazor, K. M., Simon, S. R., Yood, R. A., Martinson, B. C., Gunter, M. J., & et al. (2004). Health plan members' views about disclosure of medical errors. *Annals of Internal Medicine, 140* (6), 409-418.

McKnight, D. H., & Chervany, N. L. (2006). Reflections on an initial trust-building model. In R. Bachmann & A. Zaheer (Eds.), *Handbook of trust research* (pp. 29-51). Cheltenham, Northampton: Edward Elgar.

McKnight, D.H., Cummings, L. L., & Chervany, N. L. (1998). Initial trust formation in new organizational relationships. *Academy of Management Review, 23,* 1-18.

McLennan, S., Beitat, K., Lauterberg, J., & Vollmann, J. (2012). Regulating open disclosure: a German perspective. *International Journal of Quality in Health Care, 24* (1), 23-27.

McMullan, M. (2006). Patients using the internet to obtain health information: How this affects the patient-health professional relationship. *Patient Education and Counseling, 63* (1–2), 24-28.

McWhinney, I. (1989). The need for transformed clinical method. In M. Stewart, & D. Roter (Eds.), *Communication with medical patients* (pp. 25-40). Sage series in interpersonal communication 9. Newbury Park, London, New Delhi: Sage.

Mechanic, D. (1998). The functions and limitations of trust in the provision of medical care. *Journal of Health Politics Policy and Law, 23*, 661-686.

Mechanic, D., & Meyer, S. (2000). Concepts of trust among patients with serious illness. *Social Science and Medicine, 51* (5), 657–668.

Mechanic, D., & Schlesinger, M. (1996). The impact of managed care on pa-tients' trust in medical care and their physicians. *Journal of the American Medical Association, 275*, 1693-1697.

Medicare Australia (2014, 28 February). *Telehealth.* Retrieved from http://www.medicareaustralia.gov.au/provider/incentives/telehealth/

Mello, M. M., Senecal, S. K., Kuznetsov, Y., & Cohn, J. S. (2014). Implementing hospital-based communication-and-resolution programs: Lessons learned in New York City. *Health Affairs, 33* (1), 30-38.

Mickan, S., & Rodger, S. (2005). Effective health care teams: A model of six characteristics developed from shared perception. *Journal of Interpro-fessional Care, 19*, 358-370.

MIGA Medical Insurance Group Australia (MIGA) (2005). National open disclo-sure standard. *MIGA bulletin, 7*. Retrieved from http://www.miga.com.au/Bulletin/BulletinDetails.aspx?p=82&id=142&i=21&c=2

Miles, M., & Huberman, A. (1984). *Qualitative data analysis.* London: Sage.

Mills, J., Bonner, A., & Francis, K. (2006). Adopting a constructivist approach to grounded theory: Implications for research design. *International Journal of Nursing Practice, 12* (1), 8-13.

Misztal, B. A. (1996). *Trust in modern societies: The search for the bases of social order.* Cambridge: Polity Press.

Murray, S. L., & Holmes, J. G. (1999). The (mental) ties bind: Cognitive struc-tures that predict relationship resilience. *Journal of Personality and So-cial Psychology, 77*, 1228-1244.

Murtagh, L., Gallagher, T. H., Andrew, P., & Mello, M. M. (2012). Disclosure-and-resolution programs that include generous compensation offers may prompt a complex patient response. *Health Affairs, 31* (12), 2681-2689.

Nash, L. M., Walton, M. M., Daly, M. G., Kelly, P. J., Walter, & et al. (2010). Perceived practice change in Australian doctors as a result of medico legal concerns. *Medical Journal of Australia, 193*, 579-583.

Neuendorf, K. A. (2002). *The content analysis guidebook*. Thousand Oaks, London: Sage.

NSW Civil Liability Act 2002. Retrieved from
http://www.austlii.edu.au/au/legis/nsw/consol_act/cla2002161/

NSW Clinical Excellence Commission (2009*). Incident management in the NSW public health system 2008: January to June*. Sydney: NSW Clinical Excellence Commission. Retrieved from
http://www.cec.health.nsw.gov.au/__documents/publications/incident-management-2008_01to06.pdf

NSW Health (2006). *Profile of the medical practitioners workforce in NSW 2006. Retrieved from* www.health.nsw.gov.au

NSW Health (2007a). *Incident Management Policy*. Retrieved from
http://www0.health.nsw.gov.au/policies/pd/2007/PD2007_061.html

NSW Health (2007b). Policy directive: Open disclosure. Retrieved from
http://www0.health.nsw.gov.au/policies/pd/2007/pdf/PD2007_040.pdf

NSW Health (2007c). *Open disclosure guidelines*. Retrieved from
http://www0.health.nsw.gov.au/policies/gl/2007/pdf/GL2007_007.pdf

NSW Health (2009). *New South Wales population health survey: 2009 summary report on adult health*. Retrieved from
http://www.health.nsw.gov.au/surveys/adult/Publications/hsa_09summary.pdf

NSW Health (2011). *NSW population health survey: Health services attended in the last 12 months, adults aged 16 years and over, NSW 2010.* Retrieved from http://www.health.nsw.gov.au/PublicHealth/surveys/hsa/10pub/m_hserv/m_hserv_barresp.asp

NSW Health (2014a, 7 February). *Legislation: Acts administered by Health.* Retrieved from http://www.health.nsw.gov.au/legislation/Pages/legislation-links.aspx

NSW Health (2014b). *Open disclosure policy.* Retrieved from http://www0.health.nsw.gov.au/policies/pd/2014/PD2014_028.html

NSW Health Administration Act 1982. Retrieved at http://www.legislation.nsw.gov.au/maintop/view/inforce/act+135+1982+cd+0+N

NSW Health Administration Regulation 2010. Retrieved at http://www.legislation.nsw.gov.au/maintop/view/inforce/subordleg+427+2010+cd+0+N

NSW Health and Clinical Excellence Commission (2008*). Incident Management in the NSW Public Health System 2007: July to December.* Sydney: NSW Clinical Excellence Commission. Retrieved from http://www.cec.health.nsw.gov.au/__documents/programs/patient-safety/incident-management-2007_07to12.pdf

NSW Health Care Complaints Act 1993. Retrieved from http://www.legislation.nsw.gov.au/maintop/view/inforce/act+105+1993+cd+0+N

NSW Health Care Complaints Commission (HCCC) (2009). *Annual report 2008-09.* Retrieved from http://www.hccc.nsw.gov.au/Publications/Annual-Reports

NSW Health Care Complaints Commission (HCCC) (2013). *Annual report 2012-13.* Retrieved from http://www.hccc.nsw.gov.au/Publications/Annual-Reports

NSW Health Care Complaints Commission (HCCC) (2014a, 1 March). *About the Commission.* Retrieved from http://www.hccc.nsw.gov.au/About-Us/About-the-Commission/default.aspx

NSW Health Care Complaints Commission (HCCC) (2014b, 1 March). *Resolution Service.* Retrieved from http://www.hccc.nsw.gov.au/About-Us/Organisational-Overview/Organisation-Overview/default.aspx

NSW Health Care Complaints Commission (HCCC) (2014c, 1 March). *Complaint process.* Retrieved from http://www.hccc.nsw.gov.au/Complaints/Complaint-Process

O'Connor, E., Coates, H. M., Yardley, I. E., & Wu, A. W. (2010). Disclosure of patient safety incidents: A comprehensive review. *International Journal of Quality in Health Care, 22* (5), 371-379.

Oxford Dictionary (2014, 5 May). *Empathy.* Retrieved from http://www.oxforddictionaries.com/definition/english/empathy#empathy__22

Pearson, S. D., & Raeke, L. H. (2000). Patients' trust in physicians: Many theories, few measures, and little data. *Journal of General Internal Medicine, 15,* 509-513.

Pehm, K. (2009). Dangerous assumptions: Familiarity with long-term patients can lead to GPs missing serious complications. *Australian Doctor,* 3 July 2009, 41.

Powell-Davies, G., McDonald, J., Jeon, Y., Krastev, Y., Christl, B., & Faruqi, N. (2009). *Integrated primary care centres and polyclinics: A rapid review.* Australian Primary Health Care Research Institute, Australian National University Centre for Primary Health Care and Equity, The University of NSW.

Prokosh, H.-U. (2008). Internetnutzung zu Gesundheitsfragen (E-Health trends 2005-2007): Kontinuierlicher Anstieg [The use of internet for health related questions (E-Health trends 2005-2007): Continuous increase]. *Deutsches Ärzteblatt, 105* (50), 2712.

Readers' Digest (2013). *Australia's most trusted professions 2013.* Retrieved online http://www.readersdigest.com.au/most-trusted-professions-2013

Reason, J. (2000). Human error: Models and management. *British Medical Journal, 320,* 768-770.

Reilly, B. (2003). Physical examination in the care of medical inpatients: An observational study. *The Lancet, 362* (9390), 1100–1105.

Richards, T. (1998). Partnership with patients: Patients want more than simply information; they need involvement too. *British Medical Journal, 316,* 85-86.

Richardson, J. T. E. (1999). The concepts and methods of phenomenographic research. *Review of Educational Research, 69* (1), 53-82.

Rogers v Whitaker 175 CLR 479 (1992). Retrieved from http://www.austlii.edu.au/au/cases/cth/HCA/1992/58.html

Rotter, J. B. (1967). A new scale for the measurement of interpersonal trust. *Journal of Personality, 35,* 615-665.

Rotter, J. B. (1971). Generalized expectancies for interpersonal trust. *American Psychologist, 26,* 443-452.

Rotter, J. B. (1980). Interpersonal trust, trustworthiness, and gullibility. *American Psychologist, 35,* 1-7.

Rousseau, D. M., Sitkin, S. B., Burt, R. S., & Camerer, C. (1998). Not so different after all: A cross discipline view of trust. *Academy of Management Review, 23* (3), 393-404.

Royal Australasian College of Surgeons (2013). *Activities report for the period 1 January 2012 to 31 December 2012.* Retrieved from http://www.surgeons.org

Sächsische Landesärztekammer (2011). *Berufsordnung der Sächsischen Landesärztekammer (Berufsordnung - BO) vom 24. Juni 1998: In der Fassung der Änderungssatzung vom 23. November 2011 [Code of conduct of state medical board of Saxony of 24 June 2008: Amended version as at 23 November 2011].* Retrieved from http://www.slaek.de/de/05/aufgaben/Berufsordnung.php?lastpage=zur %20Ergebnisliste

Safran, D. G., Kosinski, M., Tarlov, A. R., Rogers, W. H., Taira, D. H., et al. (1998). The primary care assessment survey: Tests of data quality and measurement performance. *Medical Care, 36,* 728-739.

Sandberg, J. (2005). How do we justify knowledge produced within interpretive approaches? *Organizational Research Methods, 8* (1), 41-68.

Say, R., Murtagh, M., & Thomson, R. (2005). Patients' preference for involvement in medical decision making: A narrative review. *Patient Education and Counseling, 60,* 102-114.

Schiøler, T., Lipczak, H., Pedersen, B. L., Mogensen, T. S., Bech, K. B., & et al. (2001). Danish adverse event study. *DSI Institut for Sundhedsvaesen. Ugeskrift for Laeger, 163 (39),* 5370-5378.

Schneider, J., Kaplan, S. H., Greenfield, S., Li, W., & Wilson, I. B. (2004). Better physician-patient relationships are associated with higher reported adherence to antiretroviral therapy in patients with HIV infection. *Journal of General Internal Medicine, 19,* 1096–1103.

Schulz von Thun, F. (2014). Kommunikationsquadrant [communication quadrant]. Retrieved from http://www.schulz-von-thun.de/index.php?article_id=71

Schwappach, D. L. B., & Koeck, C. M. (2004). What makes an error unacceptable? A factorial survey on the disclosure of medical errors. *International Journal of Quality in Health Care, 16*, 317-326.

Seligman, A. B. (1997). *Problem of trust.* New Jersey: Princeton University Press.

Sillence, E., Briggs, P., Harris, P. R., & Fishwick, L. (2007). How do patients evaluate and make use of online health information? *Social Science and Medicine, 64* (9), 1853–1862.

Silverman, D. (2001). *Interpreting qualitative data: Methods for analysing talk, text and interaction* (2nd ed.). London, Thousand Oaks, New Delhi: Sage.

Silverman, D. (2005). *Doing qualitative research. A practical handbook* (2nd ed.). London, Thousand Oaks, New Delhi: Sage.

Skene, L., & Smallwood, R. (2002). Informed consent: Lessons from Australia. *British Medical Journal, 324*, 39-41.

Sokol, D. (2008). *A guide to the Hippocratic Oath.* Retrieved from the website of the British Broadcasting Cooperation (BBC), http://news.bbc.co.uk/2/hi/7654432.stm

Sonnenmoser, M. (2004). Ältere Patienten: Das Vertrauen gewinnen [Older patients: Gaining trust]. *Deutsches Ärzteblatt, 101* (34-35), 2348.

Statistisches Bundesamt (2014a, 7 February). *Bevölkerung auf Grundlage des Zensus 2011 [Population based on 2011 census].* Retrieved from https://www.destatis.de/DE/ZahlenFakten/GesellschaftStaat/Bevoelkerung/Bevoelkerungsstand/Tabellen/Zensus_Geschlecht_Staatsangehoerigkeit.html;jsessionid=C2C650F41EEC849624C8F4FBFE4FE9FF.cae3

Statistisches Bundesamt (2014b, 16 April). *Hospitals: Medical facilities, hospital beds and movement of patient.* Retrieved from https://www.destatis.de/EN/FactsFigures/SocietyState/Health/Hospitals/Tables/HospitalsYears.html

Stewart, M. A. (1995). Effective physician-patient communication and health outcomes: A review. *Canadian Medical Association Journal, 152* (9): 1423-1433.

Stewart, M., Brown, J. B., Donner A., McWhinney, I., Oates, J., et al. (2000). The impact of patient-centered care on outcomes. *Journal of Family Practice, 49,* 796-804.

Strauss, A., & Corbin, J. (1994). Grounded theory methodology: An overview. In N. Denzin, & Y. Lincoln (Eds.), *Handbook of qualitative research (pp. 73-885).* Thousand Oaks: Sage.

Stroud, L., McIlroy, J., & Levinson, W. (2009). Skills of internal medicine residents in disclosing medical errors: A study using standardized patients. *Academic Medicine, 84* (12), 1803-1808.

Studdert, D. M., & Brennan, T. A. (2001). No-fault compensation for medical injuries: The prospect for error prevention. *Journal of the American Medical Association, 286,* 217-223.

Studdert, D. M., Mello, M. M., Gawande, A. A., Brennan, T. A., & Wang, Y. C. (2007). Disclosure of medical injury to patients: An improbable risk management strategy. *Health Affairs 2007, 26* (1), 215-226.

Sun, F. C., Zhang, D. L., & Dong, Y. (2011*). Research on doctor-patient knowledge transfer model and management strategy based on patient trust.* Berlin, Heidelberg: Springer Verlag.

Szasz, T. S., & Hollander, M. H. (1956). A contribution to the philosophy of medicine: The basic models of the doctor-patient relationship. *AMA Archives Internal Medicine, 97* (5), 585-592.

Tajfel, H. (1978). *Differentiation between social groups: Studies in the social psychology of intergroup relations* (Vol 14). London: Academic Press.

Tajfel, H. & Turner, J. C. (1986). The social identity theory of intergroup behaviour. In S. Worchel & W. G. Austin (Eds.), *The handbook of intergroup communication* (pp. 7-24). London: Routledge.

Tang, P. C., Newcomb, C., Gorden, S., & Kreider, N. (1997). Meeting the information needs of patients: Results from a patient focus group. *Proceedings AMIA Annual Fall Symposium, 672-676.*

Tarrant, C., Stokes, T., & Baker, R. (2003). Factors associated with patients' trust in their general practitioner: A cross-sectional survey. *British Journal of General Practice, 53,* 798-800.

Tasker, R. C. (2000). Training and dealing with errors or mistakes in medical practical procedures. *Archives of Disease in Childhood, 83,* 95-98.

Teacy, L., Patel, A., Jennings, N. R., & Luke, M. (2006). TRAVOS: trust and reputation in the context of inaccurate information sources. *Autonomous Agents and Multi-Agent Systems, 12* (2), 183-198.

The National Academy of Science (2006). *Medication errors injure 1.5 million people and cost billions of dollars annually.* Retrieved from http://www8.nationalacademies.org/onpinews/newsitem.aspx?RecordI D=11623

Thom, D. H. (2001). Physician behaviors that predict patient trust. *The Journal of Family Practice, 50* (4), 323-328.

Thom, D. H., Bloch, D. A., & Segal, E. S. (1999). An intervention to increase patients' trust in their physicians. *Academic Medicine, 74,* 195-198

Thom, D. H., Hall, M. A., & Pawlson, L. G. (2004). Measuring patients' trust in physicians when assessing quality of care. *Health Affairs, 23* (4), 124-132.

Thom, D. H., Kravitz, R. L., Bell, R. A., Krupat, E., & Azari, R. (2002). Patient trust in the physician: relationship to patient requests. *Family Practice, 19* (5), 476-483.

Thom, D. H., Ribisl, K. M., Stewart, A. L., & Luke, D. A. (1999). Further validation and reliability testing of the trust in physician scale. *Medical Care, 37* (5), 510-517.

Thomeczek, C., Hart, D., Hochreutener, M. A., Neu, J., Petry, F. M., & et al. (2009). Kommunikation: Schritt 1 zur Patientensicherheit – auch nach dem unerwünschten Ereignis [Communication: Step 1 to patient safety – also after adverse events]. *Chirurgische Praxis, 70*, 691-700.

Trachtenberg, F., Dugan, E., & Hall, M. A. (2005). How patients' trust relates to their involvement in medical care. *The Journal of Family Practice, 54* (4), 344-352.

Travaglia, J., & Debono, D. (2009). Mortality and morbidity reviews: A comprehensive review of the literature. Centre for Clinical Governance Research, University of New South Wales, Sydney Australia. Retrieved from http://www.health.vic.gov.au/clinicalengagement/downloads/pasp/liter ature_review_mortality_and_morbidity_reviews.pdf

Truong, R. D., Browning, D. M., Johnson, J. A., & Gallagher, T. (2011). Talking *with patients and families about medical errors.* Baltimore: Johns Hopkins University Press.

Tuffs, A. (2005). Germany sets up a system for reporting medical mistakes. *British Medical Journal, 330*, 922.

Turjalei, A. (2008). Entwicklung und Validierung der Skala "Vertrauen in den Arzt" [Development and validation of trust in physician scale]. Dissertation. Cologne: University of Cologne.

Vaismoradi, M., Turunen, H., & Bondas, T. (2013). Content analysis and thematic analysis: Implications for conducting a qualitative descriptive study. *Nursing and Health Sciences, 15* (3), 398-405.

Wears, R. L., & Wu, A. W. (2002). Deailing with failure: The aftermath of errros and adverse events. *Annals of Emergency Medicine, 39*, 344-346.

Weston, W. W., & Belle Brown, J. (1989). The importance of patients' beliefs. In M. Stewart & D. Roter (Eds.), *Communicating with medical patients* (pp. 77-85). Sage series in interpersonal communication, 9. Newbury Park, London, New Delhi : Sage Publications.

Wojcieszak, D., Banja, J., & Houk, C. (2006). The sorry works! Coalition: Making the case for full disclosure. *Journal on Quality and Patient Safety, 32* (6), 344-350.

Wojcieszak, D., Saxton, J. W., & Finkelstein, M. M. (2007): *Sorry works! Disclosure, apology, and relationships prevent medical malpractice claims.* Bloomington, IN: AuthorHouse.

Woods, M. (2007). *Healing words: The power of apology in medicin (2nd ed.).* Oakbrook Terrace: Joint Commission resources.

World Alliance for Patient Safety (2004). *World Alliance for Patient Safety Forward Programme 2005.* Retrieved from http://apps.who.int/iris/handle/10665/43072

World Health Organisation (2005). *World alliance for patient safety: WHO draft guidelines for adverse event reporting and learning systems: From information to action.* Retrieved from http://www.who.org/patientsafety

World Health Organisation (2014, 3 February). *10 facts on patient safety.* Accessed at http://www.who.int/features/factfiles/patient_safety/en/index.html

Wu, A. W. (2000). Medical error: The second victim. *British Medical Journal, 320,* 726-727.

Wu, A. W., Huang, I-C., Stokes, S., & Provonost, P. J. (2009). Disclosing medical errors to patients: It's not what you say, it's what they hear. *Journal of General Internal Medicine, 24* (9), 1012-1017.

Zand, D. E. (1972). Trust and managerial problem solving. *Administrative Science Quarterly, 17* (2), 229-239.

Appendix A: Consent forms and participant information

A.1 Participant Information - Patients

"The role of trust and credibility in the resolution of conflicts resulting from incidents in health care"
(UTS 2009-138)

WHO IS DOING THE RESEARCH?

My name is Katja Beitat, and I am a PhD candidate under the supervision of Prof. Dr Günter Bentele, University of Leipzig, Germany. I am also an international associate researcher with the University of Technology Sydney under supervision of Prof. Rick Iedema. I have a Magister (M.A.) in Communication and Media Science from the University of Leipzig, Germany; and I hold a Master of International Business and Law by the University of Sydney.

Currently, I am employed as Communications Stakeholder Relations Officer at the NSW Health Care Complaints Commission, but I am not involved in individual complaint handling of the Commission. I am undertaking this research independent of my work for the Commission.

WHAT IS THIS RESEARCH ABOUT?

This research is to find out about factors that influence a trustful relationship between patients and their doctors. Being aware of these factors will assist in successfully resolving conflicts and thus prevent complaints in future. This research aims to help in understanding how to improve the relationship between doctors and patients in general; and in particular, how to improve the outcomes for both patient and their doctors when incidents or errors happen. An open and conflict-free relationship between doctor and patients has shown to increase patient's satisfaction, patient compliance with treatment, decrease the likelihood of similar incident happening in future and results in less time spent in emotionally draining situations.

IF I SAY YES, WHAT WILL IT INVOLVE?

If you agree to participate in the study, you would be interviewed about your experiences with an incident that led to a complaint. I will contact you to arrange for a suitable time and place to conduct the interview. Please let me know, if a suppression or non-disclosure clause applies to the complaint, as in this case you may be not able to participate in the study.

The length of the interview depends on your responses; it will take about half an hour on average. The interview will be recorded. Your answers will be transcribed after the interview. Any information that could potentially identify yourself or any other person will be de-identified. I will send you the transcript so that you can confirm that it is accurate. Your confidential interview will be anytime between now and December 2010.

ARE THERE ANY RISKS?

Talking about your experience may be distressing. Please let the interviewer know when you do not want to answer a question or feel uncomfortable talking about something. You can interrupt the interview at any time. If you feel distressed, you may contact a nominated independent conciliator, who may be able to help you in dealing with your distress. The interview and any related information, such as recordings and transcripts are strictly confidential. Any data that would identify you or any other person will be de-identified and not be disclosed to any third party, unless it would be unlawful to do so.

Your decision to participate or not participate has no consequences for the future care and treatment provided to you or your next of kin.

WHY HAVE I BEEN ASKED?

You were recently involved in a complaint about your doctor in NSW. The incident that lead to the complaint should fall in a period of 12 months before the complaint was made to accommodate an accurate recall of the events. Your complaint was either directly resolved with your doctor or was lodged with a third party, such as NSW Health Care Complaints Commission. I am interested in your view on the trustworthiness and credibility of your doctor before and after the complaint.

The study may involve an interview with your doctor to find out about their perception of the same incident. All interviews are strictly confidential and there will be no information disclosed to any other third party, including to your doctor.

DO I HAVE TO SAY YES?

You do not have to say yes. Your participation is completely voluntary and strictly confidential. You are free to withdraw your consent at any time of the study without giving reasons and without any consequences for you.

WHAT WILL HAPPEN IF I SAY NO?

Nothing. I will thank you for your time so far and will not contact you about this research again.

IF I SAY YES, CAN I CHANGE MY MIND LATER?

You can change your mind at any time and you don't have to say why. I will thank you for your time so far and will not contact you about this research again.

WHAT IF I HAVE CONCERNS OR A COMPLAINT?

If you have concerns about the research that you think I can help you with, please feel free to contact me on 0403 710 192 or send me an email to katja.beitat@uts.edu.au. If you would like to talk to someone who is not connected with the research, you may contact the Research Ethics Officer on 02 9514 9772, and quote this number 2009-138.

ETHICS APPROVAL AND ENDORSEMENT

This study has been approved by the University of Technology, Sydney Human Research Ethics Committee. The study has also received approval from the Ethics Committee of the Royal Australian College of Surgeons.

This research project is also been supported by the Projects, Research and Development Unit of the RACGP NSW; the NSW Health Care Complaints Commission and AVANT professional indemnity insurance.

A.2 Participant Consent Form - Patients

If you have any questions about the information in this consent form or about this research project in general, please contact Katja Beitat on 0403 710192 or send an email to katja.beitat@uts.edu.au.

I,_____ , agree to participate in the research project **Trust – factor in resolving conflicts that result from incidents in health care** being conducted by Katja Beitat (MA, MIntB&L), University of Leipzig /Germany and Associate Researcher at the Centre for Health Communication, at the University of Technology Sydney

(Email: katja.beitat@uts.edu.au, Phone: 0403 710 192, Address: Centre for Health Communication, University of Technology Sydney, PO Box 123, Sydney NSW 2007).

I understand that the purpose of this study is to find out about factors that influence a trustful relationship between patients and their doctors. I am aware that this research aims to help in understanding how to improve the relationship between doctors and patients in general and how to prevent conflicts and complaints in future.

I understand that my participation in this research will involve to be interviewed about my experiences with an incident that led to a complaint. I confirm that there is no non-disclosure order that applies to the incident. I will inform the interviewer prior to the interview, if any suppression or non-disclosure clause applies to the complaint. The interview will be recorded and will take about half an hour on average. My answers will be transcribed after the interview and a de-identified transcript provided for me to confirm.

I am aware that I can contact Katja Beitat, if I have any concerns about the research. I also understand that I am free to withdraw my participation from this research project at any time I wish, without consequences, and without giving a reason. I understand that my participation in this research project will not affect the ongoing provision of health services to me or any other person related to me.

I have read and understood the information sheet for participants. I agree that Katja Beitat has answered all my questions fully and clearly.

I agree to be contacted by phone by Ms Beitat for an interview. My preferred contact details are:

Phone: _____

Email: _____

Or postal address:

_____

I agree to the interview being recorded. I understand that a transcript of the interview will be provided to me via email or mail. I understand that I will be asked to confirm the accuracy of the transcript with my signature. I acknowledge that I cannot withdraw data contained in the transcript that has been previously confirmed by me.

I agree that the research data gathered from this project may be published in a form that does not identify me in any way. Any data that would identify me or any other person will be de-identified and not be disclosed to any third party, unless it would be unlawful to do so.

Please note that any information given during this interview or research would have to be released if requested by a subpoena issued by a court. Information provided during this research will not be released under a freedom of information claim, as the researcher does not fall under the jurisdiction of the *Freedom of Information Act*. Please also note that the researcher is not a registered medical practitioner and as such not subject to mandatory reporting requirements under the *NSW Medical Practices Act 1992*.

I am aware that all information collected during this research will be securely stored for a period of five years after publication of the results. After these five years, the researcher, Katja Beitat, will securely destroy any transcripts, recordings and personal data related to this research project, including this consent form.

_____   ____/____/____

Signature (participant)

_____   ____/____/____

Signature (researcher or delegate)

NOTE:

This study has been approved by the University of Technology, Sydney Human Research Ethics Committee. The study has also received approval from the Ethics Committee of the Royal Australian College of Surgeons. If you have any complaints or reservations about any aspect of your participation in this research which you cannot resolve with the researcher, you may contact the Ethics Committee through the Research Ethics Officer (ph: +61 2 9514 9772 Research.Ethics@uts.edu.au), and quote the UTS HREC reference number. Any complaint you make will be treated in confidence and investigated fully and you will be informed of the outcome.

A.3 Participant Information - Practitioners

"The role of trust and credibility in the resolution of conflicts resulting from incidents in health care" (UTS 2009-138)

WHO IS DOING THE RESEARCH?

My name is Katja Beitat, and I am a PhD candidate under the supervision of Prof. Dr Günter Bentele, University of Leipzig, Germany. I am also an international associate researcher with the University of Technology Sydney under supervision of Prof. Rick Iedema. I have a Magister (M.A.) in Communication and Media Science from the University of Leipzig, Germany; and I hold a Master of International Business and Law by the University of Sydney.

Currently, I am employed as Communications Stakeholder Relations Officer at the NSW Health Care Complaints Commission, but I am not involved in individual complaint handling of the Commission. I am undertaking this research independent of my work for the Commission.

WHAT IS THIS RESEARCH ABOUT?

This research is to find out about factors that influence a trustful relationship between patients and their doctors. Being aware of these factors will assist in successfully resolving conflicts and thus prevent complaints in future. This research aims to help in understanding how to improve the relationship between doctors and patients in general; and in particular, how to improve the outcomes for both patient and their doctors when incidents or errors happen. An open and conflict-free relationship between doctor and patients has shown to increase patient's satisfaction, patient compliance with treatment, decrease the likelihood of similar incident happening in future and results in less time spent in emotionally draining situations.

IF I SAY YES, WHAT WILL IT INVOLVE?

If you agree to participate in the study, you would be interviewed about your experiences with an incident that led to a complaint. I will contact you to arrange for a suitable time and place to conduct the interview. The length of the interview depends on your responses; it will take about half an hour on average. The interview will be recorded. Your answers will be transcribed after the interview. Any information that could potentially identify yourself or any other person will be de-identified. I will send you the transcript so that you can confirm that it is accurate. Your confidential interview will be anytime between now and December 2010.

ARE THERE ANY RISKS?

Talking about your experience may be distressing. Please let the interviewer know when you do not want to answer a question or feel uncomfortable talking about something. You can interrupt the interview at any time. If you feel distressed, you may contact a nominated independent conciliator, who may be able to help you in dealing with your distress. The interview and any related information, such as recordings and transcripts are strictly confidential. Any data that would identify you or any other person will be de-identified and not be disclosed to any third party, unless it would be unlawful to do so.

Please note that any information given during this interview or research would have to be released if requested by a subpoena issues by a court. Information provided during this research will not be released under a freedom of information claim, as the researcher does not fall under the jurisdiction of the Freedom of Information Act. Please also note that the researcher is not a registered medical practitioner and as such <u>not subject to mandatory reporting requirements</u> under the *NSW Medical Practices Act 1992*.

The study has been reviewed by AVANT, professional indemnity insurance to consider potential risks for medical practitioners who are willing to participate.

WHY HAVE I BEEN ASKED?

You are a surgeon or general practitioner practising in NSW. You were recently involved in a patient complaint about you. The incident that lead to the complaint should fall in a period of 12 months before the complaint was made to accommodate an accurate recall of the events. Your complaint was either directly resolved with the patient or was lodged with the NSW Health Care Complaints Commission. I am interested in your view about the interaction with the patient before and after the incident that led to the complaint.

The study may involve an interview with the patient who complained about you to find out about their perception of the same incident. All interviews are strictly confidential and there will be no information disclosed to any other third party, including to your patient.

DO I HAVE TO SAY YES?

You do not have to say yes. Your participation is completely voluntary and strictly confidential. You are free to withdraw your consent at any time of the study without giving reasons and without any consequences for you.

WHAT WILL HAPPEN IF I SAY NO?

Nothing. I will thank you for your time so far and will not contact you about this research again.

IF I SAY YES, CAN I CHANGE MY MIND LATER?

You can change your mind at any time and you do not have to say why. I will thank you for your time so far and will not contact you about this research again.

WHAT IF I HAVE CONCERNS OR A COMPLAINT?

If you have concerns about the research that you think I can help you with, please feel free to contact me on 0403 710 192 or send me an email to katja.beitat@uts.edu.au. If you would like to talk to someone who is not connected with the research, you may contact the Research Ethics Officer on 02 9514 9772, and quote this number **2009-138**.

Ethics approval and endorsement

This study has been approved by the University of Technology, Sydney Human Research Ethics Committee. The study has also received approval from the Ethics Committee of the Royal Australian College of Surgeons.

This research project is also been supported by the Royal Australian College of General Practitioners, NSW Projects, Research and Development Unit; the NSW Health Care Complaints Commission and AVANT professional indemnity insurance.

A.4 Participant Consent Form - Practitioners

If you have any questions about the information in this consent form or about this research project in general, please contact Katja Beitat on 0403 710192 or send an email to katja.beitat@uts.edu.au.

I,_____ , agree to participate in the research project Trust – factor in resolving conflicts that result from incidents in health care being conducted by Katja Beitat (MA, MIntB&L), University of Leipzig /Germany and Associate Researcher at the Centre for Health Communication, University of Technology Sydney (Email: katja.beitat@uts.edu.au, Phone: 0403 710 192, Address: 38 Womerah Avenue, Darlinghurst NSW 2010).

I understand that the purpose of this study is to find out about factors that influence a trustful relationship between patients and their doctors. I am aware that this research aims to help in understanding how to improve the relationship between doctors and patients in general and how to prevent conflicts and complaints in future.

I understand that my participation in this research will involve to be interviewed about my experiences with an incident that led to a complaint. The interview will be recorded and will take about half an hour on average. My answers will be transcribed after the interview and a de-identified transcript provided for me to confirm. I acknowledge that I cannot withdraw data contained in the transcript that has been previously confirmed by me.

I am aware that I can contact Katja Beitat, if I have any concerns about the research. I also understand that I am free to withdraw my participation from this research project at any time I wish, without consequences, and without giving a reason.

I have read and understood the information sheet for participants. I agree that Katja Beitat has answered all my questions fully and clearly.

I agree to be contacted by phone by Ms Beitat for an interview. My preferred contact details are:

Phone: _____

Email: _____

Or postal address:

_____

I agree that the research data gathered from this project may be published in a form that does not identify me in any way. Any data that would identify me or any other person will be de-identified and not be disclosed to any third party, unless it would be unlawful to do so.

Please note that any information given during this interview or research would have to be released if requested by a subpoena issues by a court. Information provided during this research will not be released under a freedom of information claim, as the researcher does not fall under the jurisdiction of the Freedom of Information Act. Please also note that the researcher is not a registered medical practitioner and as such not subject to mandatory reporting requirements under the NSW Medical Practices Act 1992.

I am aware that all information collected during this research will be securely stored for a period of five years after publication of the results. After these five years, the researcher, Katja Beitat, will securely destroy any transcripts, recordings and personal data related to this research project, including this consent form.

_____   ___/___/___

Signature (participant)

_____   ___/___/___

Signature (researcher or delegate)

NOTE:

This study has been approved by the University of Technology, Sydney Human Research Ethics Committee. The study has also received approval from the Ethics Committee of the Royal Australian College of Surgeons. If you have any complaints or reservations about any aspect of your participation in this research which you cannot resolve with the researcher, you may contact the Ethics Committee through the Research Ethics Officer (ph: +61 2 9514 9772 Research.Ethics@uts.edu.au), and quote the UTS HREC reference number. Any complaint you make will be treated in confidence and investigated fully and you will be informed of the outcome.

Appendix B: Guide for patient interviews

B.1 Question guide for interviews

Introduction of study and researcher– checking that consent obtained – voluntary participation –explain that interviewee can interrupt at any time – limits of confidentiality – check whether any suppression order applies – transcript will be provided for confirmation

- Before the incident, how often did you see the doctor? Over which period? What for?
- Were you referred to the doctor or was the doctor recommended to you? By whom?
- Were you confident that this doctor would be able to help you with your health problems? Why/why not?
- Did you feel you could openly talk about your health problems with the doctor?
- When you think back to first consulting the doctor with your health problems, how did you perceive the doctor during the consultation (e.g. friendly, open, respectful, understanding, concerned, stressed, pre-occupied …)
- When did the incident happen?
- Where did the incident happen?
- When the incident happened, did you know it immediately? If not, how did you find out?
- How did you feel in that moment (when you found out)?
- What did you expect from the doctor with regard to the incident?
- Did your doctor talk to you about the incident?
- Did the doctor apologise?
- Did you feel confident that the doctor wanted to help you resolving your concerns?

- Did you get all information and explanations you wanted? From whom or where?
- If you got your information from somewhere or someone else than the doctor, did the information differ? Which information did you find most convincing?
- Did you talk about the incident with someone else (e.g. partner, family member etc.)? If yes, what did they think?
- How did the doctor behave towards you after the incident? (e.g. friendly, open, respectful, understanding, concerned, stressed, pre-occupied ...)
- You complained about doctor XXXX. Please tell me, what was the reason for your complaint?
- When did you complain (immediately after the incident or some time later)?
- Why did you lodge your complaint with the Health Care Complaints Commission?
- What outcome did you seek when making your complaint?
- How did you expect the doctor to react to your complaint to the Commission?
- What was the outcome of the complaint?
- From your perspective, is your complaint resolved? Why/why not?
- Do you think that the involvement of the Commission was helpful?
- Will you take further action? If yes, which?
- Would you see this doctor again in future?
- Looking back, has what happened changed your attitude towards doctors in general? How?

During the interview, where appropriate: Trust scale before and after the incident

- At the first consultation, on a scale from 1- 5, (very much – much – neutral – not much – absolutely not), how much did you trust the practitioner?
- Immediately after the incident, on a scale from 1-5, how much did you trust the practitioner?
- At the end of the relationship/or at the time of the interview, on a scale from 1-5, how much did you trust the practitioner?

Demographics (obtained by observation or through contextual information, if possible)

Gender
- Age group: (18-30; 31-45; 46-60; over 60)
- Cultural background and family
- Occupation

General attitude

- In general, what do you think is an ideal doctor?
- In general, how to you see your relationship with a doctor? (if necessary prompt):

  o   Someone who I expect to take care of my health problems
  o   Someone who I seek advice from about my health problems
  o   Someone, I consult as an expert and who provides a service so that I am able to deal with my health problems.
  o   Other

- In general, what makes you trust a doctor? (if necessary, use following prompts?

    o   The doctor is friendly and open
    o   You believe the doctor will be able to help you
    o   The doctor will act in your best interest
    o   The doctor is competent
    o   The doctor does what he/she says

- Is there anything else that you would like to add?

Thank you.

Guide for practitioner interviews

Introduction of study and researcher– checking that consent obtained – voluntary participation – explain that interviewee can interrupt at any time – limits of confidentiality – check whether any suppression order applies – transcript will be provided for confirmation

- Before the incident, how often did you see the patient? Over which period? What for?
- Did you feel the patient did openly talk about their health problems with you?
- When you think back to the first consultation with this patient for this health problem, how did the patient behave during the consultation?
- When did the incident happen? Where did the incident happen?
- When the incident happened, did you know immediately? If not, how did you find out?
- How did you feel in that moment (when you found out)?
- What do you think the patient expected you to do with regard to the incident?
- Have you talked to the patient about the incident?
- Have you apologised?
- Were you able to give the patient all information and explanations that he/she wanted?
- Was someone else involved in your communication with the patient?
- Did you talk to someone about the incident? If yes, to whom?
- How did the patient behave towards you after the incident?
- How did the other persons involved behave towards you after the incident?
- Mr/Ms xxxx complained about you? From your perspective, what were the reasons for the complaint?
- When did the patient actually complain (immediately after the incident or some time later)?

- What do you think was the outcome the patient was seeking when making the complaint?
- How did you react to receiving a notification about the complaint from the Commission?
- What was the outcome of the complaint?
- From your perspective, is this complaint resolved? Why /why not?
- Do you believe that patient will take further action? If yes, which?
- Do you think this patient would you see you again in future?
- Looking back, has what happened changed your attitude or your practice in any way? How?

Demographics (obtained from contextual information, if possible)

- Gender
- Age group: (18-30; 31-45; 46-60; over 60)
- Cultural background and family
- Type of speciality
- Years in clinical practice

General attitude

- In general, from your perspective, what is a good doctor?
- In general, how would you describe your relationship with patients?
- How have you, or would you deal with similar incidents?
- In general, what do you think makes a doctor trustworthy?
- Is there anything you would like to add?

Appendix C: Recruitment journal for interview study

C.1 Initial recruitment strategy

Initially, in addition to incidents that resulted in a formal complaint being made, it had been planned to also recruit medical practitioners, who had directly dealt with the patient in relation to an incident, by advertising the study in newsletters of the NSW branches of the Royal Australian College of General Practitioners and the Royal Australian and New Zealand College of Surgeons. Interested practitioners could then have contacted the researcher and would have been provided with an information package about the scope and purpose of the research. If they wished to participate, they would then have been asked to sign a consent form. To recruit the patient involved in the same incident, the practitioners would also been asked to arrange for clerical staff of their practice to contact the patient to obtain their consent to participate in the study. Participant information and consent form were to be forwarded by the clerical staff to the patients.

This group was to be compared to a group consisting of patients and medical practitioners that were involved in a formal complaint handled by the NSW Health Care Complaints Commission. For this group, their consent to participate was planned to be obtained by the relevant case officer of the Health Care Complaints Commission. Information about the research project was prepared in writing and was to be forwarded to both parties that were involved in a suitable complaint, if they had indicated their interest in the study.

The initial recruitment strategy was unsuccessful. After four months, no participant was recruited. I decided to address the main barriers to obtain valid consent from both parties to a complaint and applied for a change of sample and recruitment strategy to address the issues.

Given that the initial recruitment of medical practitioners through the Colleges by using advertisements and articles in their newsletters had resulted in no responses, it appeared necessary to alter the approach. Reasons therefore included the possibly contentious nature of the subject of the study and no direct incentive for practitioners to participate. I aimed to increase the willingness of medical practitioners to participate in the study by directly approaching potential participants, for example through presenting at professional meetings, or by using direct mailings distributed by the professional body.

In regard to the initial recruitment through the Health Care Complaints Commission, case officers identified a small number of potential cases (5) over a three month period. In the majority of cases, the medical practitioner declined to participate; in one case, the patient declined. Reasons cited by medical practitioners included fear that interviewing the patient could reignite the conflict. Another reason stated by some practitioners was their limited time for face-to-face interviews. The patient declined because of being unhappy with the outcome of the complaint and not wanting the practitioner to be interviewed.

I gave several presentations to Commission staff and had repeated talks with case officers to alert them to the study and ask them to identify any other potential cases in their caseload. However, due to the high workload, the research study had a low priority for staff and it had been difficult to convince them of taking on this additional work. Particularly, as the two-tier recruitment would have required the relevant case officer to contact both parties to a complaint first and obtain their consent to be contacted by the researcher.

Even where the case officer was able to obtain the initial consent from parties to a complaint to be contacted, my follow-up phone messages or emails were repeatedly not responded to despite the initially shown interest.

Overall, the initial recruitment strategy was too limited to attract sufficient participants. There appeared to be a major barrier for medical practitioners to consent, including their fear that interviewing the patient who lodged the complaint could re-ignite the conflict and restrictions on their time to arrange for a face-to-face interview.

C.2 Changes to initial strategy

The main change to the recruitment strategy made in response to the encountered difficulties was to alter the sample of the study. In the revised sample, medical practitioners and patients did not necessarily need to have been involved in the same complaint. This was aimed to include interested participants into the study where the other side declined their consent.

In addition, a broader range of potential recruitment channels was considered, including NSW Divisions of General Practice, Professional Indemnity Insurers. I presented the study to general practitioners at several of their continuing education training events that were run by the NSw barch of the Australian College of General Practitioners.

A second alteration to the study design was to offer the option of conducting telephone interviews where this was the participants' preference. Telephone interviews had the advantage that they usually are less time consuming, more flexible in the scheduling, for example, after working hours. The phone option also helped to mitigate the risk that people may feel uncomfortable to talk about such an emotional part of their life in a face-to-face interview. Face-to-face interviews can be perceived as being more confronting than phone interviews and also can be perceived as an invasion of the personal sphere of the interviewee, as, for example, most interviews with patients were conducted at their homes. Most medical practitioners chose their consultation rooms for the interview. Again, it was difficult for them to find an uninterrupted time to conduct the interview and there were occasions where I was inclined to keep the interview brief knowing that there were patients waiting to see the practitioner.

The option of phone interviews allowed both practitioners and patients to be interviewed at the most convenient time and venue for them. Phone interviews could also easily be re-scheduled, if needed, which would limit unnecessary travel. A further advantage was that by using phone interviews, I was able to expand the geographical area of potential participants to all NSW. Prior, potential participants had to live within a two to three hour travel radius around Sydney, due to the limited resources I had available.

C.3 Recruitment through Colleges and Associations

In April 2010, through the NSW branch of the Royal Australasian College of Surgeons, I arranged a personal mail-out of information packages to 100 randomly selected surgeons. There was one response, where the surgeon wished to clarify why he had received the correspondence.

I then approached the College of Surgeons to inquire about the possibility to publish an article about the study in the College's member publications and to present at College events. This was denied by the College, who offered instead that I could advertise in the NSW Chairman's newsletter in September 2010. Again, this was unsuccessful in attracting any surgeons for the study.

In May 2010, the NSW branch of the Royal Australian College of General Practitioners agreed to distribute a personalised mail-out of information about the research study to 100 randomly selected members. There was one response, but no final consent could be obtained.

In October and November 2010, I presented at continuing professional education events, run by the NSW branch of the College. Four presentations were held. Although there was some interest amongst general practitioners at the sessions, no practitioner agreed to be formally recruited to participate in the study.

In August 2010, I approached all NSW Divisions of General Practice, a professional network of general practitioners clustered by regions, asking them to forward or publish in their member publications information about the study. After follow up, five divisions agreed to forward the information; two declined and the others did not respond. No general practitioner contacted me as a result of the information being distributed though some of the divisions.

Overall, all recruitment action that was aimed at medical practitioners in general, was unsuccessful in attracting any participants to the study. As a result, I discontinued this part of the recruitment strategy and concentrated on recruiting participants through the Health Care Complaints Commission.

C.4 Recruitment through the Health Care Complaints Commission

With the approved changes to the recruitment strategy, the Commission agreed to two mail-outs to potential candidates. The Commission decided to exclude some cases from the mail-out due to the sensitive or non-relevant nature of the subject matter. This included complaints where the issues raised by the patient related to sexual misconduct or boundary issues. Also excluded were complaints where someone else had complained on the patient's behalf, or where the patient was under-aged. Other complaints that were excluded were those raising issues that were not related to treatment or health services, such as medico-legal issues.

In January 2010, information about the study was sent to 52 patients and 62 practitioners who had been involved in suitable complaints that were finalised in the six-month period between July to December 2009. I received 15 responses, including five from practitioners and 10 from patients. There were an additional three patients who had received the correspondence and were interested to participate, but had to be excluded as they did not fit the sample criteria. Eventually, 11 interviews were conducted, of which five were with medical practitioners and six with patients.

In August 2010, the Commission agreed to a second mail-out to 345 patients and practitioners who had been involved in suitable complaints that had been finalised between January and August 2010. 32 responses were received, of which 23 resulted in interviews being conducted with seven medical practitioners and 16 patients.

The recruitment of participants through the Commission was considered successful, despite no incentive being offered to the participants and keeping in mind the common emotional impact incidents and complaints had on both patients' and practitioners' lives.

Given the explorative nature of the interview study and the fact that saturation in responses had been reached after the second round, I decided against another round of mail-out through the Commission.

Appendix D: Trust levels reported by patients

Table D1   Trust levels reported by patients relating to all practitioners

Patient	Trust level				Would you see practitioner again?
	Initially-first consultation	Immediately after incident	When complaint made/end relationship	Interview	
Patient 01	8.5 – 9	4	1	0	no
Patient 01 new GP	9	n/a	n/a	n/a	n/a
Patient 02	10	10	0	0	no
Patient 03	9	-	-	0	no
Patient 04	10	8	0	0	no
Patient 05	9	5	0	0	no
Patient 05 other GP	7	3	n/a	n/a	yes
Patient 06	8	Deteriorated, but no exact number	-	-	no
Patient 07	10	Still high, as doctor assures patient will be ok	-	0	no
Patient 08	8	-	-	-	no
Patient 08 Specialist	8	n/a	n/a	n/a	yes
Patient 08 new GP	10	n/a	n/a	n/a	n/a
Patient 09	-	-	-	-	No
Patient 09 New practitioner	10	n/a	n/a	n/a	n/a
Patient 10	10	Deteriorated, no exact rating	-	Trust remains (as family friend)	no
Patient 11	8-9	2	-	2	no

Patient	Trust level				Would you see practitioner again?
	Initially-first consultation	Immediately after incident	When complaint made/end relationship	Interview	
Patient 12	2	0	-	-	no
Patient 12 Other senior surgeon	-	n/a	n/a	n/a	yes
Patient 12 registrar	1.5	n/a	n/a	n/a	Yes (lack of alternative)
Patient 12 GP	10	n/a	n/a	n/a	yes
Patient 13	9	3	-	0	no
Patient 13 long-term GP	10	n/a	n/a	n/a	n/a
Patient 14	2	1	-	0	no
Patient 14 long-term GP	9.5	n/a	n/a	n/a	n/a
Patient 15	-	-	-	-	no
Patient 15 – usual GP	10	n/a	n/a	n/a	n/a
Patient 16	Low (2.5)	Very low	-	-	no
Patient 17	5	-	-	0	no
Patient 18	10	7	-	1	no
Patient 18 – new GP	7	n/a	n/a	n/a	n/a
Patient 19	8		0	0	no
Patient 19 – new surgeon	7-8	n/a	n/a	n/a	n/a
Patient 20	8	6	1	0	no
Patient 21	-	-	-	-	-
Patient 22*	Felt comfortable (7.5)	-	-	-	no

Appendix E: German survey of medical practitioners

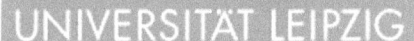 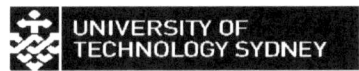

E.1 Über Fehler sprechen

Sehr geehrter Arzt,

Eine Patientenbeschwerde oder -klage zu erhalten, gehört zu den größten Ängsten im Berufsleben eines Arztes. Offene Kommunikation zwischen Arzt und Patient über medizinische Fehler oder Zwischenfälle kann einen möglichen Konflikt mildern oder sogar verhindern.

Die folgende anonyme Befragung ist Teil einer Doktorarbeit, die an der Universität Leipzig und der University of Technology, Sydney durchgeführt wird.

Der Fragebogen möchte evaluieren, wie Ärzte im derzeitigen rechtlichen, organisatorischen und beruflichen Umfeld arbeiten und ob dieses Umfeld es ihnen ermöglicht, mit Patienten über mögliche medizinische Fehler zu sprechen. Es wird auch darauf eingegangen, ob und wie Ärzte medizinische Fehler und deren Folgen in der Vergangenheit erlebt haben. Das Ziel ist es, bestehende Hürden, die eine offene Kommunikation über medizinische Fehler zwischen Arzt und Patient verhindern, besser zu verstehen und zu beseitigen. Die Kommunikation von möglichen Fehlern soll so erleichtert und die Patientensicherheit zukünftig verbessert werden.

Die vorliegende Befragung, die sowohl unter Ärzten in Sachsen als auch in New South Wales/Australien durchgeführt wird, basiert auf einer Studie, die bereits in den USA und Kanada durchgeführt wurde. Vergleichend sollen die national verschiedenen rechtlichen, organisatorischen und beruflichen Rahmenbedingungen sowie deren Auswirkungen auf die Einstellungen und Erfahrungen von Ärzten, untersucht werden. Die Untersuchungsergebnisse werden streng vertraulich und anonymisiert genutzt, um Vorschläge für Verbesserungen an bestehenden Rahmenbedingungen von Ärzten zu erarbeiten.

Zur Bearbeitung des Fragebogens benötigen Sie etwa 15-20 Minuten. Sie können den Fragebogen ausfüllen und in dem beigelegten frankierten Rückumschlag zurück senden. Sie können den Fragebogen auch online über den Link **http://surveys.uts.edu.au/index.cfm?surveyid=5888** ausfüllen. Bitte geben Sie dazu das **Passwort: Arzt** ein.

Bitte kontaktieren Sie die Studienleiterin Frau Katja Beitat (E-Mail: **katja.beitat@uts.edu.au**), falls Sie den Link zum Online-Fragebogen direkt zugeschickt bekommen möchten. Frau Beitat steht Ihnen auch gern für weitere Rückfragen und Informationen über die Studie zur Verfügung.

Vielen Dank für Ihre Unterstützung und die Beantwortung des Fragebogens.

Grundlegend für die Bearbeitung sind die folgenden Definitionen. Diese sind ebenfalls am Ende jeder Seite aufgelistet.

Medizinischer Fehler = Misslingen, eine geplante klinische Handlung wie beabsichtigt durchzuführen oder eine grundsätzlich falsche Herangehensweise, um ein Ziel zu erreichen. Ein medizinischer Fehler kann ein schwerwiegender, ein geringfügige Fehler oder ein Beinahe-Fehler sein.

Schwerwiegender Fehler = ein Fehler, der einen dauerhaften Schaden oder einen temporären, aber potenziell lebensbedrohlichen, Schaden verursacht.

Geringfügiger Fehler = ein Fehler, der einen Schaden verursacht, der weder dauerhaft noch lebensbedrohlich ist.

Beinahefehler = ein Fehler, der einen Schaden verursachen kann, aber entweder durch Zufall oder rechtzeitiges Eingreifen, verhindert werden konnte.

 Beginnen Sie hier

Sollten Sie eine der folgenden Fragen nicht beantworten können, lassen Sie diese bitte frei oder kontaktieren Sie die Studienleiterin.

Allgemeine Einstellung hinsichtlich medizinischer Fehler

1. **Medizinische Fehler sind eines der ernstesten Probleme im Gesundheitswesen.**

    ☐ Ich stimme überhaupt nicht zu
    ☐ Ich stimme nicht zu
    ☐ Ich stimme zu
    ☐ Ich stimme voll und ganz zu

2. **Wie viele von jeweils 100 Patienten in Ihrem medizinischen Fachgebiet erleben Ihrer Meinung nach einen:**

Schwerwiegenden Fehler:

___ von 100 Patienten

Geringfügigen Fehler:

___ von 100 Patienten

Beinahefehler:

___ von 100 Patienten

3. **Wie viele von jeweils 100 Ärzten in Ihrem medizinischen Fachgebiet werden Ihrer Meinung nach innerhalb des nächsten Jahres:**

Eine Beschwerde erhalten: ___

Wegen Unterlassung oder Fehlverhalten verklagt werden: ___

4. **Für wie wahrscheinlich halten Sie, dass Sie innerhalb des nächsten Jahres:**

Eine Beschwerde erhalten: ___%

Wegen Unterlassung oder Fehlverhalten verklagt werden: ___%

5. **Ihrer Meinung nach werden medizinische Fehler normalerweise verursacht durch:**

☐   Systematische Fehler in der Behandlung von Patienten
☐   Individuelle Fehler des behandelnden Arztes
☐   Eine Kombination aus individuellen und systematischen Fehlern
☐   Andere Gründe (bitte angeben):

_____

_____

Möchten Sie etwas zum Thema allgemeine Einstellung hinsichtlich medizinischer Fehler ergänzen?

_____

_____

_____

Über medizinische Fehler mit Patienten sprechen

6. Beinahefehler sollten dem Patienten mitgeteilt werden.

    ☐ Ich stimme überhaupt nicht zu
    ☐ Ich stimme nicht zu
    ☐ Ich stimme zu
    ☐ Ich stimme voll und ganz zu

7. Geringfügige Fehler sollten dem Patienten mitgeteilt werden.

    ☐ Ich stimme überhaupt nicht zu
    ☐ Ich stimme nicht zu
    ☐ Ich stimme zu
    ☐ Ich stimme voll und ganz zu

8. Schwerwiegende Fehler sollten dem Patienten mitgeteilt werden.

    ☐ Ich stimme überhaupt nicht zu
    ☐ Ich stimme nicht zu
    ☐ Ich stimme zu
    ☐ Ich stimme voll und ganz zu

9. Dem Patienten einen schwerwiegenden Fehler mitzuteilen, würde dessen Vertrauen in meine Kompetenz beeinträchtigen.

    ☐ Ich stimme überhaupt nicht zu
    ☐ Ich stimme nicht zu
    ☐ Ich stimme zu
    ☐ Ich stimme voll und ganz zu

10. Dem Patienten einen <u>schwerwiegenden Fehler</u> **mitzuteilen, würde es weniger wahrscheinlich machen, dass sich der Patient über mich beschwert.**

☐ Ich stimme überhaupt nicht zu
☐ Ich stimme nicht zu
☐ Ich stimme zu
☐ Ich stimme voll und ganz zu

11. Dem Patienten einen schwerwiegenden Fehler mitzuteilen, würde es weniger wahrscheinlich machen, dass der Patient mich verklagt.

☐ Ich stimme überhaupt nicht zu
☐ Ich stimme nicht zu
☐ Ich stimme zu
☐ Ich stimme voll und ganz zu

12. Welche der folgenden Faktoren würde es weniger wahrscheinlich machen, dass Sie einem Patienten einen schwerwiegenden Fehler mitteilen? (Bitte kreuzen Sie alle zutreffenden Möglichkeiten an)

☐ Falls der Patient nicht wüsste, dass ein Fehler passiert ist.
☐ Wenn ich glaube, dass der Patient über den Fehler nichts wissen möchte.
☐ Wenn ich glaube, dass der Patient ärgerlich werden würde, wenn ich es ihm mitteile.
☐ Wenn ich den Patienten nicht sehr gut kenne.
☐ Wenn ich denke, ich könnte verklagt werden.
☐ Wenn ich glaube, dass der Patient es nicht verstehen würde, was ich ihm mitzuteilen habe.
☐ Andere Gründe (bitte nennen Sie diese):

_____

Möchten Sie etwas zum Thema *über medizinische Fehler mit Patienten sprechen,* **ergänzen?**

_____

_____

_____

Erfahrung mit medizinischen Fehlern

13. **In welche Art von medizinischen Fehlern waren Sie schon persönlich involviert ?** (Bitte kreuzen Sie alle zutreffenden Möglichkeiten an)

☐ In Beinahefehler
☐ In geringfügige Fehler
☐ In schwerwiegende Fehler
☐ Ich war noch nie in einen Fehler involviert.

14. **Haben Sie jemals einem Patienten gegenüber einen** <u>**schwerwiegenden**</u> <u>**Fehler**</u> **offengelegt?**

☐ Nein (bitte gehen Sie direkt zu Frage 18)
☐ Ja

15. **Für den jüngst zurückliegenden Fall, in dem Sie einen schwerwiegenden Fehler einem Patienten gegenüber offengelegt haben, wie zufrieden waren Sie mit dem Patientengespräch?**

☐ Sehr unzufrieden
☐ Eher unzufrieden
☐ Eher zufrieden
☐ Sehr zufrieden

16. **Wie hat sich die Offenlegung des** <u>**schwerwiegenden Fehlers**</u> **auf Ihre Beziehung zum Patienten ausgewirkt?**

☐ Sehr negativ
☐ Eher negativ
☐ Keine Auswirkung
☐ Eher positiv
☐ Sehr positiv

17. **Ich war erleichtert, nachdem ich mit dem Patienten über diesen Fehler gesprochen hatte.**

☐ Ich stimme überhaupt nicht zu
☐ Ich stimme nicht zu
☐ Ich stimme zu
☐ Ich stimme voll und ganz zu

18. Haben Sie jemals einem Patienten gegenüber einen <u>geringfügigen Fehler</u> offengelegt?

☐ Nein
(Bitte gehen Sie direkt zu Frage 22)
☐ Ja

19. Für den jüngst zurückliegenden Fall, in dem Sie einen <u>geringfügigen Fehler</u> einem Patienten gegenüber offengelegt haben, wie zufrieden waren Sie mit dem Patientengespräch?

☐ Sehr unzufrieden
☐ Eher unzufrieden
☐ Eher zufrieden
☐ Sehr zufrieden

20. Wie hat sich die Offenlegung des <u>geringfügigen Fehlers</u> auf Ihre Beziehung zum Patienten ausgewirkt?

☐ Sehr negativ
☐ Eher negativ
☐ Keine Auswirkung
☐ Eher positiv
☐ Sehr positiv

21. Ich war erleichtert, nachdem ich mit dem Patienten über diesen Fehler gesprochen hatte.

☐ Ich stimme überhaupt nicht zu
☐ Ich stimme nicht zu
☐ Ich stimme zu
☐ Ich stimme voll und ganz zu

Möchten Sie zum Thema *Erfahrung mit medizinischen Fehlern* etwas ergänzen?

_____

_____

_____

Mit medizinischen Fehlern umgehen

22. **Wurden Sie in irgendeiner Form darin geschult oder trainiert, wie Sie Fehler gegenüber Patienten kommunizieren?**

    ☐ Nein
    ☐ Ja, vor _____ Jahren

23. **Wie sehr wären Sie an einer entsprechenden generellen Schulung oder einem Training interessiert?**

    ☐ Überhaupt nicht interessiert
    ☐ Etwas interessiert
    ☐ Sehr interessiert

24. **Nachdem ein** <u>schwerwiegender Fehler</u> **aufgetreten ist, wie sehr wären Sie daran interessiert, Unterstützung von einem auf Patientenkommunikation spezialisierten Experten zu erhalten?**

    ☐ Überhaupt nicht interessiert
    ☐ Etwas interessiert
    ☐ Sehr interessiert

25. **Wen würden Sie um Unterstützung bitten, um einen** <u>schwerwiegenden Fehler</u> **offenzulegen?** (Bitte kreuzen Sie alle zutreffenden Möglichkeiten an)

    ☐ Die Geschäftsleitung des Krankenhauses, der Klinik oder Praxis, in der ich arbeite
    ☐ Vorgesetzte
    ☐ Kollegen
    ☐ Familie/Freunde
    ☐ Haftpflichversicherung

☐ Ärztekammer
☐ Berufsorganisation/Verband
☐ Rechtsanwalt
☐ Andere (Bitte nennen Sie diese):

_____

☐ Ich würde Niemanden um Unterstützung bitten

26. **Haben sich medizinische Fehler, in die Sie persönlich involviert waren, negativ auf einen oder mehrere Ihrer folgenden Lebensbereiche ausgewirkt?** (Bitte kreuzen Sie alle zutreffenden Möglichkeiten an)

☐ Meine Zufriedenheit mit meinem Beruf
☐ Mein Vertrauen in meine Fähigkeiten als Arzt
☐ Meinen professionellen Ruf
☐ Meinen Umgang mit anderen Patienten
☐ Meine Angst vor zukünftigen Fehlern
☐ Meine Schlafqualität
☐ Andere (Bitte nennen Sie diese):

_____

☐ Der Fehler hatte keinerlei Auswirkungen

27. **Wie sehr wären Sie am Zugang zu psychologischer Beratung interessiert, wenn Sie in einen schwerwiegenden Fehler involviert wären?**

☐ Überhaupt nicht interessiert
☐ Etwas interessiert
☐ Sehr interessiert
☐ Ich habe bereits Zugang zu psychologischer Beratung nach schwerwiegenden Fehlern

28. **Welche der folgenden Gründe würden verhindern, dass Sie psychologische Beratung ersuchen?** (Bitte kreuzen Sie alle zutreffenden Möglichkeiten an)

☐ Ich habe keine Zeit, die ich von meiner Arbeit freinehmen kann.
☐ Ich habe Bedenken, dass im Falle einer Klage, das was ich sage nicht vertraulich bleibt.
☐ Ich habe Bedenken, dass die Inanspruchnahme von psychologischer Hilfe in meiner Personalakte vermerkt wird.

☐ Ich habe Bedenken, dass die Inanspruchnahme von psychologischer Beratung Auswirkungen auf meine Haftpflichtversicherung hat.

☐ Ich habe Bedenken, dass mich meine Kollegen negativ beurteilen, wenn ich psychologische Beratung in Anspruch nehme.

☐ Ich glaube, dass psychologische Beratung nicht hilfreich wäre.

☐ Andere Gründe (Bitte nennen Sie diese):

☐ _____

☐ Keiner der genannten Punkte würde verhindern, dass ich psychologische Hilfe in Anspruch nehme.

Möchten Sie zum Thema *mit medizinischen Fehlern umgehen* etwas ergänzen?

_____

_____

_____

Über medizinische Fehler mit anderen sprechen

29. Um die Patientensicherheit zu verbessern, sollten Ärzte <u>schwerwiegende Fehler</u> ihrem Krankenhaus, ihrer Klinik oder ihrer Praxis melden.

☐ Ich stimme überhaupt nicht zu
☐ Ich stimme nicht zu
☐ Ich stimme zu
☐ Ich stimme voll und ganz zu

30. Um die Patientensicherheit zu verbessern, sollten Ärzte <u>geringfügige Fehler</u> ihrem Krankenhaus, ihrer Klinik oder ihrer Praxis melden.

☐ Ich stimme überhaupt nicht zu
☐ Ich stimme nicht zu
☐ Ich stimme zu
☐ Ich stimme voll und ganz zu

31. Um die Patientensicherheit zu verbessern, sollten Ärzte <u>schwerwiegende Fehler</u> mit ihren Kollegen besprechen.

☐ Ich stimme überhaupt nicht zu
☐ Ich stimme nicht zu
☐ Ich stimme zu
☐ Ich stimme voll und ganz zu

32. Um die Patientensicherheit zu verbessern, sollten Ärzte geringfügige Fehler mit ihren Kollegen besprechen.

- ☐ Ich stimme überhaupt nicht zu
- ☐ Ich stimme nicht zu
- ☐ Ich stimme zu
- ☐ Ich stimme voll und ganz zu

33. Insofern geschehen: Was haben Sie bei der Offenlegung eines Fehlers getan? Ich habe: (Bitte kreuzen Sie alle zutreffenden Möglichkeiten an)

- ☐ es einem Kollegen mitgeteilt
- ☐ es einem Vorgesetzten mitgeteilt
- ☐ es der Geschäftsleitung des Krankenhauses, der Klinik oder der Praxis mitgeteilt
- ☐ einen Bericht über den Vorfall geschrieben oder jemanden gebeten, einen Bericht zu schreiben
- ☐ die Haftpflichtversicherung informiert
- ☐ es dem Patienten oder dessen Familie mitgeteilt
- ☐ Andere (Bitte nennen Sie diese):

_____

34. Bitte schildern Sie kurz das Ergebnis Ihrer Offenlegung.

_____

_____

_____

35. Insofern relevant: Was haben Sie bei der Offenlegung eines Fehlers, den ein Kollege begangen hat, getan?

Ich habe: (Bitte kreuzen Sie alle zutreffenden Möglichkeiten an)

- ☐ es einem Kollegen mitgeteilt
- ☐ es einem Vorgesetzten mitgeteilt
- ☐ es der Geschäftsleitung des Krankenhauses, der Klinik oder der Praxis mitgeteilt
- ☐ einen Bericht über den Vorfall geschrieben oder jemanden gebeten, einen Bericht zu schreiben
- ☐ die Haftpflichtversicherung informiert
- ☐ es dem Patienten oder dessen Familie mitgeteilt
- ☐ Der Ärztekammer gemeldet

☐ Andere (Bitte nennen Sie diese):

_____

36. Bitte schildern Sie kurz das Ergebnis Ihrer Offenlegung.

_____

_____

_____

Möchten Sie etwas zum Thema _über medizinische Fehler mit anderen sprechen_ ergänzen?

_____

_____

_____

_____

Informationen über medizinische Fehler erhalten

37. Um die Patientensicherheit zu verbessern: Welche der folgenden Eigenschaften müsste ein Meldesystem haben, um Ihre Bereitschaft zu erhöhen, Fehler zu melden?
(Bitte kreuzen Sie alle zutreffenden Möglichkeiten an)

☐ Das Melden dauert weniger als zwei Minuten
☐ Das System ist lokal.
☐ Das System ist einfach zugänglich und einfach in der Benutzung.
☐ Das Melden hat keine negativen Konsequenzen für mich.
☐ Das System ist anonym.
☐ Informationen werden vertraulich behandelt und sind Anwälten nicht zugänglich.
☐ Es gibt Nachweise, dass die Meldungen für systematische Verbesserungs-maßnahmen genutzt werden.
☐ Es besteht eine Meldepflicht.
☐ Andere Gründe (Bitte nennen Sie diese):

_____

38. Um die Patientensicherheit zu verbessern, müssen Ärzte über medizinische Fehler, die in ihrem Krankenhaus, Klinik oder Praxis auftreten, informiert werden.

☐ Ich stimme überhaupt nicht zu
☐ Ich stimme nicht zu
☐ Ich stimme zu
☐ Ich stimme voll und ganz zu

39. Derzeit erhalte ich Informationen über medizinische Fehler durch: (Bitte kreuzen Sie alle zutreffenden Möglichkeiten an)

☐ Medizinische Sitzungen, Tagungen oder Kongresse
☐ Qualitätszirkel, Ärztestammtische
☐ Informelle Gespräche mit Kollegen
☐ Krankenhaus/Klinik/Praxispatienten-sicherheitsprogramm
☐ Apotheken
☐ Pharmaindustrie
☐ Haftplichtversicherungen
☐ Berufs(fach-)verbände, -organisationen
☐ Ärztekammer
☐ Fachliteratur
☐ Webseiten über Patientensicherheit
☐ Andere Quellen (Bitten nennen Sie diese):

_____

40. Die derzeitigen Wege, um Ärzte über medizinische Fehler zu informieren, sind ausreichend.

☐ Ich stimme überhaupt nicht zu
☐ Ich stimme nicht zu
☐ Ich stimme zu
☐ Ich stimme voll und ganz zu

41. Welche Informationen über <u>schwerwiegende medizinische Fehler</u> würden Sie gern erhalten? (Bitte kreuzen Sie alle zutreffenden Möglichkeiten an)

☐ Ich möchte keine Informationen erhalten
☐ Information über schwerwiegende Fehler, die meine eigenen Patienten betreffen

☐ Information über schwerwiegende Fehler, die ähnliche Patienten betreffen

☐ Information über schwerwiegende Fehler, die alle Patienten betreffen

☐ Wie man schwerwiegende Fehler, die häufig auftreten, verhindern kann

☐ Andere Informationen (bitte geben Sie diese an):

_____

42. Welche Informationen würden Sie gern über geringfügige Fehler erhalten?

☐ Ich möchte keine Informationen erhalten

☐ Information über geringfügige Fehler, die meine eigenen Patienten betreffen

☐ Information über geringfügige Fehler, die ähnliche Patienten betreffen

☐ Information über geringfügige Fehler, die alle Patienten betreffen

☐ Wie man geringfügige Fehler, die häufig auftreten, verhindern kann

☐ Andere Informationen (bitte geben Sie diese an):

_____

43. Woher würden Sie diese Informationen gerne bekommen? Von: (Bitte kreuzen Sie alle zutreffenden Möglichkeiten an)

☐ Medizinischen Sitzungen, Tagungen oder Kongressen

☐ Qualitätszirkeln, Ärztestammtischen

☐ Informellen Gesprächen mit Kollegen

☐ Krankenhaus/Klinik/Praxissicherheits-programmen

☐ Apotheken

☐ Pharmaindustrie

☐ Haftplichtversicherungen

☐ Berufsverbänden, -organisationen

☐ Ärztekammer

☐ Fachliteratur

☐ Webseiten über Patientensicherheit

☐ Andere Quellen
(Bitten nennen Sie diese):

_____

Möchten Sie etwas zum Thema *Informationen über medizinische Fehler erhalten* ergänzen?

_____

_____

_____

_____

Über Ihre Person

Ihr Alter: ___ Jahre

Ihr Geschlecht

☐ Männlich
☐ Weiblich

Seit wann praktizieren Sie?

Seit ___ Jahren

Wo praktizieren/arbeiten Sie vorrangig?

☐ Öffentliches Krankenhaus / Klinik
☐ Privates Krankenhaus / Klinik
☐ Einzelpraxis
☐ Gemeinschaftspraxis
☐ Andere Einrichtungen
    (Bitte nennen Sie diese): _____

In welcher Fachrichtung praktizieren Sie?

Ich praktiziere als:

☐ Allgemeinmediziner
☐ Praktischer Arzt
☐ Hausärztlich tätiger Internist
☐ Chirurg, generell
☐ Chirurg, mit speziellem Fachgebiet
    (Bitte nennen Sie dieses): _____

☐ Arzt in einer anderen Fachrichtung
(Bitte nennen Sie diese): _____

Bitte teilen Sie Ihre Arbeitszeit auf: Wie viel Prozent Ihrer Tätigkeit entfällt auf klinische Arbeit im Vergleich zu administrativer oder akademischer Arbeit.

☐ 0%
☐ 1-25%
☐ 26-50%
☐ 51-75%
☐ 76-100%

Falls Sie im Krankenhaus oder in einer Klinik tätig sind: Wie viel Prozent Ihrer Zeit arbeiten Sie direkt am Patienten?

☐ 0%
☐ 1-25%
☐ 26-50%
☐ 51-75%
☐ 76-100%

Vielen Dank.

Bitte senden Sie den Fragebogen in dem beigelegten, frankierten Umschlag zurück.

Appendix F: Australian survey of medical practitioners

UNIVERSITÄT LEIPZIG 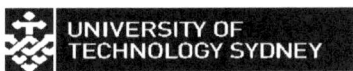 UNIVERSITY OF TECHNOLOGY SYDNEY

F.1 Communicating about medical errors

Dear practitioner,

Receiving patient complaints and medico-legal action are two major concerns in the professional life of medical practitioners. Open communication about medical errors or incidents can prevent or lessen a conflict that results from such incidents.

This anonymous survey is part of a doctoral study at the University of Leipzig/Germany and the Centre for Health Communication at the University of Technology, Sydney.

The survey aims to understand how medical practitioners work in the current legal, organisational and professional environment with regard to safely communicating with patients about medical incidents. It asks if and how you have experienced medical errors in the past and whether there are barriers to open communication about medical errors between practitioners and patients. The results of this survey are intended to improve the communication between practitioners and patients, as well as patient safety in future.

The survey, which is based on a previous study in the USA and Canada, is part of an international study that will be conducted among general practitioners and surgeons in NSW/Australia and Saxony/Germany. The survey will compare the legal, organisational and professional environment in which doctors' work, and how these circumstances may impact on their attitudes and experiences with medical incidents.

The survey will take approximately 15-20 minutes to complete. For every response received, $10 will be donated to a nominated charity. You can choose to complete the enclosed questionnaire and return it in the provided reply-paid envelope. Alternatively, you can also complete the survey online at http://surveys.uts.edu.au/index.cfm?surveyid=7402.

The information you provide is anonymous and will be used to recommend and design improvements to the current working environments of medical practitioners.

If you have any questions about the purpose of the research, what it involves, possible risks and benefits, or anything else, please contact the **researcher, Ms Katja Beitat, on 0403 710 192 or by email to** katja.beitat@uts.edu.au.

Thank you for your assistance in completing this survey. Please return it in the enclosed reply-paid envelope.

Please use the following definitions when completing the survey. These definitions are also listed at the bottom of each page.

Medical error = the failure of a planned action to be completed as intended or the use of a wrong plan to achieve an aim. A medical error includes serious errors, minor errors, and near misses.

Serious error = error that causes permanent injury or transient but potentially life threatening harm.

Minor error = error that causes harm which is neither permanent nor life threatening.

Near miss = an error that could have caused harm but did not either by chance or timely intervention.

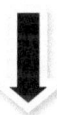 **Start here**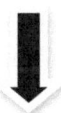

If you cannot answer one of the following questions, please leave it blank, or contact the researcher, if you have any questions.

General attitude to medical errors

1. Medical errors are one of the most serious problems in health care.

    ☐ Strongly disagree
    ☐ Disagree
    ☐ Agree
    ☐ Strongly agree

2. **For every 100 patients in your area of practice, how many do you think will experience one of the following:**

    Serious error: __ of 100 patients
    Minor error:__ of 100 patients
    Near miss: __ of 100 patients

3. **For every 100 medical practitioners in your speciality, how many do you think within the next year will:**

    Receive a complaint about them:

    _____ of 100 practitioners

    Be sued for malpractice or negligence:

    _____ of 100 practitioners

4. **What do you think is the likelihood that within the next year <u>you</u> will:**

    Receive a complaint: __%

    Be sued for malpractice or negligence: __%

5. **In your opinion, medical errors are most likely caused by:**

    ☐ Failures of care delivery systems
    ☐ Failures of individuals
    ☐ A combination of system and individual failures
    ☐ Other reasons (please specify):

    _____

Would you like to add anything else in relation to *general attitudes to medical errors*??

_____

_____

_____

Communicating about medical errors with patients

6. **<u>Near misses</u> should be disclosed to patients.**

    ☐ Strongly disagree
    ☐ Disagree
    ☐ Agree
    ☐ Strongly agree

7. <u>Minor errors</u> should be disclosed to patients.

   ☐ Strongly disagree
   ☐ Disagree
   ☐ Agree
   ☐ Strongly agree

8. <u>Serious errors</u> should be disclosed to patients.

   ☐ Strongly disagree
   ☐ Disagree
   ☐ Agree
   ☐ Strongly agree

9. Disclosing a <u>serious error</u> would damage the patient's trust in my competence.

   ☐ Strongly disagree
   ☐ Disagree
   ☐ Agree
   ☐ Strongly agree

10. Disclosing a <u>serious error</u> would make it less likely that the patient would complain about me.

   ☐ Strongly disagree
   ☐ Disagree
   ☐ Agree
   ☐ Strongly agree

11. Disclosing a <u>serious error</u> would make it less likely that the patient would sue me.

   ☐ Strongly disagree
   ☐ Disagree
   ☐ Agree
   ☐ Strongly agree

12. **Which of the following factors would make it less likely that you would disclose a <u>serious error</u> to a patient? (choose all that apply)**

   ☐ If the patient is unaware that the error had happened.
   ☐ If I think the patient would not want to know about the error.
   ☐ If I think that the patient would become angry with me if I did so.
   ☐ If I didn't know the patient very well.
   ☐ If I think I might get sued.
   ☐ If I think the patient would not understand what I was telling him or her.

Would you like to add anything else in relation to *communicating about medical errors with patients*?

_____

_____

_____

Experience with medical errors

13. **Which medical errors have you personally been involved with? (choose all that apply)**

   ☐ A near miss
   ☐ A minor error
   ☐ A serious error
   ☐ None

14. **Have you ever disclosed a <u>serious error</u> to a patient?**

   ☐ No (please go to question 18)
   ☐ Yes

15. **For the most recent <u>serious error</u> you disclosed, how satisfied were you with how the disclosure conversation went?**

   ☐ Very dissatisfied
   ☐ Somewhat dissatisfied
   ☐ Somewhat satisfied

☐   Satisfied

16. **How did disclosing this <u>serious error</u> impact on your relationship with the patient?**

    ☐   Very negatively
    ☐   Somewhat negatively
    ☐   No change
    ☐   Somewhat positively
    ☐   Very positively

17. **I experienced relief after disclosing this error to the patient.**

    ☐   Strongly disagree
    ☐   Disagree
    ☐   Agree
    ☐   Strongly agree

18. **Have you ever disclosed a <u>minor error</u> to a patient?**

    ☐   No (Please go to question 22)
    ☐   Yes

19. **For the most recent <u>minor error</u> you disclosed, how satisfied were you with how the disclosure conversation went?**

    ☐   Very dissatisfied
    ☐   Somewhat dissatisfied
    ☐   Somewhat satisfied
    ☐   Satisfied

20. **How did disclosing this <u>minor error</u> impact on your relationship with the patient**

    ☐   Very negatively
    ☐   Somewhat negatively
    ☐   No change
    ☐   Somewhat positively
    ☐   Very positively

21. I experienced relief after disclosing this error to the patient.

☐ Strongly disagree
☐ Disagree
☐ Agree
☐ Strongly agree

Would you like to add anything else in relation to your *experience with medical errors*?

_____

_____

_____

Dealing with medical errors

22. Have you received any education or training on how to disclose errors to patients?

☐ No
☐ Yes, _____ years ago

23. How interested would you be in receiving general education or training on how to disclose errors to patients?

☐ Not at all interested
☐ Somewhat interested
☐ Very interested

24. After a <u>serious error</u> occurred, how interested would you be in receiving support/coaching from an error disclosure expert on how to disclose the error to the patient?

☐ Not at all interested
☐ Somewhat interested
☐ Very interested

25. **From where would you seek support when disclosing a <u>serious error</u>? (choose all that apply)**

    ☐ Hospital or organisation I work for
    ☐ Supervisor
    ☐ Colleagues/Peers
    ☐ Family/friends
    ☐ Medical indemnity insurer
    ☐ Medical board
    ☐ College/association
    ☐ Lawyer
    ☐ Nobody
    ☐ Others (please specify):_____

26. **Have errors that you have been involved with negatively impacted on any of the following areas of your life? (choose all that apply)**

    ☐ My job satisfaction
    ☐ My confidence in my abilities as a doctor
    ☐ My professional reputation
    ☐ My interaction with other patients
    ☐ My anxiety about future errors
    ☐ My ability to sleep
    ☐ Other (please specify): _____
    ☐ The error had no impact.

27. **How interested would you be in having access to counselling if you were involved with a <u>serious error</u>?**

    ☐ Not at all interested
    ☐ Somewhat interested
    ☐ Very interested
    ☐ I already have access to counselling after serious errors

28. **Which of the following reasons would prevent you from seeking counselling? (choose all that apply)**

    ☐ Not wanting to take time away from my work
    ☐ Concern that what I say would not be kept confidential if I were sued
    ☐ Concerns that talking to a counsellor would be placed on my permanent record

☐ Concern that talking to a counsellor would affect my medical indemnity insurance
☐ Concern that my colleagues would judge me negatively if I receive counselling
☐ Belief that the counsellor would not be helpful
☐ Other (please specify): _____
☐ None of the above reasons would prevent me from seeking counselling

Would you like to add anything else in relation to *dealing with medical errors*?

_____

_____

_____

Communicating about medical errors with others

29. **To improve patient safety, practitioners should report <u>serious errors</u> to their hospital or health care organisation.**

   ☐ Strongly disagree
   ☐ Disagree
   ☐ Agree
   ☐ Strongly agree

30. **To improve patient safety, practitioners should report <u>minor errors</u> to their hospital or health care organisation.**

   ☐ Strongly disagree
   ☐ Disagree
   ☐ Agree
   ☐ Strongly agree

31. **To improve patient safety, practitioners should discuss <u>serious errors</u> with their colleagues.**

   ☐ Strongly disagree
   ☐ Disagree
   ☐ Agree
   ☐ Strongly agree

32. To improve patient safety, practitioners should discuss minor errors with their colleagues.

- ☐ Strongly disagree
- ☐ Disagree
- ☐ Agree
- ☐ Strongly agree

33. Which of the following, if any, have you used to disclose a serious error made by you? (choose all that apply)

- ☐ Told a colleague
- ☐ Told a supervisor or manager
- ☐ Told an executive of the hospital or health organisation
- ☐ Made an incident report, or asked someone to complete an incident report
- ☐ Notified the medical indemnity insurer
- ☐ Told the patient, or their family
- ☐ Other (please specify): _____

34. What was the outcome?

_____

_____

35. Which of the following, if any, have you used to disclose a serious error by someone else?

- ☐ Told a colleague
- ☐ Told a supervisor or manager
- ☐ Told an executive of the hospital or health organisation
- ☐ Made an incident report, or asked someone to complete an incident report
- ☐ Notified the medical indemnity insurer
- ☐ Told the patient, or their family
- ☐ Notified the medical board/council or health care complaints commission
- ☐ Other (please specify):
- ☐ _____

36. What was the outcome?

_____

_____

Would you like to add anything else in relation to _communicating about medical errors with others_?

_____

_____

_____

Receiving information about medical errors

37. Which of the following features of a reporting system would increase your willingness to report errors to improve patient safety? (choose all that apply)

☐ Takes less than 2 minutes to report
☐ System is local
☐ System is easy to access and use
☐ System is non-punitive
☐ System is anonymous
☐ Information is confidential and not discoverable by lawyers
☐ Evidence that reports are used for system improvements
☐ Reporting is mandatory
☐ Other (please specify):

_____

38. To improve patient safety, practitioners need to know about medical errors that occur in their hospital or health organisation.

☐ Strongly disagree
☐ Disagree
☐ Agree
☐ Strongly agree

39. **I currently receive information about medical errors from: (choose all that apply)**

   ☐ Medical meetings or conferences
   ☐ Quality round tables, including M&M
   ☐ Informal discussions with colleagues
   ☐ Hospital/health organisation safety program
   ☐ Pharmacy
   ☐ Pharmaceutical industry
   ☐ Medical indemnity insurers
   ☐ Professional college/association
   ☐ Medical board/health complaints commission
   ☐ Medical literature
   ☐ Patient safety websites
   ☐ Others (please specify): _____

40. **Current mechanisms to inform practitioners about medical errors are adequate.**

   ☐ Strongly disagree
   ☐ Disagree
   ☐ Agree
   ☐ Strongly agree

41. **What information would you like to receive about <u>serious errors</u>?**

   ☐ No information wanted
   ☐ Serious errors that occur in my patients
   ☐ Serious errors that occur in patients like mine
   ☐ Serious errors that occur in all patients
   ☐ How to prevent serious errors that commonly occur
   ☐ Other information (please specify):

   _____

42. **What information would you like to receive about <u>minor errors</u>?**

   ☐ No information wanted
   ☐ Minor errors that occur in my patients
   ☐ Minor errors that occur in patients like mine
   ☐ Minor errors that occur in all patients
   ☐ How to prevent minor errors that commonly occur

☐ Other information (please specify):

_____

43. **From where would you like to receive this information? (choose all that apply)**

☐ Medical meetings or conferences
☐ Quality round tables, including M&M
☐ Informal discussions with colleagues
☐ Hospital/health organisation safety program
☐ Pharmacy
☐ Pharmaceutical industry
☐ Medical indemnity insurers
☐ Professional college/association
☐ Medical board/health complaints commission
☐ Medical literature
☐ Patient safety websites
☐ Other (please specify): _____

Would you like to add anything else in relation to *receiving information about* *medical errors*?

_____

_____

_____

Demographics

What is your age?

____ years

What is your gender?

☐ Male
☐ Female

How long have you been a medical practitioner?

____ years

Are you primarily working:

- ☐ in public hospitals
- ☐ in private hospitals
- ☐ as a sole practitioner
- ☐ In a joint practice with other practitioners
- ☐ Other (please specify): _____

What is your speciality?

- ☐ General practice
- ☐ General medicine (Physician)
- ☐ Surgery, general
- ☐ Surgery, speciality: _____
- ☐ Other, (please specify): _____

What percentage of your time is spent in clinical practice as opposed to health administration or academic practice?

- ☐ 0%
- ☐ 1-25%
- ☐ 26-50%
- ☐ 51-75%
- ☐ 76-100%

What percentage **of your time is spent to care for hospitalised patients?**

- ☐ 0%
- ☐ 1-25%
- ☐ 26-50%
- ☐ 51-75%
- ☐ 76-100%

Thank you for completing this survey.

Please nominate a charity to which $10 will be donated for your response:

- ☐ Médecins Sans Frontières
- ☐ Save the Children